For Jan Roth and her brother Dave Urquhart,
and for Ed and Fay Wojtowicz

Contents

Preface: Comments from the Centers for Disease Control and Prevention

Anemia is often preventable, and its severe complications are typically avoidable or fairly easy to treat. Yet anemia remains a major public health problem throughout the world. Why? Many of us who obtain information mostly from our popular media may overlook the significance of age-old problems that continue to harm hundreds of millions of people throughout the world. Still others of us in medicine and public health tend to specialize by organ systems and assume that anemia is the job of the hematologists, while failing to remember that the oxygen-carrying capacity of hemoglobin and normal oxygen delivery to tissues is a mission we should all embrace. Regardless of the reasons, the science explaining the importance of normal iron balance has far outpaced our clinical and public health activities. This book, like the literature it references, is a call to action for all of us.

Today as I sit in a rural region of a developing country, I see the many faces of iron deficiency—mostly unrecognized and unaddressed. Barefoot children, whose diets are iron deficient, unknowingly donate some of their precious iron stores to the parasites growing within their intestines as they experience growth failure and intellectual difficulties that will follow them throughout their lives. Their mothers, anemic after multiple bouts of malaria in childhood, entered their reproductive years already anemic—preconception care opportunities lost, and themselves at increased risk of death from postpartum hemorrhage since they are severely anemic before the bleeding begins. Their anemia, progressing in severity from one pregnancy to the next, helps place their youngest children at the highest risk of preventable disease, with even higher rates of growth failure and preventable intellectual disabilities. Indeed, anemia and iron deficiency contribute to the cycle of poverty and disease throughout the developing world.

Back home in the United States, the association between poverty and iron deficiency plays a role in our own cycle of poverty and poor health. While none of us should minimize the impact of social determinants of disease, we should also not minimize the importance of treating iron deficiency in order to give our citizens the opportunities to take advantage of economic opportunities. The faces of anemia must be recognized in developed countries too, and their problems addressed in order to improve the health of those in richer countries.

As the readers of this book will learn, almost all of us at some time in our lives will be at risk for anemia. As our population ages, as we do a better job treating chronic diseases, and as we hopefully enhance access to health care for all Americans, anemia will be more commonly recognized as a co-morbidity. We in the United States have long underestimated the burden of sickle cell anemia in our society; now with improved newborn screening and better treatment and prevention options, improving the lives of people with sickle cell anemia is a moral imperative. Hemophilia and other bleeding disorders, although rare, are important both because of the very high cost of inadequate treatment, and because we have now proven that we can enhance the longevity and improve the quality of life among people with hemophilia. While we address the bigger public health problems worldwide associated with iron deficiency, we must maintain and enhance our efforts in these less common, but critically important, blood disorders.

Just as we are all at risk for anemia, the job of preventing and treating anemia is a job for all of us. Preventing and treating anemia worldwide is too big a job for just one medical specialty. Certainly blood disorders experts, such as the contributors to this book, and specialty organizations in the field of anemia and hematology, should help lead prevention and treatment efforts. But only when preventing and treating anemia and its complications becomes a mandate for all of us in medicine and public health will we likely achieve the improvements in health that we all desire. Congratulations to the authors and to the Iron Disorders Institute for producing this important book. Now it is time for all of us to use these pages to improve health.

Edwin Trevathan, MD, MPH
Director, National Center on Birth Defects and
Developmental Disabilities
Centers for Disease Control and Prevention (CDC)
Atlanta, Georgia
USA

Acknowledgments

The Iron Disorders Institute Guide to Anemia was made possible because of the work of exceptional people such as those listed here. Each one mentioned below gave generously of his or her time—in spite of demanding schedules. These individuals helped to read, write, or review, or they graciously permitted the reprinting of text or images for the book:

Eugene Weinberg, PhD; Herbert Bonkovsky, MD; P. D. Phatak, MD; Barry Skikne, MD; Jim Connor, PhD; John Beard, PhD; Graydon Funke, MD; Paul Reisberg, PhD; Peter Kouides, MD; Ernest Beutler, MD; Molly Cogswell, RN, DrPH.; Jane A. Rubey, MPH, RD; Johan Bolaert, MD; Chris Kieffer; David Garrison; Randy Lauffer, PhD; Gary Moore; J. Fawcett, PhD; Sherri Wick; Erin O'Rourke; Deb and Eli Hill; Cheryl Mellan; Jim Hines; Arthur Callahan; Linda Alongi; Brian Pearlman, MD; Harold S. Ballard, MD; Susanne Hiller-Sturmhöfel; Donna Perry; Thomas Nifong, MD; Susan Leitman, MD; Zubair Baloch, MD; Adrianna Vlachos, MD; Trish Linke; Connie Anderson; Doug Smith, MD, Jeremy E. Kaslow, MD; Susan Lang; Jere Douglas Haas, PhD; Emily Pualwan; Leah Robin; Deborah Judy; Marilyn Baker; Neal Young, MD; Bruce Camitta, MD; Yvette Ju, MD; Jaroslaw Maciejewski, MD, PhD; David Araten, MD; Barbara Acosta; Craig Butler; Gargi Paduah; Carolyn Rooney; Isabel Bedell; Alan Powell; Priscilla Savary; Eddie Leigh; Rebecca Gaskin; Jan Roth; George M. Rodgers, MD; Joseph Cranston,

MD; Raymond J. Browne, MD, MPH; Mo Mayrides, MD; Martha Liggett; Dudley Pennell, MD; Marion Nestle, PhD, MPH; Joseph Murray, MD, MPH; David Brandhagen, MD; Robert Means, MD; Charles Peterson, MD; Jackie Fiedler; Robin McDowell; Mary Jane Thomson; Sandra Buchan; Elliott Vichinsky, MD; MaryAnn Foote, PhD; Paul Sakiewicz, MD; Bruce Gore; Mary Sanford; Lisa Taylor; Ron Pitkin; Paul Milos; Regan Blinder; Robert Stuart, MD; Chip Mainous, PhD; Robert T. Means Jr., MD; Gerry Koenig; Lee Woods; Peggy Clark; Angela Cole; Susan Geiger; Lodovico Balducci, MD; Tomas Ganz, PhD, MD; and Sukirti Bagal, MD, MPH; Mark Wurster, MD; Ann Fagan; James Bentley; Angela Parks; Carol Rooney; Jackie Spencer MSW; Jerome A Bailey; Nicole Schaefer; Christopher Parker; Ed Trevathan, MD; Bud Brown; Isabel Bedell; Caroline Alexander; Carol Jordan; Adam Tanner; Sheryll Stewart; Eric J. Norman, PhD; Ellis Neufeld, MD, PhD; and Paul Scribner.

* * *

For updates on iron balance and *The Iron Disorders Institute Guide to Anemia*, visit our website: www.irondisorders.org.

Foreword

Anemia is common and the word is fairly familiar to most of us; nevertheless, the complexities of its causes and consequences are not always understood. Yet for the person with anemia and the clinician considering treatment, the proper diagnosis of the cause of the disorder in a given individual is one of the critical requirements of clinical medicine.

Anemia is not a complete diagnosis; it is a sign of a problem, just like a fever, chronic cough, headache, or pain. From the moment a physician determines that his or her patient is anemic, what happens thereafter will determine a correct diagnosis, appropriate treatment, and improved or impaired health for this patient. If anemia remains the diagnosis, the physician has stopped short of the complete picture. Because anemia can arise from so many different kinds of medical problems, it is imperative to find the cause before beginning treatment.

Sometimes the cause is quite simple and treatment can begin immediately. Sometimes the cause is complicated and requires all the skills and talents of the person with the anemia along with medical professionals to establish the proper diagnosis and allow treatment to begin. Thus the informed patient may often provide the crucial clue to the diagnosis and ultimately the proper therapy. *The Iron Disorders Institute Guide to Anemia*, therefore, will be useful to all members of the healthcare team—including patients and clinicians.

We now have the technology to travel the Internet, a wondrous place where we can learn or where we can be misinformed. It is important that all of us learn how to distinguish the difference between information that has been substantiated by science and information that is speculation, which may or may not be valid. The deeper one's knowledge base, the more valuable a tool like the Internet can become. Information gathered from the Internet can be made much more valuable when combined with the wonderful foundation this book provides. Nevertheless, as science and medicine become more complex, almost anyone, physician or patient, needs guidance and, more often than not, an advocate, in order to navigate the healthcare system. Thus while many feel that books may soon be obsolete, the present effort attests to both the informational and advocacy roles that a good book can provide. Perhaps the need for such books is greater than ever.

We now are perfecting the technologies to view life in its most basic forms. We are also learning about other new cures and therapies that will benefit patients with every form of anemia. Nevertheless, anemia remains a challenge. The complexities of therapies are creating multiple new reasons for people to become anemic, while many of the old causes of anemia remain to be solved. For example, while malaria no longer exists in this country as a public health problem, in many parts of the world the anemia that accompanies malaria remains a major predictor of death and disability, especially for women and children.

The National Institutes of Health maintain an ongoing interest in the causes and treatments of the various forms of anemia because these issues remain a constant challenge. In medical school, physicians are taught to look at causes based on evidence. By the time a physician finishes the requirements to begin his or her practice, much of what was learned in medical school is obsolete.

To quote Dr. John Clough, editor-in-chief of the *Cleveland Clinic Journal of Medicine,* "Given the short life expectancy of medical truth, physicians have no choice but to be lifelong students." Until the latter part of the last century, nutritional anemias were common and often treated without making a diagnosis. Now this approach can be dangerous, as is illustrated by the fact that iron-deficiency anemia is becoming much less common in the United States, while recognition of the genetic causes of iron overload is becoming almost as common as the deficiency state. Thus it is more critical than ever to know the iron status of someone before administering iron for anemia. *The Iron Disorders Institute Guide to Anemia* was written for the patient and patient's family. It is a reference tool that can help the patient understand the importance of when and when not to take iron supplements or other medicines, supplements, vitamins, or recommendations when diagnosed with anemia.

Most physicians welcome and encourage the well-informed patient. Feel free to share the contents of this book with your physician and other medical personnel. The worst that will happen is that everyone on the care team will gain in knowledge and be able to better care for you and those you care about. Likewise, all who practice medicine come to a point in a given case where "we don't know…" At these times another opinion is welcome, and you as the patient should feel free to recommend this approach if the answer does not seem right or fit your case as you know it. Ultimately it is you who must live with the diagnosis and the treatment, and you should feel comfortable with both in order to get the best from your medical care.

—Charles M. Peterson, MD, MBA
Director, Division of Blood Diseases and Resources,
National Heart Lung Blood Institute,
National Institutes of Health (retired)

Introduction from the National Anemia Action Council

Government statistics indicate that 3.5 million Americans are anemic, but the actual number of people suffering from anemia is probably far greater. Anemia is associated with a wide array of health problems, including a reduced life expectancy, decreased ability to live independently, increased risk of cardiovascular diseases, and worsening of dementia. Anemia may also be the first sign of a serious underlying disease such as cancer or nutritional deficiency. Unrecognized and untreated, these diseases can have serious consequences, including death. Most causes of anemia are reversible if treated appropriately and in a timely manner. Etiologies of anemia include anemia of iron deficiency due to chronic bleeding or dietary disorders, anemia of chronic renal insufficiency due to decreased production of erythropoietin, and anemia related to endocrine and metabolic disorders. Unfortunately, anemia is often overlooked.

Anemia due to iron deficiency is the most common type of anemia. In the United States, 7 percent of toddlers ages one to two years old and 9 to 16 percent of menstruating women are iron deficient. In the economically deprived countries in the world, 30 to 70 percent of the people have iron-deficiency anemia. Based on such statistics and a myriad of scientific publications regarding the prevalence of anemia among patients with chronic diseases, the National Anemia Action Council (NAAC) has identified anemia as an underdiagnosed public health concern that requires concerted attention and action.

The council applauds the Iron Disorders Institute for understanding that need and answering that call for action. *The Iron Disorders Institute Guide to Anemia* provides readers with a basic overview of the pathophysiology of anemia, some of the conditions that cause anemia, as well as some available options for treatment. The purpose of this guide is to educate physicians, healthcare professionals, and patients about anemia and the resulting health problems that can occur. It is designed to help initiate and facilitate open dialogue between healthcare professionals and patients regarding anemia. As emphasized, anemia is a condition that affects people across the age spectrum, from the newborn to the elderly. While anemia is not as recognized a diagnosis as cancer, for example, it has far-reaching implications on cardiovascular and overall health. Many individuals, including physicians, erroneously consider anemia to be a benign condition when, in fact, anemia can reduce quality of life and increase the risk of death.

The anemia experts on the National Anemia Action Council are committed to fulfilling our mission of raising the awareness of healthcare professionals and the public regarding the prevalence, symptoms, consequences, and treatment options of anemia. *The Iron Disorders Institute Guide to Anemia* is another step forward in this effort, and we at NAAC appreciate this work. We encourage readers to visit the Iron Disorders Institute's and NAAC's websites for more information, and to join in the effort to educate healthcare professionals, patients, and the general public in this important area of health.

—Lodovico Balducci, MD
President, National Anemia Action Council

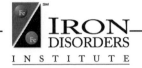

PART ONE

Anemia—The Basics

1

Iron Out-of-Balance

Iron has been used for centuries as a cure for anemia, but only in the most recent decades have physicians and scientists realized the full potential of this metal. As the findings from comprehensive studies of iron emerge, we are learning that when iron is out of balance a whole host of symptoms and illnesses are possible.

Nearly half the world's population has a health concern caused or worsened by an iron imbalance. The severity of symptoms that result can vary from mild and almost unnoticeable to extreme and incapacitating. The most widely recognized iron imbalance is iron-deficiency anemia, which is estimated conservatively to affect more than one-third of the world's population. Iron overload, another iron imbalance, is believed to affect more than thirty-five million people globally. Countless unknown numbers of people worldwide are coping with simultaneous iron overload and anemia. These patients can have excessive iron in the tissues, but their bodies cannot access it. The organs of these patients literally rust away because of the extraordinary accumulation of iron, while the symptoms of anemia such as chronic fatigue and weakness prevail due to the lack of iron in their hemoglobin.

Ironically, an iron imbalance in certain situations can protect a person against disease. In this scenario, iron

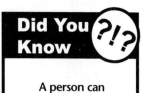

Did You Know

A person can have anemia and iron overload at the same time.

accessibility is limited for a time because the body detects the presence of harmful bacteria or cancer cells that depend on iron for survival.

Iron alone is not enough to assure that iron balance in the body remains constant. Genetics, medications, diet, environmental and economic factors, blood loss, disease, therapies such as blood transfusion, and a host of nutrients all play a crucial role in the body's ability to regulate iron levels.

Did You Know ?!?

Iron, once absorbed, cannot be excreted. Iron is the only essential mineral with this distinction.

For certain, too much iron or too little iron can be harmful to our health. The difficulty with an iron imbalance is in determining why the imbalance exists at all. Before we can be sure of iron's role in chronic disease, we must thoroughly investigate and understand the beneficial and destructive qualities of this metal and the numerous factors that affect its balance in the body.

Many people with iron imbalances are not aware that they have a potential problem. Imbalances such as iron deficiency without anemia and iron overload are often missed in routine physical exams, where iron pills might be inappropriately prescribed. In a 1996 U.S. Centers for Disease Control and Prevention Hemochromatosis/Iron Overload Patient Survey to which 2,851 people with HHC responded, 17 percent reported that they had been prescribed iron supplements by their doctor, and another 18 percent reported they had taken iron supplements for their health. These patients most likely took the iron supplements as a remedy for the chronic fatigue that accompanies iron overload disease; but fatigue is also the most prevailing symptom for people with anemia.

A variety of nutrients and body conditions play a role in iron absorption and transport. Vitamins A, B, C, D, and E, and minerals copper, zinc, and calcium can all cause problems of iron metabolism, red blood cell production, early blood cell destruction, or impaired bone marrow response. The various causes of anemia are detailed in other chapters. This chapter

4

focuses on iron and how easily mistaken some people can be about this metal.

Our one-sided view of iron

It is nearly universal for people to equate fatigue or anemia with a need for iron. No doubt this bias exists because of one of the most successful marketing campaigns of the twentieth century.

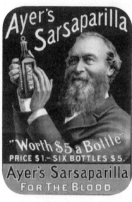

J. B. Williams Company, one of the smaller drug companies of the 1950s, needed a gimmick to sell one of its products, a multivitamin called Geritol®. Instead of selling it for what it was, a nutritional supplement for iron deficiency, the company decided to sell it as a "quick fix" remedy for fatigue, a known symptom of iron-deficiency anemia. Even though the medical community knew fatigue could be a symptom of any number of conditions, a large portion of the public did not. By using the prefix *geri*, as in geriatric, the company was in effect pushing iron to one of the groups that probably needed it least.

Though ads selling Geritol® as a remedy for fatigue ran only six years and were eventually banned in 1969 by the Federal Trade Commission, Americans were hooked. The Geritol® success sensitized the nation to iron deficiency. No matter how objective a person might be, those incessant commercials had an effect. "Tired blood" and "My wife, I think I'll keep her" are phrases still familiar to millions of Americans some thirty years later.

With repeated claims that "Geritol® contains twice the iron as a pound of calves' liver!" and the notion that "tired blood is iron-poor blood," it was only a matter of time before the medical community was influenced. Many physicians were prompted to write prescriptions for iron at the patient's first mention of fatigue.

Though iron supplementation may be necessary in confirmed cases of iron-deficiency anemia, it is not automatically appropriate for those whose number-one complaint is "fatigue."

Our need for iron

Iron is a metal so essential that without it most life on this planet would cease to exist. Plants would wither and die; animals and human beings would suffocate. Plants require iron to make chlorophyll. Plants, animals, and human beings require iron to make DNA, which encodes all life. Animals and humans also need iron to make hemoglobin, which delivers oxygen to the body; also, we need iron to make myoglobin in muscles. Myoglobin is a protein like hemoglobin, except that it is an oxygen-storage protein contained in muscles of the body. We call upon the oxygen stored in myoglobin when we use our muscles to walk, run, climb, or move in any way.

On the other hand, iron can be so deadly that 450 milligrams can poison a small child. Too much iron absorbed from diet, injections, or repeated blood transfusions can accumulate to levels that "rust" vital organs and cause them to fail. Remember that streak of iron in the bathtub? That's rust or iron oxide; the same thing can be present in your liver, joints, pancreas, heart, brain, lungs, and skin if too much iron gets into your system.

So what is this magical but potentially lethal metal? Where does it come from, and how do we get it? Iron is a metallic element that can be found in plants, animals, soil, meteorites, and rocks, including ones found on the surface of the moon. Here on earth, plants absorb iron through their root systems; animals eat these plants; and humans consume these plants and animals.

Some people refer to iron as a heavy metal, but this is incorrect. Heavy metals include lead, arsenic, mercury, cadmium, thallium, gold, and platinum. Iron is a micronutrient.

Iron is an essential *micro*nutrient because the body requires only small amounts: one milligram per day as compared with macronutrients such as oxygen, nitrogen, phosphorus, potassium, magnesium, and calcium. On the Periodic Chart of the Elements, which is used in chemistry, the symbol for iron is Fe.

What is iron?

Remember high school chemistry when you learned about atoms? What are they? Atoms are the basic units of all the elements. For example, everyone has heard of carbon (symbol C) or hydrogen (symbol H). If you had a chunk of carbon and you cut it into smaller and smaller pieces until you couldn't cut it any smaller, you would have one atom of carbon.

Iron is the same, like pure iron that makes the railroad rail or Granny's skillet. If you chopped either into smaller and smaller pieces about a billion times you would eventually get iron atoms. Think of it this way: you could lay 26,000 bacterial cells end to end and they would form a chain an inch long. Inside each of those you could lay a chain of iron atoms about 10,000 long. That means you could lay down a chain of about 260 million atoms and it would only be one inch long.

Compare Atomic Weights	
Iron	55.8
Lead	207.2
Arsenic	74.9
Mercury	200.5
Cadmium	112.4
Thallium	204.3
Gold	196.9
Platinum	195.0

NATIONAL INSTITUTES OF STANDARDS AND TECHNOLOGY

Each atom is a little ball. Actually, most of each atom is empty space, kind of like the solar system. At the center is the nucleus, made of neutrons and protons. Spinning around the outside, like the planets, are the negatively charged electrons. Those electrons orbit at the speed of light—so fast that they appear solid—like a little solid ball.

The interesting thing about atoms is that the number of negatively charged electrons (planets) equals the number of positively charged protons in the nucleus—they cancel each other out, so most atoms aren't charged like little magnets. If you remove an electron, the protons outnumber the electrons and the atom gains a positive charge; do it twice and it gets a double positive charge; remove three and it gets a triple positive charge, and so on. The same thing can happen in reverse, too, resulting in negatively charged atoms.

When an atom is charged it acts like a little magnet and sticks to stuff. Like in love, opposites attract. So atoms that are positively charged stick to negatively charged atoms. When atoms are charged we call them ions. Iron has two kinds of ions. Both are positively charged; one has two plus charges (ferrous ion) and the other has three plus charges (ferric ion).

Iron must be changed to be absorbed

Iron cannot be absorbed by the body; it must be oxidized, or changed by being united with oxygen. Bound with oxygen, iron becomes ferric oxide or common rust. The body cannot absorb iron in this form either. Iron must be changed into ferrous iron, which occurs when ferric oxide is exposed to an acidic environment. This is accomplished in the stomach when ferric oxide mixes with adequate hydrochloric acid (HCL or stomach acid).

Iron is ready to be absorbed and transported

Iron moves out of the stomach into the duodenum, the portion of the small intestine where the majority of absorption will take place. Ferrous iron is able to be absorbed in the duodenum. With the exception of another possible opportunity for a small amount of absorption that can take place later in the digestive system, all other iron will continue on to be excreted. Absorbed iron is grabbed by fingerlike projections called villi, which line the surface of the intestinal wall called the mucosa. Villi can pull iron into cells that then pass the metal into the bloodstream where it is met by a transport protein molecule called transferrin. Each molecule of transferrin can bind with and carry two atoms of iron.

Villi illustration adapted with permission from *The Visual Dictionary of the Human Body,* DK Publishing, New York, NY

Image adapted from National Cancer Institutes www.cancer.gov

Transported, controlled, and utilized

Scientists have been studying iron transport since the early 1940s. Two New York scientists, A. L. Schade and L. Caroline, noted an anti-infective agent in human plasma. They called it siderophilin; the name was later changed to transferrin. The term "siderophilin" also applies to lactoferrin. Transferrin and lactoferrin form a unique class of proteins. Transferrin remains the best-known transporter protein for iron, though other proteins such as DMT1 (divalent metal transporter 1) and ferroportin (also known as IREG1, MTP1) have been identified. Gene Weinberg describes the iron withholding defense system, seen in patients with inflammation. The body limits the amount of iron available for hemoglobin production to levels just sufficient for function, while the balance of the iron supply is placed in containment. Early clinicians observed this response but did not fully understand it.

At first, these physicians assumed that these altered ways of handling iron during illness were detrimental to the patients. Therefore, the patients were fed and injected with additional iron! Not surprisingly, the increased iron made the diseases worse, so within about ten years, the mistaken practice was discontinued.

During the 1970s and 1980s, several of the hormones (cytokines) that regulate the shift in iron metabolism were found by cell biologists. These chemicals include various interleukins and interferons. However, the compounds have a variety of actions not only on iron but on many other body processes as well. Biologists and biochemists, therefore, continued to search for more specialized hormones that might have a very specific action on iron itself and thus might be developed into useful drugs.

In 2000, such a hormone was discovered. It is a small peptide (a chain of 25 amino acids) called hepcidin. The name was coined because the compound is produced mainly by liver cells (hep) and can weakly inhibit growth of bacteria and yeasts in laboratory culture (cidin). The main effect of hepcidin is to lower the iron content of blood by trapping iron inside macrophages and inhibiting dietary iron transfer into blood from duodenal intestinal cells. Normally, when hepcidin is made in small amounts, macrophages and duodenal intestinal cells transfer iron into blood using the iron exporter protein ferroportin. When hepcidin amounts are high, hepcidin binds to ferroportin and causes ferroportin to be taken up into the cells and destroyed, thereby inhibiting the transfer of iron into the blood.

During infections, a cytokine called interleukin-6 signals the patient's hepatocytes to produce hepcidin. The peptide circulates in the bloodstream and suppresses (a) duodenal cell release of absorbed dietary iron into blood, and (b) macrophage release of iron from recycled red blood cells. Because hepcidin is a small peptide molecule, it is excreted into urine by the kidneys. Nevertheless, as long as the infection emergency persists, the patient's hepatocytes continue to form more hepcidin under the influence of interleukin-6.

Remarkably, hepcidin synthesis is increased not only in response to microbial invasion but also during iron overloading. Conversely, the production of the hormone is decreased in iron deficiency. In the very near future, hepcidin assays may be commercially available. Such a test would be helpful in distinguishing between iron overload, iron deficiency, and anemia of inflammatory or chronic disease.

Lactoferrin binds with iron, and its primary role is defense related. Lactoferrin is found in human secretions such as tears, perspiration, vaginal fluid, seminal fluid, and mother's milk. Lactoferrin can withhold iron from invading microorganisms, with few exceptions. *H. pylori*, a cause of gastric ulcer, actually seeks out lactoferrin-bound iron contained in the lining of the stomach. Lactoferrin-bound iron gives *H. pylori* its initial nourishment, enabling the microorganism to bore through the stomach wall, where it then obtains iron directly from hemoglobin.

Normally, transferrin is 25 to 35 percent saturated with the iron, but when there is too much iron for transferrin to carry, this transporter becomes unstable. Transferrin molecules that are heavily saturated lose the ability to tightly bind iron. Unbound or free iron is highly destructive and dangerous. Unbound iron can trigger free-radical activity, which can cause cell death and destroy DNA. Free iron can also provide nourishment for pathogens such as Yersinia, Listeria, and Vibrio bacteria. These bacteria are harmless for people with normal iron levels, but when transferrin is highly saturated with iron, Yersinia, Listeria, and Vibrio (contained in raw shellfish such as oysters) can be deadly.

Some microorganisms are skilled in other ways in obtaining iron from human hosts. Staph, for example, can break open red blood cells and extract the iron it needs. Another pathogen, the protozoan that causes malaria, can get into the red blood cell to obtain iron necessary to thrive. And finally, there are bacteria such as the one that causes tuberculosis that grow best inside macrophages that are iron loaded. Macrophages are white blood cells that protect us against disease; they scavenge for harmful invaders that enter our bloodstream. Iron-loaded macrophages are helpless to defend us against opportunistic infection and disease.

When working normally, transferrin binds to iron and transports it to all tissues, vital organs, and bone marrow so that normal metabolism, DNA synthesis, and red blood cell production can take place. Current research has discovered that transferrin does not work completely alone in the transport of iron. Ceruloplasmin, a protein that binds with copper, is involved in iron transport. Iron needs adequate amounts of copper to reach some of its intended destinations, such as the brain.

Some scientists theorize that there is more than one pathway through which iron is transported. They speculate that since there are different types of iron, perhaps different pathways are available for transport. In any event, absorbed iron that is not needed for metabolism, production of DNA, or hemoglobin synthesis is placed within cells in ferritin.

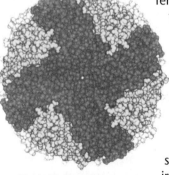

Ferritin is a protein that is produced by nearly every cell of the body. It is a huge molecule; one ferritin molecule alone can hold up to 4,500 atoms of iron. Ferritin serves as a containment device for the metal when iron is in ample quantity or when iron has the potential to be harmful to one's health. Elevated serum ferritin is an indicator that disease, or potential disease causing factors, may be present. Elevated serum ferritin is also an indicator of iron overload.

Model of ferritin molecule courtesy of Dr. James Bashkin, Maureen J. Donlin, Regina F. Frey, Christopher Putnam, and Jody K. Proctor, Department of Chemistry, Washington University, St. Louis, MO

Like transferrin, ferritin can also become unstable and ineffective. Think of ferritin like a big sink; when this sink gets full, ferritin and its iron can be changed into a precipitate called hemosiderin.

Hemosiderin is like rust and can accumulate in cells of the heart, liver, lungs, pancreas, and other organs, restricting their ability to function. For example, when beta cells (insulin-producing cells of the pancreas) are loaded with hemosiderin, these cells become unable to produce or store adequate amounts of the hormone insulin, which results in diabetes mellitus.

Scientists can obtain small amounts of tissue with a needle biopsy, stain it, and see hemosiderin in cells. For hemosiderin to be removed, it must be placed back into ferritin, which then may be released to transferrin, which is then available for hemoglobin.

Clearly, inadequate amounts or excessive accumulation of iron endangers health, but unbound iron can be harmful to a person's health in yet another way.

Oxidative stress or free-radical activity

Iron can reduce or change oxygen in two ways: As a chemical component of heme in hemoglobin, iron is capable of carrying oxygen throughout the body. Behaving in this way, iron is a lifesaver. However, "free" or unbound iron can produce free radicals, which may damage cells.

Free radicals (FR) are normal byproducts of human metabolism as oxygen is utilized. FRs are atoms or a group of atoms that have at least one unpaired electron. More stable and less reactive chemical structures as a rule have their electrons all paired to one another. Free radicals are on the hunt for an additional electron and are highly reactive with other chemicals in the body.

Programmed from its creation to find its missing part, the FR steals electrons from anywhere in the body to make up for its missing partner. The free radical can steal from any cell in any organ, including the heart, pancreas, brain, liver, joints, etc. Free radicals can also change the structure of DNA. Once DNA is changed or mutated, it is passed on in this mutated form for all future generations. The free radical doesn't care about preserving a human cell or DNA; it only wants its missing part. Ravaged atoms within the cell are now also missing a part, which creates a chain reaction unleashing free-radical activity at increasing speed.

Examples of oxidation include rotting foods or rust you might see on a car

IRON DISTRIBUTION	males 4 grams females 3.5 grams children 3 grams
Hemoglobin	70%
Myoglobin and Enzymes	15%
Ferritin	14%
In transit in serum	1%

or lawn furniture. Often, as in the case of the oxidation of fats, this sets off chain reactions, with one radical causing the destruction of hundreds or thousands of previously normal molecules. Iron-triggered free-radical activity can contribute to liver disease, pancreatic "burn out" (type II diabetes), joint disease, heart disease, neurological problems, and acceleration of aging, to name a few of the consequences of oxidative stress on the body.

Antioxidants protect the body from free-radical damage. An antioxidant donates or gives up the sought-after electron to a free radical and renders it harmless. Our bodies contain antioxidants obtained from fresh fruits and vegetables in our diets. When our diets lack fresh fruits and vegetables or are high in fats and sugars we can have an overabundance of free-radical activity.

Iron that is not absorbed

For those with normal iron metabolism, unabsorbed iron, about 90 percent of iron ingested through diet, is taken up by specific cells in the intestinal tract called enterocytes. These cells become engorged with iron, die, drop off, and are excreted in feces. The portion of iron that gets absorbed is in the form of heme from the meat one consumes, nonheme from the plants we eat, and inorganic or chelated iron from supplements and food additives. Each of these represents a form of iron.

How much iron is in the body?

Males have about 4 grams of iron in their body; females about 3.5 grams; children will usually have 3 grams or less. These 3 to 4 grams are distributed throughout the body in hemoglobin, tissues, muscles, bone marrow, blood proteins, enzymes, ferritin, and hemosiderin, and transported in plasma.

The greatest portion of iron in a normal human is in hemoglobin. Except in cases of great blood loss, pregnancy, or growth spurts, where larger amounts of iron are required, our bodies only need about 1 to 1.5 milligrams of iron per day to replace what is lost. Normal daily excretion of iron through urine, vaginal fluid, sweat, feces, and tears total about 1 to 1.5 milligrams or the equivalent of what most of us require per day to function normally. Tiny amounts of iron can also be lost because of blood loss that can occur when medicines such as aspirin are used regularly.

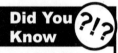

Did You Know

People with iron overload can actually set off metal detectors.

With normal iron regulatory processes working properly, iron balance is maintained. Iron is one of the few metals that cannot be excreted. When iron is absorbed in amounts beyond the body's normal iron regulatory processes, the only way to remove the metal is with blood loss or with pharmaceuticals that are formulated specifically to remove iron from ferritin.

On a whimsical note, people with iron overload have been known to set off metal detectors. "What sets off airport metal detectors is the metal itself. Iron is, after all, a metal," explains Eugene Weinberg, PhD, Professor emeritus, Microbiology, Indiana University.

2

Looking Back at Anemia

In their quest for improved health, ancient peoples ingested and applied to their bodies a wide variety of herbs and potions containing potentially toxic chemicals. They would try anything their "medicine man" dreamed up. Modern medicine had thousands of years of experience with human guinea pigs from which to select promising treatments. Many of these treatments have turned out to make sense in the light of modern science, but others were only fanciful.

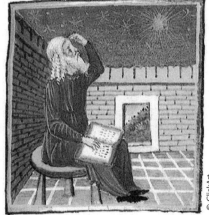

© ClickArt

Since iron was thought of as the "metal of heaven"—some scholars think this was because of the high iron content found in meteorites that had fallen from the sky—it was only a matter of time before someone tried it as a medicine.

The first "prescription" for iron can be found in the oldest recorded document, the Egyptian medicine book *Ebers Papyrus*, which dates back to about 1500 B.C. It is, oddly enough, a prescription for a potion—along with some magic words—to treat baldness:

Parts of this chapter are excerpts from *Iron and Your Heart* © 1991 St. Martin's Press and are reprinted with permission of the author, Randy Lauffer, PhD.

> "O shining One, thou who hoverest above!
> Xare! O disc of the sun!
> O protector of the divine Neb-Apt!"
> *to be spoken over:*
> *~ Iron ~ Red lead ~ Onions ~ Alabaster ~ Honey ~*
> *make into one and give against.*

In the Greco-Roman period, iron was regarded as a gift of the god of war, known to the Greeks as Ares and to the Romans as Mars. Iron was often applied directly to battle wounds, since it was believed that the contact with the original weapon would aid healing.

The first use of orally administered iron to obtain strength appears to be in Greek mythology. Legend has it that Jason and his Argonauts would sharpen their iron swords, letting the filings drop into red wine. It was supposed to be the savage power of the weapon that gave the wine its empowering force. But we now know that some of the iron would dissolve in the acidic wine, providing, at most, an iron supplement.

Another Greek legend purported that a similar potion cured the mythical Prince Iphylus of impotence. The prince was unable to beget a child and consulted his local medicine man. Using a method that would delight Freudians, the doctor had the prince talk about his childhood. It turned out that the prince had suffered a severe emotional blow as a child. He had watched his father perform the gelding of a lamb and was haunted by the blood-covered knife. The knife remained both in the prince's mind and at the site of the operation, for his father had driven the bloody knife into a nearby oak tree. Doctors today might say the prince was suffering from castration anxiety. While the prince's medicine man may have had a different term for it, his recommended treatment seemed right on the mark: the prince was to confront his fears by chopping down the oak tree, recovering the knife, and preparing a potion of wine mixed with filings from the rusty knife. In the end, the prince was cured, his manhood restored, and the royal lineage was maintained. Though it was only indirectly responsible for the "cure" in this case, iron and its magical effects had nevertheless found their way into the folklore of the time.

Curing green virgins with iron

We now know that the only justified medical use of iron is in the treatment of true iron-deficiency anemia. A sustained lack of iron leads to anemia, a reduced capacity of the blood to carry oxygen, which makes its victims pale and listless. For this condition, iron is indeed a miracle drug. The story behind the discovery of iron as a treatment for anemia is rich with amusing misdiagnoses and cures.

For thousands of years, iron-deficiency anemia was common among girls after the onset of puberty. These adolescent girls failed to get enough iron to keep up with the dual demands of growth and iron loss through menstruation.

Their pale faces, for unknown reasons, often had a greenish-yellow tint, leading to the popular term "green sickness" and the medical term "chlorosis" (from the Greek word for green). Writers from Hippocrates to Shakespeare mentioned this curious disease, and several artists, particularly seventeenth-century Dutch artists, captured the image of chlorotic women in oil paintings.

The first medical description of chlorosis was by the Dutch physician Johannes Lange. In 1554, Lange wrote to a friend who had a sick daughter, surprised that no other doctor had diagnosed her properly:

> You complain to me... that your eldest daughter, Anna, is now marriageable, and has many eligible suitors, all of whom you are obliged to dismiss on account of her ill health, the cause of which no doctor can discover... Wherefore you entreat me by our ancient friendship to give an opinion on her case, with advice as to marriage, and you send me an excellent account of her symptoms. Her face which last year showed rosy cheeks and lips, has become pale and bloodless, her heart palpitates at every moment, and the pulse is visible in the temporal arteries; she loses her breath when

17

dancing or going upstairs, she dislikes her food, especially meat, and her legs swell towards the ankles. I marvel that your physicians have not diagnosed the case from such typical symptoms. It is the affection, which the women of Brabant call the "white fever," or love sickness, for lovers are always pale…

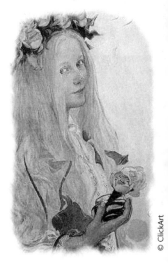

© ClickArt

It was quite common to regard this condition as a "love sickness" because it seemed frequently to affect young, unmarried women, particularly those thought to have suffered unrequited love. (One of the famous Dutch paintings by Gerrit Dou was actually entitled *Mal d'Amour*, or "Love Sickness.") The wistful mood of these poor damsels is best captured in Shakespeare's description of Viola in *Twelfth Night*:

> She never told her love
> But let concealment, like a worm in the bud
> Feed upon her damask cheek; she pined in thought
> And, with a green and yellow melancholy
> She sat, like patience on a monument.

What was the cure in those days? Marriage was often thought to be the best medicine. Johannes Lange, the first to identify "the sickness of virgins," offered this commonsense advice in the letter referred to earlier: "I therefore say, I instruct, virgins afflicted with this disease, that as soon as possible they live with men and copulate."

Why were some women so iron deficient? Modern-day nutrition sleuths have conjectured that these girls were not getting enough meat, the best source of iron. For example, the squeamish Victorians actually thought that spicy foods and meats aroused sexual appetites; these dishes were often with-held from young girls to keep their yearnings at bay. This prac-tice was especially popular in cities and towns. Country girls, on the other hand, apparently had a more natural, balanced diet and, according to some medical historians, had less of a problem with chlorosis. Even before the Victorian age, "natural girls" from the country were thought to have had some special charm, as expressed in this passage from Izaak Walton's *The Compleat Angler* (1653):

> I married a wife of late,
> The more's my unhappy fate:
> I married her for love
> As my fancy did me move,
> And not for a worldly estate.
> But oh! the green-sickness
> Soon changed her likeness;
> And all her beauty did fail.
> But 'tis not so
> With those that go
> Thro' frost and snow
> As all men know
> And carry the milking pail.

Eventually certain folk remedies, including iron filings dis-solved in wine, were identified as more effective treatments for chlorosis than marriage or certain other activities. These, of course, actually solved the iron-deficiency problem, though physicians at that time had no idea why the treatments were working. One of the more interesting customs passed on from mother to daughter involved sticking a number of nails into an apple, removing the nails after a few hours and eating the apple. We now believe that trace amounts of iron must have dissolved into the apple, bringing color back into the girls' cheeks.

The man credited with discovering iron as a specific remedy for chlorosis was Thomas Sydenham of London. In the late 1600s, he wrote a classic description of the effects of a "steel tonic":

> I comfort the blood and the spirits belonging to it by giving [iron] thirty days running... The pulse gains strength and frequency, the surface warmth, the face (no longer pale and deathlike) a fresh ruddy color... Next to steel in substance, I prefer a syrup. This is made by steeping iron or steel filings in cold Rhenish wine. When the wine is sufficiently impregnated, strain the liquor; add sugar; and boil to the consistency of syrup.

As science marched on, it was discovered that iron is an important constituent of blood. When most of the iron in blood was found to be part of the oxygen-carrying protein molecule called hemoglobin, the treatment of anemia with supplemental iron finally made complete sense. When the body is deficient in iron, the dark red hemoglobin molecules cannot be synthesized; lower hemoglobin levels in the blood lead to poor oxygen delivery and the pale cheeks of anemia.

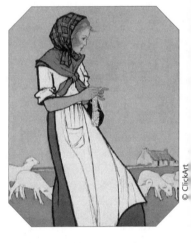

© ClickArt

Though it took a great deal of convincing, doctors finally agreed that chlorosis was caused by iron deficiency. However, many still thought it was a female nervous disorder and that iron was an effective placebo. Persuasive evidence was offered in 1893 by Ralph Stockman, a lecturer at the School of Medicine in Edinburgh, Scotland. He showed clearly that the hemoglobin levels in chlorotic women were raised after iron treatment. He also performed one of the first nutritional analyses focused on iron: he found that his own diet provided approximately 9 milligrams of iron per day; that of a normal, healthy young woman, 8 milligrams per day; and that of two chlorotic girls, 1.3 to 3.4 milligrams per day. The sick girls were obviously not getting enough iron to replace their average daily losses.

Soon after these discoveries, simple iron supplements became available for medicinal purposes. In addition, iron-deficiency anemia could be detected earlier by measuring hemoglobin levels in blood. These factors combined to wipe "green sickness" off the medical map.

> *Gold is for the mistress—silver for the maid*
> *Copper for the craftsman cunning at his trade.*
> "Good!" said the Baron, sitting in his hall,
> "But Iron—Cold Iron—is master of them all.
> So he made rebellion 'gainst the King his liege,
> Camped before his citadel and summoned it to siege.
> "Nay!" said the cannoneer on the castle wall,
> "But Iron—Cold Iron—shall be master of you all!"
> Woe for the Baron and his knights so strong,
> When the cruel cannon-balls laid 'em all along;
> He was taken prisoner, he was cast in thrall,
> And Iron—Cold Iron—was master of it all!
> Yet his King spake kindly (ah, how kind a Lord!)
> "What if I release thee now and give thee back
>   thy sword?"
> "Nay!" said the Baron, "mock not at my fall,
> For Iron—Cold Iron—is master of men all."
> *"Tears are for the craven, prayers are for the clown—*
> *Halters for the silly neck that cannot keep a crown."*
> "As my loss is grievous, so my hope is small,
> For Iron—Cold Iron—must be master of men all!"
> Yet his King made answer (few such Kings there be!)
> "Here is Bread and here is Wine—sit and sup with me.
> Eat and drink in Mary's Name, the whiles I do recall
> How Iron—Cold Iron—can be master of men all!"
> He took the Wine and blessed it. He blessed and
>   brake the Bread,
> With His own Hands He served Them, and presently
>   He Said:

"See! These Hands they pierced with nails, outside
　　My city wall,
Show Iron—Cold Iron—to be master of men all:
"Wounds are for the desperate, blows are for the strong.
Balm and oil for weary hearts all cut and bruised
with wrong.
I forgive thy treason—I redeem thy fall—
For Iron—Cold Iron—must be master of men all!"
"Crowns are for the valiant—sceptres for the bold!
Thrones and powers for mighty men who dare to take
and hold."
"Nay!" said the Baron, kneeling in his hall,
"But Iron—Cold Iron—is master of men all!
Iron out of Calvary is master of men all!"

—Rudyard Kipling's "Cold Iron" from
Rewards and Fairies (1910)

3

Definition of Anemia, Risk Factors, and Symptoms

What is anemia?

Definitions vary. If you search the Internet or refer to medical dictionaries and encyclopedias you will find a number of different definitions for anemia. Following are just a few.

Anemia is

- a condition in which the number of red blood cells is below normal
- a reduction in total circulating red blood cell mass, diagnosed by a decrease in hemoglobin concentration
- a hemoglobin level below 12 g/dl in women or 13 g/dl in men
- any condition resulting from a significant decrease in the total body erythrocyte mass
- a decrease in the circulating red blood cell mass and a corresponding decrease in the oxygen-carrying capacity of the blood
- decreased ability of the red blood cells to provide adequate oxygen supplies to body tissues
- a reduction in the hemoglobin concentration to below 13.5 g per deciliter in an adult male and below 11.5 g/dl in an adult female
- any condition characterized by an abnormal decrease in the body's total red blood cell mass

- when either red blood cells or the amount of hemoglobin (oxygen-carrying protein) in the red blood cells is low
- a condition where a person has inadequate amounts of iron to meet body demands
- a decrease in the amount of red cells in the blood caused by having too little iron
- having less than the normal number of red blood cells or less hemoglobin than normal in the blood
- decreases in numbers of red blood cells or hemoglobin content caused by blood loss, deficient erythropoiesis, excessive hemolysis, or a combination of these changes
- a blood disorder that results from a shortage of hemoglobin in the red blood cells, the disk-shaped cells that carry oxygen to all parts of the body
- an abnormal reduction in red blood cells
- when the amount of red blood cells or hemoglobin (oxygen-carrying protein in the blood) becomes low, causing the tissues of the body to be deprived of oxygen-rich blood
- a reduction in the number of red blood cells in the body
- a condition in which the blood is low on healthy red blood cells
- a blood problem
- the reduction of circulating red blood cells per cubic millimeter, the amount of hemoglobin per 100 ml, or the volume of packed red cells per 100 ml of blood

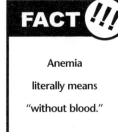

FACT!!!

Anemia

literally means

"without blood."

- when hemoglobin levels are too low to provide for the oxygen demands of the body
- decreased or absent iron stores; decreased serum ferritin; low serum iron; low transferrin saturation; increased iron-binding capacity of hypochromic, microcytic, erythrocytes
- a decreased amount of hemoglobin in the blood
- a reduction in hemoglobin
- below-normal hemoglobin

Even though all of these definitions of anemia are correct to some extent, none of them is a complete definition. If one takes into consideration the enormous number of variables that can result in anemia, providing one definition is practically impossible. Anemia literally means "without blood," but this definition is absurd; after all, we could not live without blood. One problem with a precise definition is trying to determine what "normal" is. For example, it is usual for hemoglobin to be slightly decreased in anemia of chronic disease (ACD). Anemia of chronic disease is explained in greater detail in chapter 10, but people who have ACD will have a naturally lowered hemoglobin that is perfectly "normal," given the situation.

Further, "normal" ranges for hemoglobin, hematocrit, and other red blood cell indices vary from lab to lab, between healthcare providers and healthcare policy makers. Some health agencies consider a person anemic when his or her hemoglobin value falls below 12.0 g/dL or 13.2 g/dL for women or men, respectively. These levels, however, are perfectly normal for some people. Other agencies use the term "cutpoint," where a person with a hemoglobin value of 11.0 g/dL is not anemic but at 10.9 g/dL he or she is. Some females can function just fine with hemoglobin values at 10.9 g/dL and even lower. Males, on the other hand, might have symptoms of anemia when their hemoglobin levels drop 2 or 3 points below what they are accustomed to, yet still be within a "normal" range. Hemoglobin values differ for age, gender, and ethnicity; with so many different definitions and variables to consider, it is easy to see why anemia is widely misunderstood. Within the general population, if you ask what is the number-one symptom of anemia, most will reply "fatigue." When you ask what is the remedy for fatigue, almost without exception, the response will

Reference Ranges

hemoglobin	Adult Males	Adult Females
Normal Range	13.5-17.5 g/dL	12.0-16.0 g/dL
Adolescents, Juveniles, Infants, and Newborns of normal height and weight for their age and gender		
Age 6-18 years 10.0-15.5 g/dL	Age 2-6 mos 10.0-17.0 g/dL	
Age 1-6 years 9.5-14.0 g/dL	Age 0-2 weeks 12.0-20.0 g/dL	
Age 6 mos-1 year 9.5-14.0 g/dL	Newborn 14.0-24.0 g/dL	

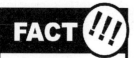

FACT

Anemia is not a *diagnosis*. It is a *symptom* of some underlying condition.

be "iron." If you ask what causes anemia, the most common reply is "not enough iron." This thinking is not limited to the general population. Anemia is still considered a diagnosis by some physicians and synonymous with a need for iron pills.

To better understand what anemia is, it might be easier to define what it isn't. Anemia is not a diagnosis; it is a symptom of some underlying condition or health event. When anemia is present, a physician must find out why.

Healthcare providers use evidence-based strategies (e.g., blood chemistries, diagnostic aids, biopsy) to investigate the underlying cause for anemia. They will rule out the most common or frequently known causes first and then pursue the more rare causes. Examples of underlying causes include (but are not limited to):

- nutritional deficiencies (iron, zinc, B$_{12}$, folate)
- increased demand for iron (pregnancy, growth spurt)
- blood loss (menstruation, childbirth, surgery, injury)
- disease (infections, autoimmune, inflammatory bowel, cancer, bleeding disorders)
- hormone imbalances (hypothyroidism)
- bone marrow function (leukemia, aplastic anemia)
- chronic hemolysis (premature destruction of red blood cells)
- poisoning (lead and other heavy metals)
- medications (aspirin, anticonvulsants)
- genetics (inherited blood-forming diseases)

Sometimes the underlying cause of anemia is realized quickly. Conversely, sometimes the puzzle is solved after the tedious pursuit of a very complex set of clues. The findings of blood chemistries, diagnostic aids, biopsy, a patient's report of symptoms or presence of disease, family history, and genetics are all pieces of the puzzle. Often, these pieces will generate enough clues for the healthcare provider to make a complete diagnosis and move toward a cure, when possible. The clues can also prompt the need for additional tests, procedures, and consultations with a specialist.

Symptoms of anemia

Symptoms vary depending upon what is causing the anemia, but the most frequently reported symptom for people with anemia is chronic fatigue.

Fatigue can be caused by a number of conditions such as hormone imbalances, infection, or disease; but the fatigue that accompanies anemia is generally due to a lack of oxygen.

Iron in hemoglobin binds with oxygen and carries it throughout the body to vital organs. When there is inadequate iron, there is inadequate oxygen. Oxygen-deprived organs cannot function properly and may even fail if deprived of oxygen-rich blood for a prolonged length of time.

Besides fatigue, weakness is a common experience for people with anemia. Weakness is due to the body straining to acquire more oxygen; muscles stressed to function without sufficient blood flow become progressively weaker and eventually may begin to spasm. Twitching, flinching, or an uncontrollable urge to move the legs is a condition called restless legs syndrome (RLS).

Restless legs syndrome, although until recently little recognized, is a prevalent disorder affecting between 5 to 15 percent of the adult population. The accepted diagnostic criteria for RLS is based on the following four clinical symptoms:

1) A strong urge to move the extremities, usually the legs, frequently accompanied by dysesthesia (abnormal sensation on the skin, such as numbness, burning, prickly, or cutting feeling).

2) Restless movements of the extremities made to relieve the urge to move and sometimes occurring spontaneously.

3) Onset or exacerbation of symptoms when at rest and relief with movement, particularly walking. The onset may occur after some period of rest, but the relief is almost immediate with movement and persists as long as the movement continues.

4) Symptoms have a marked circadian pattern, becoming worse at night with a peak severity usually in the middle of the night.

While much of the clinical intervention for RLS has focused on the dopaminergic system (caused by dopamine, a chemical synthesized by the adrenals), there is a growing body of literature that suggests a significant role for iron. Iron deficiency has been recognized as a significant contributing cause of RLS.

Pallor, or pale skin, is often observed in a person with anemia; the person may have a ghostly pale appearance. Other areas that will be pale include the inside of the eyelids, inside of the mouth, cheeks, and tongue, the fingernail beds, and the palms of the hands. Paleness occurs as the body diverts oxygen-rich blood from less vital areas to the heart, lungs, and brain. Blue sclera may be present in the white part of the eye, which takes on a bluish tint, similar to the color of skim milk. The skin color of someone who is anemic can also be a gray-green or pale yellow.

Tongue problems can be a consequence of prolonged anemia, especially pernicious anemia, which is a vitamin-B_{12} deficiency. Lack of sufficient nutrients can cause a loss of tongue papillae, or the tiny fingerlike projections that cover the tongue. Hyposalivation, an abnormal or decreased supply of saliva (dry mouth), often accompanies tongue problems. Candida, more commonly known as a yeast infection, seems to proliferate with some forms of anemia. Candida can cause a painful tongue or mouth and is often seen as "thrush," which appears as a whitish coating on the tongue. The exact reason Candida flourishes in people who are anemic is not known; Candida needs iron to survive and proliferate. It gets its iron supply from free iron, that is, unbound iron.

Lactoferrin is a protein contained in body fluids such as saliva, tears, and vaginal secretions. Lactoferrin provides a defense function because it binds with iron and withholds the iron from pathogens such as Candida. When lactoferrin levels are low, Candida can proliferate on the free iron. Studies of patients with Sjogren's disease, which is a chronic condition of dryness in the eyes and mouth, found that many of these patients had chronic Candida infections of the eyes and mouth. These patients also had deficiencies in vitamin B, especially vitamin B_{12}, which is a prominent cause of anemia, and complaints of sore tongue. Since lactoferrin is found in fluids such as saliva, patients with reduced amounts of saliva would also have a reduced amount of lactoferrin present in the mouth. Candida could flourish in such an environment, which may provide one reason for the sore tongue often reported by patients with anemia caused by nutritional deficiencies.

Brittle or spoon nails (koilonychia) can be observed in people with iron deficiency. Koilonychia is the dystrophy or malformation of the fingernail in which the nails are concave and raised on the edges.

NOTE: buckling, shiny, raised, or depressed areas on the nail surface

Koilonychia

Image courtesy of The National Institutes of Health. Copyright © 2002 A.D.A.M., Inc.

Pica, or the desire to eat nonfood items such as glue, hair, paint, clay, or dirt, is a symptom of iron deficiency that can be seen in any age, but pica is most often seen in children. In adults pica might manifest itself as a craving for ice, especially a need to chew ice.

Headache, dizziness, drowsiness, shortness of breath, and syncope (loss of consciousness) occur when too little oxygen is available to the heart and the brain. This lack of oxygen can also bring on tachycardia (rapid heartbeat) and chest pain. Shortness of breath is due to air hunger, or need for oxygen. Air hunger is compensation by the respiratory system to take in more oxygen quickly with rapid, shallow breaths. Weakness is due to insufficient oxygen to muscles.

An enlarged spleen (splenomegaly) or enlarged or inflamed liver (hepatomegaly) can be present with hemolytic anemias such as combined sickle cell disease, thalassemia, hemoglobin C disease, or in some viral infections such as viral hepatitis and AIDS.

Symptoms not generally thought to accompany anemia include stomach pain, acid reflux, vomiting, diarrhea, rash, and fever. These symptoms can be a result of infection with a wide variety of germs, such as harmful bacteria, viruses, and intestinal parasites. If not treated, these invaders can cause blood loss from the digestive tract and iron deficiency eventually develops.

How is anemia detected?

Children are routinely checked for iron deficiency with or without anemia at the ages of six, nine, and twelve months. Iron deficiency with or without anemia is determined by the level of hemoglobin and serum ferritin. A person can be iron deficient (low iron stores in ferritin) but not be anemic because of the hemoglobin concentration being within a normal range. Iron deficiency with anemia occurs when both the hemoglobin and serum ferritin are below normal. Later in this chapter, hemoglobin and serum ferritin are discussed in greater detail.

Others routinely checked for iron deficiency anemia are those who are in high-risk groups, such as young women of childbearing age, pregnant females, and ethnic groups where inherited anemia is common.

As iron deficiency is only one cause of anemia, specific tests are used to differentiate between these causes. When hemoglobin values are below the established normal range for age and gender, a complete blood count is the first set of tests a healthcare provider may order. Findings from the complete blood count will yield basic information such as red blood cell size, shape, weight, quality, and quantity, which enables the physician to classify the anemia present in the patient.

Anemia is classified by measuring the size, weight, and hemoglobin content of red blood cells. Mean corpuscular volume (MCV) is the measure of the average volume or size of a single red blood cell. When MCV is decreased, red blood cells are abnormally small or microcytic; conversely, when the red blood cells are abnormally large they are macrocytic.

Red blood cell distribution width (RDW) also contributes information about cell size—mostly it helps compare the differences in size between cells. Mean corpuscular hemoglobin (MCH) expresses how much color is contained in a red blood cell. Hypochromic are pale in color; hyperchromic are dark. Mean corpuscular hemoglobin concentration (MCHC) is the percentage of hemoglobin contained within a single red blood cell.

Red blood cells can also be normal in size (normocytic) and color (normochromic) and the patient still be anemic. Normocytic-normochromic anemia can be seen in early stage iron deficiency, anemia of chronic disease, and acute blood loss. Microcytic-hypochromic anemia can be seen in late stage iron deficiency, thalassemia, and lead poisoning. Microcytic-normochromic anemia can be seen in renal disease. Macrocytic-normochromic anemia can be seen in vitamin B_{12} or folate deficiency and in some chemotherapy patients. This latter classification is also called megaloblastic anemia.

Causes of Anemia	
Iron Deficiency	Not enough meat in the diet Increased demand for iron growth spurts, pregnancy Blood loss due to: heavy menstruation, parasites, tumors or fibroids, lesions, ulcers, tumor or cancer; drinking cow's milk before age of two
Problems of Absorption	H.pylori infection Crohn's Achlorhydria
Vitamin & Mineral Deficiencies	B6 due to alcoholic abuse Vitamin A, B, C, E, K, zinc, copper or iron B12 due to lack of intrinsic factor
Early Hemolysis (Premature destruction of red blood cells)	Inherited hemolytic anemias Acquired or mechanical hemolytic anemias Enzyme deficiencies Misshapen red blood cells Autoimmune disease
Problems with Erythropoiesis (Red blood cell production)	Kidney failure Bone marrow failure (Aplastic Anemia) Cancer Thalassemia Sideroblastic Anemia
Bleeding Disorders	von Willebrand's PNH Hemophilia

The retic count or reticulocyte index is another test that is used to determine the cause of anemia. This test tells a physician how well the bone marrow is responding to the anemia. If the retic count is elevated, the bone marrow is responding appropriately. If the retic count is low there is inadequate response. In this case a bone marrow aspiration may be necessary to examine the cells directly for more serious and complicated diseases such as sideroblastic anemia or leukemia.

Complete Blood Count

	Findings	Possible Cause
Red Blood Cell Indices	MCV <80fL (microcytic)	Iron-Deficiency Anemia Anemia of Chronic Disease Thalassemia
	MCV >100fL (macrocytic)	Vitamin B12, B6 or Folate Deficiency
	MCV Normal (normocytic)	Renal Insufficiency Thyroid Disease Liver Disease
White Blood Cell	Increased	Infection Inflammation
	Decreased	Bone marrow problem Autoimmune Disease Drug Toxicity
Platelets	Increased	Malignancy Iron-Deficiency Anemia Rheumatoid Arthritis
	Decreased	Hemorrhage Leukemia Pernicious Anemia Hemolytic Anemia Infection

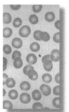
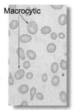
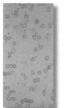

Macrocytic

Normal red blood cells   Red blood cells   Microcytic red blood cells

Images courtesy of the American Society of Hematology.

A fecal exam can often detect occult (hidden) blood loss from the digestive tract or the lung. Blood that is coughed up and swallowed or bleeding caused by inflammation due to ulcer, infection, or inflammatory bowel disease will cause the test to be positive.

Iron studies

Hemoglobin measures the functional iron, which is the iron that is circulating and delivering oxygen to tissues throughout the body. Iron is also contained in stores; serum ferritin is used to determine this value. Iron can also be free (unbound) or in transit, bound to transferrin.

Transferrin is the transport protein that binds with iron and carries it to various sites in the body such as the liver and bone marrow. Transferrin and serum iron are evaluated to determine how much iron is in transport in the body. Together, these values help a physician determine iron deficiency anemia and anemia of chronic disease. This is determined by calculating the transferrin iron saturation percentage (TS%) by dividing serum iron by TIBC (total iron binding capacity) and multiplying by 100 percent. Normal TS% is 25 to 35 percent; in anemia of chronic disease TS%

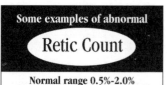

Some examples of abnormal

Retic Count

Normal range 0.5%-2.0%

 Increased retic count

Hemolytic anemia
Sickle cell anemia
Hemorrhage
Pregnancy

Decreased retic count

Pernicious anemia
Folic acid deficiency
Aplastic anemia
Chronic infection
Marrow failure
Leukemia

can be 15 to 25 percent and in iron deficiency anemia the TS% is 15 or below.

Serum transferrin receptor (sTfR) is another iron-related test, although it is not widely used by healthcare providers. The sTfR is not affected by inflammation or infection as is serum ferritin, and therefore can help the physician distinguish between iron deficiency anemia, anemia of chronic disease, and iron overload. Furthermore, the sTfR is elevated between the stages of iron deficiency even before hemoglobin drops below normal and is therefore a better way to diagnose true cases of iron deficiency anemia, especially subclinical cases that might not be identified until symptoms manifest.

Another test used to determine iron deficiency is the reticulocyte hemoglobin content (CHr). This test is a direct measurement of young red blood cells (reticulocyte) in hemoglobin. It may identify iron-deficient states earlier when compared to traditional parameters for iron deficiency (serum iron <40 mcg, TS<15%, serum ferritin <20 ng/mL, or hemoglobin <11.0 g/dL). CHr is especially helpful in pediatric cases, where early intervention can take place.

A family practice physician or physician's assistant is qualified to perform basic iron panel tests and address most causes of iron deficiency. If the cause of anemia is complicated the family physician will refer the patient to a specialist, where a more comprehensive set of tests and procedures will be performed.

Important Ferritin Reference Ranges *ferritin*	Adult Males	Adult Females
Normal Range	up to 300 ng/mL	up to 200 ng/mL
In treatment*	below 100 ng/mL	below 100 ng/mL
Ideal maintenance	25-75 ng/mL	25-75 ng/mL
Adolescents, Juveniles, Infants, and Newborns of normal height and weight for their age and gender		
Male ages 10-19 23-70 ng/mL	Infants 7-12 months 60-80 ng/mL	
Female ages 10-19 6-40 ng/mL	Newborn 1-6 months 6-410 ng/mL	
Children ages 6-9 10-55 ng/mL	Newborn 1-30 days 6-400 ng/mL	
Children ages 1-5 6-24 ng/mL		

*In treatment applies only to patients with hereditary hemochromatosis undergoing therapeutic phlebotomy

As a general rule, when the anemia is suspected to be due to problems of the digestive system, the patient is referred to a gastroenterologist. If renal disease is suspected, a urologist, nephrologist, or gastroenterologist can be consulted. When the problem is with the blood or blood-forming organs, the patient may be referred to a hematologist. All specialists may deal with cancers related to their fields, but often when cancer is diagnosed the patient is referred to a hematologist/oncologist for treatment.

These specialists are not the only types of physician that might be consulted. Internists, cardiologists, neurologists, pediatricians, gynecologists, pulmonary specialists, endocrinologists, infectious disease specialists, and surgeons also may be involved in the diagnosis and treatment of anemia.

Who is at risk for anemia?

Nearly 3.5 million Americans have some form of anemia, and this is probably a conservative estimate when all causes of anemia are taken into consideration. Worldwide estimates of anemia range from 2 to 3 billion. This makes anemia one of the world's leading health concerns. Anemias can affect young children, toddlers, juveniles, adolescents, teens, young women, young men, adults, expectant mothers, the elderly, all ethnic groups, active people, inactive people, people of all shapes and sizes.

4

The Normal Blood Cell Cycle

Blood accounts for nearly 7 percent of the body's total weight. When we lose blood or blood cannot be produced normally, we become anemic. As blood is pumped out of the heart, it circulates through arteries, capillaries, and veins, bringing oxygen, electrolytes, hormones, vitamins, antibodies, and nutrients to tissues of the body. From these tissues blood carries metabolic waste to the kidneys and the liver to be excreted and carbon dioxide to the lungs to be expelled through exhalation.

Liquid components of blood
About half of the blood volume is composed of blood cells; the other half consists of a liquid called plasma. Plasma is mostly water, which contains dissolved salts, sugars, hormones, electrolytes, fats, minerals, vitamins, and proteins such as albumin. Plasma also contains antibodies called immunoglobulins and clotting proteins, which control bleeding. Plasma represents a little more than half of the total blood volume. Besides being a transport vehicle for blood cells, plasma cools and warms the body as needed and provides a reservoir of water for the body that prevents blood vessels from collapsing or clogging. Plasma also helps to maintain blood pressure and circulation throughout the body.

Cellular components
Cells such as red blood cells, white blood cells, lymph cells, and platelets make up about 40 to 45 percent of the total volume of the blood. Erythrocytes, which are red blood cells (RBCs),

contain hemoglobin, a protein that enables the blood to transport oxygen and carbon dioxide. Leukocytes are white blood cells (WBCs), which make up approximately 1 percent of the blood volume, in a ratio of about 1 white blood cell to every 600 to 660 red blood cells. White blood cells defend the body against the invasion of harmful pathogens, such as bacteria, viruses, fungi, and cancer cells. Lymphocytes are released into blood from the lymphatic system and work with certain white blood cells as part of the immune and defense system.

How cells are made

All blood cells begin as stem cells produced by the bone marrow, which is contained in the sternum, vertebrae of the spine, ribs, hips, and skull. A stem cell is called pluripotent because it has the potential to be many types of cells. Stem cells are released from marrow based on need, such as blood loss or inflammation. If a lymph cell is needed, stem cells are released to the lymphatic system to become B-cells or T-cells. If a blood cell is needed, stem cells become part of the myeloid system where cells become platelets, macrophages, granulocytes, or red blood cells.

Red blood cells contain hemoglobin, which can bind with gases such as oxygen and carbon dioxide. Hemoglobin carries up to four atoms of oxygen to the tissues and exchanges them for two atoms of carbon dioxide (CO_2). CO_2 is then carried by hemoglobin to the lungs, where the CO_2 is expelled upon exhalation. When the number of circulating red blood cells drops below a certain level, the person is deprived of oxygen and carbon dioxide builds to toxic levels in the body.

Normal red blood cells are disc-shaped, concave on both sides. They are very pliable so that they can squeeze through the smallest capillaries.

normal red
blood cell

White blood cells can be classified into three general types: granulocytes, which are characterized by enzyme-containing granules that can be seen with a microscope; monocytes/macrophages; and lymphocytes. Lymphocytes and monocytes do not normally contain cytoplasmic granules visible by light microscopy.

There are three types of granulocytes: neutrophils, eosinophils, and basophils. Each type of white blood cell responds to a particular invader. For example, neutrophils respond to bacterial and fungal infections; eosinophils respond to allergic reactions, kill parasites, and attack cancer cells; basophils also respond to allergies.

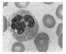
neutrophil

Immature neutrophils are called band cells; when they mature their nuclei become segmented (polymorphonuclear—PMN). Normally, neutrophils account for 50 to 70 percent of all leukocytes. If the count exceeds this percentage, the cause is usually due to an acute infection such as appendicitis, smallpox, or rheumatic fever. If the count is considerably less, it may be due to a viral infection such as influenza, viral hepatitis, or measles.

Eosinophils kill parasites, destroy cancer cells, and are involved in allergic responses. This granulocyte has large granules that contain digestive enzymes that are particularly effective against parasitic worms in their larval form. These cells also phagocytize antigen–antibody complexes.

eosinophil

These cells account for fewer than 5 percent of the WBCs. Increases beyond this amount may

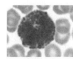
basophil

be due to parasitic diseases, bronchial asthma or hay fever, or other allergies. Eosinopenia (low eosinophils) may occur when the body is severely stressed.

Basophils play a central role in inflammatory and immediate allergic reactions. Basophils are the smallest circulating granulocytes and contain histamines (cause vasodilation) and heparin (anticoagulant).

In a differential WBC count we rarely see these as they represent less than 1 percent of all leukocytes. If the count showed an abnormally high number of these cells, a myeloproliferative syndrome or an immunologic/inflammatory disorder may be suspected.

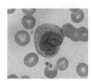
monocytes

The monocyte, pictured at the right, is the largest of the leukocytes and is agranular. The nucleus is most often "U"- or kidney bean–shaped because it is folded over. Monocytes become macrophages in response to cytokines released into the bloodstream when a harmful pathogen has invaded the body. As a macrophage, these cells are phagocytic, which means they ingest things as they function to defend the body against viruses, bacteria, and other invaders. These cells account for 3 to 9 percent of all leukocytes. In people with malaria, endocarditis, typhoid fever, and Rocky Mountain spotted fever, monocytes increase in number.

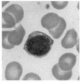

lymphocyte

Lymphocytes originate in bone marrow and myeloid tissue and are carried in the bloodstream to the lymph nodes, spleen, and tonsils. There are two types of lymphocytes: T-cells and B-cells. These cells play an important role in our immune response. The T-lymphocytes act against virus-infected cells and tumor cells. The B-lymphocytes produce antibodies.

Platelets (thrombocytes) are small fragments of blood cells that contain clotting factors that are responsible for blood coagulation. Platelets control bleeding by gathering at a bleeding site in a sticky clump that plugs up the open wound.

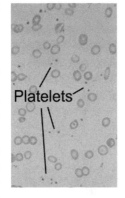

Platelets

When any complication in the process of blood cell production occurs, such as renal failure, bone marrow failure, nutritional deficiencies, problems of absorption, inherited or acquired blood disorders, and problems of hemolysis (early destruction of red blood cells), anemia is the consequence.

We appreciate the contribution of images to this chapter made by: Professor of Biology Dr. J. Fawcett, University of Nebraska at Omaha; the American Society of Hematologists; Sherri Wick for the images of blood cells; the National Institutes of Alcohol Abuse and Alcoholism; Harold S. Ballard, MD, Associate Chief of Hematology and Oncology at the New York Department of Veterans Affairs Medical Center, New York, New York, for the illustration of the blood cell development.

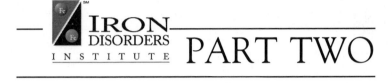

PART TWO

Iron-Deficiency Anemia—Most
Common Cause

5

Anemia in Newborns, Infants, and Toddlers

"In 1993 it was estimated that the prevalence of iron-deficiency anemia among children younger than five years was less than 3 percent and most cases were mild; however, among high-risk groups, the prevalence may be 10 to 30 percent. Increased prevalence of iron-deficiency anemia occurs among blacks, American Indians, Alaska Natives, persons of low socioeconomic status, preterm and low–birth weight infants, immigrants from developing countries, and infants whose primary nutritional source is unfortified cow's milk."

—*Martin C. Mahoney, MD, PhD, "Screening for Iron-Deficiency Anemia Among Children and Adolescents,"* American Family Physician, *2000*

Elaine Gunther did not know why her twenty-month-old son, Ryan, looked so pale; his eyes were hollow and sunken, with dark circles underneath. Everyone who saw Ryan commented on how ghostly he looked or how tired he seemed. Elaine had noticed this too. Even though Ryan slept all night, he wasn't as playful; normally he was very busy and curious, yanking open drawers or slamming cabinet doors. Also, she was puzzled by his habit of putting pennies into his mouth. She feared he would swallow one of the coins, but every time she took the pennies away from him, he would find something else to stick in his mouth. If he couldn't find a coin, he seemed to like chewing on paper.

Elaine took Ryan to the clinic. The doctor examined the baby and remarked that Ryan was normal height and weight for his age, but agreed he was very pale. The physician noted that the insides of Ryan's eyelids were also pale and the whites of his eyes had a blue tint. The doctor noted that Ryan had a few cavities, tachycardia (rapid heartbeat), and a bit of a murmur. Ryan's stool was normal in color but positive for blood; his liver and spleen were not enlarged. Ryan did not have a fever and he had not had a fever or any symptoms of an infection within the previous two weeks.

The physician ordered a complete blood count and while waiting for the results she asked Elaine a few more questions about Ryan. Elaine described Ryan as normally very active, cruising at four months and walking (toddling) at seven months. Elaine had breast-fed Ryan for the first four months. He pushed away from the breast and so she began feeding him milk from a bottle. She introduced foods one by one starting with soupy cream of wheat. When she mixed some sugar in it, he enjoyed the cereal and ate it well. She tried giving Ryan some beef and then some chicken, but he didn't care for either. Elaine frowned as she explained that Ryan became very hard to please and was a picky eater. She had tried giving him fruits and vegetables, but Ryan just spit them out, shivered, and shook his head "no." The only thing he enjoyed was milk. He drank the milk without a problem; he liked milk a lot. In fact, Ryan drank six to eight bottles a day; drinking the last bottle as he fell asleep.

The doctor said that she suspected Ryan had iron-deficiency anemia due to the early introduction of cow's milk. She explained that children younger than two just cannot handle some of the proteins in cow's milk. Their immature guts bleed as a result of these undigested proteins and iron-deficiency anemia is the consequence. She also explained to Elaine that children should not be given a bottle to fall asleep with; this may be the reason for Ryan's cavities. The physician suggested that Elaine stop the milk for a while, again, try to feed Ryan some meat, and give him a daily vitamin with iron. The doctor asked that Elaine bring Ryan back in four weeks.

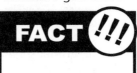

FACT !!!

Cow's milk should not be given to children younger than two years of age.

When the results of Ryan's blood work came back, the findings confirmed for the physician that Ryan's condition was iron-deficiency anemia. Ryan's hemoglobin value was 6.5 g/dL, which is below normal for his age (9.5–14.0 g/dL). His hematocrit was also low, 19.5 percent; his platelet count was elevated, and his white blood cell count was normal. Mean corpuscular volume (MCV) was below normal. His reticulocyte count was normal, and the lab reported microcytic-hypochromic red blood cells with mild anisocytosis (small, pale, and different sizes of red blood cells).

Upon the return visit four weeks later, Ryan's hemoglobin had improved. The physician recommended following the same therapy for two months and then returning for a recheck of the hemoglobin value.

Iron deficiency in newborns, infants, and toddlers

The case study of Ryan Gunther illustrates one of the most common reasons for iron-deficiency anemia in children younger than two. In newborns and infants up to the age of six months who are of normal birth weight, iron-deficiency anemia is quite rare even though the demand for iron during this time is enormous. Right before birth, the mother delivers a huge amount of iron through the placenta to her unborn child. Studies of the timing of cord clamping demonstrate that when clamping of the umbilical cord is delayed (up to two minutes versus immediate clamping), more placental blood is available to the newborn. Infants who have had the benefit of delayed cord clamping are less likely to become iron deficient as they mature. The additional blood contains additional iron, which is placed in a ferritin or bound to transferrin. The natural third-trimester infusion of iron, along with the added benefit of additional placental iron, prepares the infant for the growth

---

Iron-deficiency anemia is rarely seen in infants younger than six months.

---

that will take place in the first weeks and months of life. Normal birth weight newborns and infants have a naturally high serum ferritin and transferrin-iron saturation percentage. These levels demonstrate the elegant and natural ability of humans to assure adequate iron for normal growth, development, and survival in the first months of life.

A full-term newborn weighing eight pounds has about 300 milligrams of iron in its body. In contrast, the normal adult male body can have as much as 4,000 milligrams of iron. Nearly three-quarters of this body iron is in hemoglobin; the remaining iron is in other blood proteins, such as myoglobin,

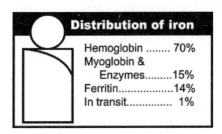

Distribution of iron

Hemoglobin 70%
Myoglobin &
    Enzymes.........15%
Ferritin...................14%
In transit............... 1%

transferrin, and ferritin. Myoglobin supplies oxygen to muscles so they can move. Transferrin is the protein that binds with iron and carries it to the bone marrow, the liver, and to ferritin. Iron stored in ferritin will be used during the first six months of growth when the demand for iron is great.

Beyond six months of age, the risk of iron-deficiency anemia increases. Iron stores are decreased and must be replenished from the diet. If adequate iron during this time is not available, developmental delays, cognitive impairment, decreased motor skills, and decreased attention span can result. Studies of test scores of older children who were iron deficient during these key developmental periods of time did not improve when the anemia was addressed later on, indicating that once a child is iron deficient some of the damage cannot be reversed. Therefore it is imperative that a child get adequate iron during these early years.

Investigators Hurtado, Claussen, and Scott of the Department of Psychology, University of Miami, report that "by age ten, the age at which the rate of educational handicaps peak, children who had suffered anemia early in life were more likely to have been placed in special education classes for children with mild to moderate mental retardation than were children without a history of anemia."

Consequences for children attributed to iron deficiency
- learning disabilities
- hyperactivity

Iron deficiency can have long-term consequences that are often irreversible. Several studies have found that reversal of the anemia did *not* improve standardized test scores, suggesting that adequate iron during the first years of life is crucial to mental development.

- decreased attention span
- impaired muscle and skeletal development
- delayed growth
- precocious puberty (early development, such as early onset of menstruation for young girls)
- mild mental retardation

Causes of iron-deficiency anemia (IDA)
Early introduction of cow's milk (an inappropriate substitute for breast milk or formula), increased iron demands during growth spurts, blood loss, and lead poisoning are the primary causes of iron-deficiency anemia in young children.

Diet
Cow's milk contains proteins that are difficult for the immature intestine to digest and should not be given to a child younger than two. Also inappropriate are substitutes for breast milk or formula, which include some health food store beverages such as rice milk, and some soy milks that may not contain adequate nutrients for an infant. Any substitute for breast milk or infant formulas should be discussed in detail with a pediatrician or family physician.

Children over the age of six months can become iron deficient if their diets do not include some meat. Meat can be introduced to some children as young as four months of age but is generally given around the age of six months or when the child develops teeth. Meat contains heme iron, a form of iron easily absorbed by the body. Nonheme iron is the type of iron we get from plants, such as grains, nuts, fruits, and vegetables. This type of iron is not as easily absorbed. Iron in fortified foods or vitamin supplements, well water, soil, or cooking utensils is also nonheme iron.

Vitamin B_{12}, B_6, folate, C, zinc, iron, and beta-carotene are essential to red blood cell production. Insufficient amounts of these nutrients can result in iron deficiency anemia. These nutrients can be obtained from meat and some plant sources, such as nuts, grains, potatoes, avocados, cereal, fruits, and leafy green vegetables.

Besides vitamin deficiencies, certain foods and substances can inhibit the absorption of plant-based or nonheme iron. These foods are: tea, coffee, dairy products, chocolate, eggs, bran fiber, apple juice, antacid products, and calcium. When consumed in amounts greater than 500 milligrams, calcium can inhibit the absorption of both nonheme and heme iron.

Growth spurts

Growth and development takes place at an astonishing rate during the first years of life, especially for a newborn. Ample iron is essential to these episodes of rapid growth. Insufficient iron during this time can result in developmental delays, learning disabilities, behavioral problems, and decreased immune function. As an infant grows, more red blood cells are needed to supply larger organs and expanding red blood cell and muscle mass. This need for iron is reflected in a naturally high transferrin-iron saturation percentage and high serum ferritin values of newborns and infants.

A parent should note that physicians do not routinely measure transferrin-iron saturation and serum ferritin of newborns and infants. A child's levels of these two iron tests will be dramatically higher than levels of older children or adults. The very high levels of transferrin-iron saturation percentage and serum ferritin are normal for newborns and infants and not a cause for concern.

Blood loss

Blood loss from the digestive tract in infants and toddlers is generally due to the early consumption of cow's milk. Undigested proteins from cow's milk can cause inflammation and eventually lead to bleeding from the intestinal tract. However, conditions of inflammation such as colitis or celiac disease can also result in anemia for small children. Another cause of blood loss is from infection with bacteria, protozoa, or parasites. Among the common culprits that can infect children are H. pylori, E. coli, G. lamblia, S. enteritidis (commonly known

Normal Ranges	TS%	Ferritin
Newborn up to six months	76-90%	6-410 ng/mL
Infant 7-12 months	18-25%	60-80 ng/mL
Child 1-5 years	22-30%	6-24 ng/mL

TS% = transferrin iron saturation percentage
Ferritin = serum ferritin

as salmonella), or parasites such as roundworm or hookworm. Behavior that can increase the risk of infection includes walking barefoot in an area contaminated by animal feces or urine (usually a pet's), eating pet droppings (sandboxes), drinking contaminated water (lakes or streams), eating contaminated foods (usually foods that are not fully cooked or have been stored at improper temperatures—e.g., meats, pastas, or beans), or improperly handling foods (i.e., insufficient hand washing or cross contamination of raw meats (especially poultry) with uncooked foods).

Poisoning

Children can be poisoned by any number of things, but when iron-deficiency anemia (IDA) is diagnosed in a child, lead poisoning is high on the list of suspects, especially if the child lives

---

Lead can be inhaled or ingested by both adults and children. Many states have laws about lead, especially for paint used in homes built prior to 1978.

---

in an older home where lead-based paints were used. Lead poisoning can mimic and also cause iron deficiency. When both iron deficiency and lead poisoning are present simultaneously, anemia can become quite severe. Children with IDA can absorb up to 50 percent more lead than children with normal hemoglobin levels.

Some physicians use the zinc protoporphyrin (ZPP) test

when lead poisoning is suspected. Elevated ZPP results are seen in both early and late iron deficiency, anemia of chronic disease, and in chronic lead poisoning. Measuring blood lead levels is a better way to determine lead poisoning because ZPP levels are not usually elevated in lead poisoning until blood lead levels are greater than 25 µg/dL. Nerve damage, hearing loss, and hypertension (high blood pressure) could already be underway. Another test, Reticulocyte Hemoglobin Content (cHr), can be used to predict iron deficiency before anemia is present.

Other causes—rare and exceptional

Problems relating to red blood cell production, such as hemoglobin diseases, abnormal bone marrow function, and red blood cell destruction (hemolysis—hemolytic anemia), are some of the less common, albeit severe, causes of anemia in children.

Hemolytic anemia can occur because of certain medications, especially antiseizure medicines, or because of infections, usually due to the antibiotics given to treat the infection. In a study of children given either sulfa antibiotics or beta-lactam antibiotics who were infected with *E. coli*, investigators found that hemolytic-uremic syndrome (HUS) developed in five of the nine (56 percent) children who were given these antibiotics.

Hemolytic anemia can also be inherited. The most common forms are sickle cell disease and thalassemia major. Read about these conditions in chapters 21 and 22; both of these types of hemolytic anemia affect children.

Bone marrow failure

Bone marrow failure, or aplastic anemia, is very rare in children; it is a serious life-threatening condition. Aplastic anemia occurs when the bone marrow is unable to produce sufficient numbers of blood cells. This may be due to an inherited defect, such as in Fanconi anemia, which affects all three blood cell types (red, white, and platelets) or in Diamond-Blackfan anemia, which affects red blood cell levels. Among the more common causes of aplastic anemia is an exposure to certain toxic chemicals, antibiotics, antiseizure medicines, cancer medications (chemotherapy), or radiation.

Leukemia

In youths nearly all leukemias are acute, such as acute lympho-cytic leukemia (ALL), which involves the cells of the lymphatic system, or acute non-lymphocytic leukemia (ANLL), which involves specific white blood cells called lymphocytes (also known as T-cells and B-cells). ANLL is sometimes called acute myelogenous leukemia (AML). Together, leukemias account for about 25 percent of cancers in children. ALL generally affects children ages two to four, although this type of leukemia can occur in children as old as eight. AML may occur in newborns or infants but is somewhat rare until the teens. Read more about leukemia in the chapter on cancers.

There are some rare but serious causes of iron-deficiency ane-mia that occur primarily in very young children. Hirschsprung's disease is a condition that leads to intestinal blood loss because portions of the colon become dilated and impacted.

Pulmonary hemosiderosis due to Heiner's syndrome, which is a group of symptoms including allergies to cow's milk, can result in blood loss. The American Academy of Family Physicians states that Heiner syndrome is "an uncommon syndrome of infancy… characterized by an immune reaction to cow's-milk proteins… resulting in… pulmonary hemosiderosis (iron over-load in the lungs), anemia, recurrent pneumonia, and failure to thrive." Children with this condition will have repeated respira-tory problems, coughing, sometimes coughing up blood, and iron-deficiency anemia due to the blood loss from the lung. They might also run a fever and vomit.

Dorr G. Dearborn, PhD, MD, Pediatric Pulmonary Division, Case Western Reserve University School of Medicine, an expert in pulmonary hemosiderosis (PH), recommends that "if your infant or child has chronic cough and chest congestion and is anemic, ask your physician to consider the possibility of pulmonary hemosiderosis among all the other more common diagnostic possibilities."

Anemia of inflammation or chronic disease

Anemia of chronic disease (also called the anemia of inflamma-tion) is a condition that results from inflammation. It is more fully explained in chapter 10; however, when this condition is present in young children, it is likely due to some common ailments, such as a head or chest cold, ear infection, tonsillitis, or stomach or intestinal flu. Other lesser known causes include bowel diseases. In one New York clinical setting, ninety-three children younger than age five (58% boys and 42% girls) with inflammatory bowel disease were studied. Principal investigator Clare Ceballos, MA, APRN-BC, PNP, WOCN, reported that the average age at diagnosis was 3.2 years. Sixty-two percent of the children had ulcerative colitis and 38 percent had Crohn's disease. Growth failure was observed in 10 percent of the children; otherwise, these children eventually achieved or exceeded growth for their percentile.

Infectious diseases in older children can include tonsillitis, mononucleosis, strep throat, and urinary tract infections, as well as bacterial infections such as *H. pylori*. These children also can experience inflammatory bowel disease. Many of these conditions are easily treatable, but some require more specialized attention by a physician expert in gastroenterology, hematology, or other pediatric specialties. In anemia of chronic disease, a mild drop in hemoglobin with an elevated serum ferritin distinguishes this transient type of anemia from iron-deficiency anemia. When the child becomes healthy again, this transient form of anemia will be corrected and the hemoglobin will return to normal. Iron supplementation is not appropriate for children with anemia due to an inflammatory response, especially if the child has a fever.

In children of any age who have slightly lower than normal hemoglobin values, anemia of chronic disease should be ruled out before supplemental iron is given. A physician can determine the difference between anemia of chronic disease and iron-deficiency anemia by measuring serum ferritin.

iron panel	IRON PANEL TESTS					
	Serum Iron	Serum Ferritin	Transferrin Iron Saturation Percentage	Total Iron Binding Capacity (TIBC)	Transferrin	Serum Transferrin Receptor
Anemia of Chronic Disease (ACD)	⬇	⬆ OR NORMAL	⬇	⬇	⬇	NORMAL
Iron Deficiency Anemia	⬇	⬇	⬇	⬆	⬆	HIGH

If the anemia persists once an illness is corrected, the doctor will want to investigate further for a secondary underlying cause of anemia that may be more serious.

Risk factors for anemia in small children
- genetics
- income level
- exposure to toxins or medications
- low birth weight
- premature clamping of the umbilical cord
- drinking cow's milk too soon or drinking formulas with inadequate nutrients
- not being breast-fed

Signs and symptoms of anemia in newborns, infants, and toddlers
Some of the first indications that anemia may be present in a child are paleness, lack of energy, and fatigue, especially when there has been adequate sleep. Other common signs include irritability, shortness of breath or frequent sighing (taking short but deep breaths), headache, and pica (the eating of non-food items).

Diagnosing anemia in children
Family doctors, pediatricians, nurses, and physician assistants are among the healthcare providers who may suspect and then determine anemia in a small child. However, if the healthcare provider informs you that your child is anemic, ask why or what is causing the anemia. If the anemia is described as "idiopathic" or no cause is given, further investigation is warranted. A visit to a specialist, such as a pediatric hematologist or gastroenterologist, to determine the causal factor of the anemia may be necessary. The child may very well need supplemental iron, but it is important to determine the cause of anemia and rule out inflammation before supplemental iron is consumed.

Young children especially cannot always articulate descriptions of symptoms such as headache, fatigue, or pain. Adults must be observant and look for signs that a child is anemic. Checking the insides of eyelids for paleness (pallor) is one way to identify youths who may have iron-deficiency anemia. Pallor is indicative of anemia, but not of what is causing the anemia. Some children may not exhibit pallor until hemoglobin values are quite low (< 7.0 g/dL). Other areas that can be checked for pallor include the inside of the mouth, cheeks, tongue, and palms of the hands. The tongue may be smooth, pale, and glossy, and seem smaller than usual in size. The fingernails may be pale, have indentations, or they can be spoon shaped, a condition known as koilonychia. Blue sclerae may be present in the white part of the eye, which takes on a bluish tint, similar to the color of skim milk.

Severe anemia, usually due to acute or sudden blood loss or drop in red blood cells, can result in syncope, which is fainting or a loss of consciousness. This is quite serious and requires immediate medical attention.

The diagnostic process is like putting together pieces of a puzzle to get a picture. In determining the cause of anemia, pieces of information are collected, studied, and put into place to form a conclusion. Each piece of information by itself is not likely to be enough to determine the cause, but collectively the pieces will help the physician to rule out conditions one by one.

A parent or caregiver may take their sick child to see a pediatrician. Keeping good notes about symptoms, behavior, and nutrition can be invaluable to finding the problem that is causing the anemia. Next, a thorough physical examination will be performed. Body temperature, weight, height, blood pressure, reflexes, and eyes will be checked. Also during the physical examination, the physician will look for physical clues such as those mentioned previously.

A parent's notes should include information about what symptoms he or she has observed in the child such as vomiting, diarrhea, breathing problems, tugging or pulling on the ears, level of activity, mood, what the child has eaten including supplements, whether or not pica was observed, and something about the home, especially the age of the home.

Another procedure the physician may do during the physical exam is a digital rectal exam (DRE). With a gloved finger inserted into the rectum the doctor obtains a fecal matter sample. From this sample blood loss can be detected; also, the sample can be further studied for worms, parasites, or certain bacteria.

hemoglobin	
Infants, Newborns, and Toddlers of normal height and weight for their age and gender	
Newborn: birth-2 weeks 12.0-20.0 g/dL	Age 6 mos-1year 9.5-14.0 g/dL
Newborn 3 weeks-2 mos14.0-24.0 g/dL	Age 1-6 years 9.5-14.0 g/dL
Age 2-6 mos 10.0-17.0 g/dL	

The first blood tests a physician might order included complete blood count (CBC), differential count, and a reticulocyte count. A simple finger stick can be used to obtain blood for these tests. If blood must be taken from the arm, a needle called a butterfly needle can be used. This needle is smaller than standard needles used to obtain blood from the arm. The CBC is a very important test because a great deal of information can be gained about the cause of anemia from the results. A CBC includes red blood cell count, hemoglobin, hematocrit, and information about the color, size, weight, and shape of red blood cells, details about white blood cell activity and platelets. The retic count or retic index provides some basic information about bone marrow function.

Pediatric ranges for hemoglobin and iron studies such as transferrin iron saturation percentage and serum ferritin are quite different from older children or adults. The differences can be seen in the normal ranges panel, where these levels are very high in the newborn and drop dramatically in the one- to five-year-old child. Abnormalities in any of these findings will be meaningful and may bring the physician closer to finding the cause of anemia. Once the cause is determined, therapy can begin.

Treatment for iron-deficiency anemia in children

Treatment will vary depending upon the underlying cause of anemia. Physicians will generally rule out iron deficiency due to lack of iron in the diet and recommend a trial of supplemental iron for one month. If there is a response in the hemoglobin value, supplementation will generally continue for another month or two, until hemoglobin is in the normal range.

In newborns and infants the very best source of iron is breast milk. Mothers are encouraged to nurse their babies for at least the first six months of life and ideally up to one year. Mother's milk serves as the infant's first immunization against numerous life-threatening diseases. Her milk contains more than sixty different enzymes, antibodies, proteins, hormones, electrolytes, vitamins, and minerals including a type of iron that is easily absorbed by her infant. Cow's milk and formulas can be fortified with vitamins and minerals, but they lack natural antibodies, hormones, and enzymes contained in breast milk. Even though breast milk is considered low in iron, the iron in mother's milk is highly bioavailable to the nursing infant. Infants absorb nearly 50 percent of the iron in breast milk compared with only 4 percent of the iron in formula.

Mother's milk also contains a high amount of lactoferrin, which is not in formulas. Lactoferrin is protein that binds with free iron to assure that harmful pathogens do not gain access to this metal. In the most current policy statement on breast-feeding, the American Academy of

> **Breast-feeding has been shown to have a positive effect on intelligence.**

Pediatrics addresses iron and infection: "The proposed mechanism is that the higher iron content of iron-fortified formulas may saturate lactoferrin, a protein important in protecting the intestine from overgrowth with *Escherichia coli* (*E. coli*). Infants fed iron-fortified formula, partially breast-fed infants supplemented with iron-fortified formula, and exclusively breast-fed infants who receive iron supplements may have a higher prevalence of *E. coli* in the fecal flora compared with exclusively breast-fed infants who receive no iron supplementation. In the latter, lactobacillus predominates."

According to recommendations by the American Academy of Pediatrics, there is strong evidence that human milk decreases the incidence or severity of diarrhea, lung infection, ear infections, bacterial infections (including bacterial meningitis), botulism, urinary tract infection, and damage to the intestinal mucosa, the lining through which all nutrients are absorbed. Additionally, there are a number of studies that show a possible protective effect for infants fed human milk against sudden infant death syndrome, Type I diabetes, which is the type that requires insulin, cancer of the lymph system, allergies,

Iron Absorption
Breast Milk • Formulas • Cow's Milk

Substance	Iron Content (mg/L)	Bioavailable iron (%)	Absorbed iron (mg/L)
Nonfortified formula	1.5--4.8	about 10%	0.15--0.48
Iron-fortified formula*	10.0--12.8	about 4%	0.40--0.51
Whole cow's milk	0.5	about 10%	0.05
Breastmilk	0.5	**about 50%**	0.25

* The average iron content is 6.8 milligrams of iron per liter of formula.

celiac sprue, Crohn's disease, ulcerative colitis, and other chronic and inflammatory bowel diseases.

Breast-feeding has also been shown to have a positive effect on intelligence. An article in the October 1999 issue of *The American Journal of Clinical Nutrition* provides that breast-fed infants tested 5.2 IQ points higher than formula-fed infants. The study, performed by Anderson, Johnstone, and Remley of the Metabolic Research Group, Veterans Affairs Medical Center, was comprehensive and involved mothers of more than 7,000 children. According to the article about the study, "Some researchers believe the link is based on the fact that well-educated, wealthier women breast-feed far more than poor and less-educated women. Consequently, breast-fed children will be found to test better for all the reasons that wealthier children from high social classes test better on standardized tests." To address this bias, Anderson's group weighted and mathematically controlled for the effects of fifteen factors from their study, such as maternal smoking and education, birth weight, birth order, and family income. After all these factors were removed, the researchers still found that breast-fed babies tested 3.1 IQ points higher than formula-fed babies.

The American Academy of Pediatrics (AAP) recommends breast-feeding exclusively for an infant's first six months. Unfortunately the continued choice to breast-feed declines for many mothers once they leave the hospital. An AAP survey provides that "in 1995, 59.4 percent of women in the United

States were breast-feeding either exclusively or in combination with formula feeding at the time of hospital discharge; only 21.6 percent of mothers were nursing at 6 months, and many of these were supplementing with formula... The highest rates of breast-feeding are observed among higher-income, college-educated women older than 30 years of age living in the Mountain and Pacific regions of the United States."

More reasons to breast-feed

Mother's milk is sterile, just the right temperature, and readily available as long as Mom consumes adequate amounts of fluid. The interaction between mother and child during breast-feeding provides an immeasurable bonding activity. Also, mothers who breast-feed their babies return to prepregnancy weight more readily and get the benefit of brain chemicals released during the nursing process. This is not to suggest that bonding will not take place if a mother chooses to bottle feed her infant.

Nutritionists in the Department of Nutrition at the University of California, Davis, state that "breast-feeding is sufficient to maintain adequate iron nutrition for most, if not all, of the

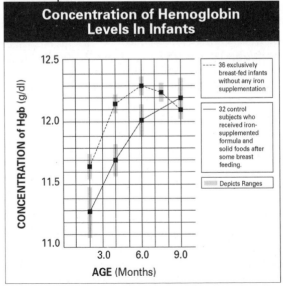

Concentration of Hemoglobin Levels In Infants

CONCENTRATION of Hgb (g/dl)

AGE (Months)

- - - - 36 exclusively breast-fed infants without any iron supplementation

——— 32 control subjects who received iron-supplemented formula and solid foods after some breast feeding.

▓▓ Depicts Ranges

Image adapted from Siimes, MA, "Hematopoeisis and Storage of Iron in infants." In *Iron Metabolism in Infants*, edited by B. Lonnerdal, 34–62. CRC Press: Boca Raton, FL, 1990.

first year of life. Infants fed fortified formula containing 10–14 mg/L of iron are receiving as much as 24 times more iron per day than what breast-fed infants consume." This suggests that these formulas may contain more iron than the infant needs.

Studies have shown that the amount of iron in breast milk cannot be increased by giving iron supplements to the mother. These studies show that anemic women taking iron supplements have levels of iron in their milk that are similar to those of non-anemic women, suggesting that the amount of iron the breast fed infant receives is highly regulated by the mother's body.

There are some situations in which breast-feeding is not in the best interest of the infant. One case involves infants with galactosemia, an inherited enzyme deficiency whereby the baby cannot metabolize galactose, an enzyme needed by the liver to produce glucose or blood sugar. Other exceptions for breast-feeding include mothers who use illegal drugs, have untreated active tuberculosis, or have been infected with the human immunodeficiency virus (HIV). These drugs and diseases can be transmitted to an infant through breast milk.

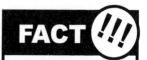

FACT !!!

Low-iron formula is defined by the U.S. Food and Drug Administration (FDA) as containing less than 6.7 milligrams of iron to one liter of formula.

When an infant is not breast-fed, formula fortified with at least 4.5 up to 10 milligrams of iron per liter of formula is recommended. The attending family physician or pediatrician will determine an individual child's needs within this range. There are milk-based and soy-based formulas from which to choose. Again, individual needs must be assessed based on circumstances, such as whether or not the formula is the only source of food, the formula is supplemental to some amount of breast milk, the child is being raised as a vegetarian, or if the child has allergies. All of these factors along with general health and growth rate of the child will help the physician to determine the right formula.

According to the American Academy of Pediatrics 1999 Committee on Nutrition Policy Statement, "Numerous studies have documented the unequivocal reduction in iron deficiency... in infants fed iron-fortified versus low-iron formula."

Prior to the 1970s, when iron-deficiency anemia in the United States was significantly higher, infant formulas were often homemade using evaporated milk, which contained about 2 mg/L of iron. In the early 1970s, when manufacturers of infant formulas increased iron fortification up from 10 mg/L to 12 mg/L of iron, the rate of iron-deficiency anemia in the United States dropped dramatically from more than 20 percent to less than 3 percent, where it has remained to date.

Weaning off breast milk

Some infants will wean themselves from the breast as early as four months of age but the average weaning takes place around six to nine months. A mild anemia is observed in breast-fed babies at about nine months. This is a normal phenomenon and might be suggestive of the natural weaning process. As an infant matures, the need for sucking decreases and the need to develop muscles for chewing arises. During this period of transition it is probably time to supplement mother's milk with other food sources such as meats, grains, fruits, and vegetables.

At the age of four to five months babies can be introduced to cereals and pureed vegetables, fruits, and meats. It is best to introduce foods one at a time rather than in combination because of the possibility of intolerance and allergic reaction to some foods.

Young children who are weaned from breast milk are usually fed iron-fortified cereals. Rice cereal mixed with a bit of breast milk is the first choice because rice contains no gluten and is better tolerated by the immature digestive systems of young children. Oatmeal is a fairly good source of iron and often well tolerated.

Next, pureed vegetables are added to the diet, such as carrots, yams, and green beans, and then fruits are introduced. Vegetables and fruits high in beta-carotene are excellent choices as beta-carotene improves the absorption of dietary iron. Vitamin C also improves the absorption of iron but vitamin C is destroyed in cooking and must be added as a supplement to foods. Juices that are fortified with vitamin C are fine if used sparingly and only given from a cup. Though it has no effect on the absorption of iron, juice should not be given in baby bottles. Drinking from a cup can protect a child from cavity-causing bacteria that multiply rapidly in the sugary juices confined to a baby bottle.

Foods that inhibit the absorption of iron **in kids**	
Milk & Dairy	Tea
Eggs	Coffee
Grape Juice	Chocolate
Bran Fiber	

Foods that increase the absorption of iron
Meat, Vitamin C, Beta–carotene, Sugar (NOTE: honey should not be given to an infant or child younger than age one.)

When trying to maximize the amount of iron your child can get from these new foods, keep in mind the combinations of foods eaten together. Certain foods and substances can inhibit or improve the absorption of iron. No nutritional food should be eliminated from a child's diet, unless there is an allergy to that food.

Sugar improves the absorption of iron, but parents should be cautioned against using refined sugars or honey. Refined sugar, also called white sugar, can result in damage to developing teeth, decay, and cavities, and refined sugar contains no nutrients whatsoever. Honey should not be given to babies because of a Botulism bacterium that can be dangerous and even deadly to a young child. Honey can be safely given to children after the age of one.

Pureed or finely chopped dried fruits, such as apricots, and fresh fruits, such as peaches and pears, are good choices. Also, blackstrap molasses, which is rich in iron, can be used to sweeten cereals. When dried fruits or blackstrap molasses are added to cereal, a half-cup serving can contain as much as 7 milligrams of iron. Cereals are best eaten without milk (except for breast milk), because milk can inhibit the absorption of iron due to its calcium and phosphate content.

Taking action: prevention is key

- Breast-feed for the first six to nine months if possible.
- When using infant formulas, especially low-iron choices, see a pediatrician for regular checkups to assure adequate levels of iron are available for red cell production.
- Watch for changes in your child, such as paleness of skin, eyelids, and insides of the mouth, irritability, or unusual sleepiness.
- Do not give iron to a child with a fever or a child who is vomiting or who has diarrhea or who is in pain.
- Only give iron supplements as directed by a doctor.

Resources

Numerous resources are available through the National Institutes of Health Library of Medicine, www.nlm.nih.gov; also, there are organizations that address specific disorders—look for them on the Internet or in other chapters of this book. While compiling *Guide to Anemia*, the editors found these resources particularly helpful: American Academy of Pediatrics, www.aap.org; the American Academy of Family Physicians magazine and their website www.aafp.org; National Organization of Rare Diseases (NORD), www.rarediseases.org; and www.cdc.gov, www.nih.gov, www.kidshealth.org, and www.nemours.org.

6

Anemia in Juveniles, Adolescents, and Early Teens

"As many as 20 percent of children in the United States will be anemic at some point by the age of eighteen."

—Joseph J. Irwin, MD, and Jeffrey T. Kirchner, DO, "Anemia in Children," American Academy of Family Physicians, October 2001

Sixteen-year-old Annie Porter fainted during math class. Her teacher rushed to the office and called the emergency medical service. Upon arrival the emergency attendant noted that Annie's blood pressure was low, her breathing shallow, her pulse weak, and her heartbeat erratic. They immediately took her to the emergency room. Numerous tests were performed, including a complete blood count and serum ferritin. The tests revealed that Annie was severely anemic and quite iron deficient. Her hemoglobin was a dangerous 5.9 g/dL and her serum ferritin was 4 ng/mL. She was given 2 units of blood and admitted to the hospital.

For several months prior to the incident, Annie had not felt well. She was very thin, tired most of the time, and had vicious and frequent headaches. She was also very pale. Annie was quite popular in school and involved in many activities. She disregarded the symptoms and went on with her busy schedule. Often, she had felt dizzy but didn't tell anyone. She ate on the run, frequently eating only an apple or drinking chocolate milk at mealtimes.

While in the hospital her family doctor visited with her and was able to determine that Annie had serious problems with her menstrual cycle. She had her first period at age eleven and from onset to the age of fifteen her periods were never regular. In the past few months the situation had worsened. Her periods were occurring sometimes every two weeks and often were very heavy.

The physician prescribed oral iron supplements, 325 milligrams twice a day and a birth control pill to regulate Annie's menstrual cycle. The doctor also recommended that Annie eat more regularly and include meat in her diet. Annie had reported that she was a vegetarian.

At her first follow-up visit, Annie's hemoglobin was 12.6 g/dL, a dramatic improvement. After six months on the birth control pills, Annie discontinued taking them. Her cycle had become regular and she no longer had symptoms.

Iron deficiency in youths

Iron-deficiency anemia is relatively uncommon in youths, especially males, but it is the most common cause of anemia in young females, especially those who have erratic or heavy menstrual cycles. Otherwise, when anemia is seen in older children, it is usually anemia of chronic disease due to inflammation from an infection. Infection can be as mild as a simple chronic ear infection or a more serious infection such as viral hepatitis B or C, or bacterial infections such as *Helicobacter pylori* (*H. pylori*). People with infections that are not addressed can develop iron-deficiency anemia, generally from blood loss, or poor absorption.

Estimates of iron-deficiency anemia (IDA) among U.S. children range between 2 and 10 percent, but they are as high as 80 percent in developing countries. Poverty and disease such as malaria and intestinal parasites top the list for causes of anemia among children of these developing countries.

Causes of anemia in juveniles, adolescents, and teens

Increased demands for iron: the growth spurt
In normal growth, cells of the muscles, bones, brain, heart, lungs, sex organs, and even skin all grow at a rate that keeps each body system compatible in size. Requirements for proper

growth include a number of nutrients. Some of the most critical to growth include adequate protein, vitamins B_{12} and B_6, folate, calcium, zinc, copper, magnesium, and iron. These nutrients are dependent upon one another to assure the proper rate of growth takes place. An imbalance in any of these nutrients at any moment in the growth process can result in poor mental development and brain function, underdeveloped bodies, short stature, low weight, bone deformities, muscle wasting, and poor sexual development. Other problems of iron deficiencies during this growth period include attention deficit disorder, hyperactivity, and in extreme cases of iron deprivation, mental retardation.

A growth period begins as the youngster sleeps, when the anterior lobe of the pituitary releases a hormone appropriately named the growth hormone (GH) into the bloodstream. Growth hormone is not only essential to how the body grows but it is also necessary for normal metabolism of protein, lipids, carbohydrates, and minerals.

The growth hormone makes its way through the bloodstream to bind to receptors on the surface of the liver. Receptors work just like a key fits into a lock. The liver is stimulated to produce another type of growth hormone called IGF-1 or somatomedin, which is released into the bloodstream where it is carried to receptors on bones, the heart, lungs, brain, and sex organs so that each of these organs can begin to grow in unison.

While growth takes place, there is an increase in red blood cell and muscle mass, a decrease in body fat, and an increase in the metabolic rate. Organs become greater in size and additional iron is needed to supply oxygen to the larger organs and support the increase in the amount of red blood cells. Considering that this growth spurt involves the entire body and its systems, it is easy to see why huge amounts of iron are required during periods of rapid growth. Control of growth is managed by the hypothalamus, a gland at the base of the brain that regulates the pituitary. When adequate growth has taken place, the hypothalamus signals the anterior pituitary to slow down production of the growth hormone and healthy growth is observed.

In preparation for these episodes of tremendous growth, the

human body first steps up production of transferrin, a protein that binds with and transports iron. Then the body increases absorption of iron from the intestines. For this reason, a temporary increase in transferrin iron saturation percentage may be present in these youths. The level should return to normal range once the growth spurt has slowed. One other test that can be naturally elevated during a growth spurt is the enzyme ALP (alkaline phosphatase). The ALP increases in youths that are undergoing rapid bone growth changes. In these youths GGT (gamma glutamyl transpeptidase) will be normal, which is how a physician distinguishes between liver disease and normal bone growth activity.

Episodes of growth are somewhat predictable in all children even though youths mature at different rates. Periods of rapid growth and development occur just before birth, the first six months of life, at toddler age, at juvenile age, as an adolescent, and in the early to middle teenage years. Eventually, all healthy children will achieve height and weight within a normal range given their genetic makeup.

Anemia of chronic disease

In young children, anemia of chronic disease is likely due to some chronic condition such as a head or chest cold, ear infection, tonsillitis, stomach flu, or intestinal flu. In older children infectious diseases such as measles, mumps, roseola, chickenpox, rhinovirus adenovirus, mononucleosis, strep throat, urinary tract infections, and *H. pylori* are among the more common conditions associated with anemia of chronic disease.

> **IMPORTANT**
>
> In children who are growing, the ALP can be naturally elevated because of bone growth. This natural elevation should not to be misinterpreted as iron overload disease.

Most of these conditions are treatable and when the child becomes healthy again the anemia will disappear. If the anemia persists once an illness is corrected, the doctor will want to investigate further for a secondary underlying cause of anemia that may be more serious.

Anemia of chronic disease can be present in serious conditions such as peptic or duodenal ulcer, cancer, leukemia, inflammatory bowel disease, cystic fibrosis, pulmonary hemosiderosis, biliary disease, liver disease, such as viral hepatitis B or C, AIDS, pancreatic disease, diabetes, arthritis, and renal failure, which are among the less common causes of anemia in youths.

Blood loss in youths

Blood loss in youths can be caused by inflammatory bowel disease such as celiac sprue or Crohn's disease, an infection in the respiratory or digestive tract. Human parvovirus B-19, also known as fifth disease and "slapped-face" disease, or viral hepatitis B or C are among the viruses that can result in blood loss. Bacterial infections with *Helicobacter* (*H. pylori*), *E. coli*, *S. enteritidis* (salmonella), or parasites such as roundworm, hookworm, or *G. lamblia* are among the types of infections that can cause blood loss.

Since infection with most of these organisms results in symptoms of diarrhea, fever, and vomiting, the blood loss is acute and will very likely be identified and corrected early by the attending physician. One germ called *Helicobacter* might slip by unnoticed. A child infected with *Helicobacter* might complain frequently of a stomach ache, which is often mistakenly attributed to improper diet or stress (such as not wanting to go to school).

Historically, infection with *Helicobacter* was not thought to occur in children. In a 1999 *American Family Physician* article, Dr. Alan Lake, Johns Hopkins University School of Medicine, writes, "Exposure to the bacterium (*H. pylori*) increases during childhood, infecting approximately 11 percent by the age of five, 20 percent by the age of ten and as much as 45 percent by the late teens." More recently, scientists at the Department of Medicine, Veterans Affairs Medical Center and Baylor College of Medicine, Houston, completed a study that confirmed earlier findings, determining the prevalence of *H. pylori* in children to be high.

In the study, published in the March 16, 2002, issue of *Lancet*, Dr. Hoda Malaty and her colleagues tested blood samples from 224 children who were participating in a Louisiana-based heart study. Malaty's team of investigators found that among the participants, 8 percent of children aged one to three had antibodies against *H. pylori* as compared to 13 percent of black children and 4 percent of white children. The rate of infection continued to increase more rapidly among black children. By the time these children reached eighteen to twenty-three years of age, nearly 25 percent of them were

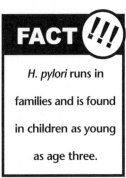

FACT !!!

H. pylori runs in families and is found in children as young as age three.

infected. The investigators found that the incidence of *H. pylori* infection was highest among children ages four to five and that black children were three times more likely to be infected with *H. pylori* than whites. Nearly 50 percent of the black children were infected as compared with 8 percent of the white children. Canadian investigators found a low prevalence of infection among Canadian children tested, while Chinese investigators' findings were similar to Malaty's reports.

Chronic stomach pain is the most prominent symptom associated with *H. pylori* infection. Undetected *H. pylori* infection can eventually result in a peptic or duodenal ulcer and acute blood loss.

Blood loss in young females

At the onset of menses, the start of a monthly period, a female can become quite iron deficient if her stores are not adequate to offset iron loss. A female will increase absorption of iron right before beginning her cycle, but if periods become heavy (menorrhagia), more frequent than once a month (metrorrhgia), or prolonged (hypermenorrhea), this can deplete iron stores and result in iron-deficiency anemia.

A normal or average menstrual cycle or period lasts about three to five days. Blood loss is a little more than one ounce, which contains about 13 milligrams of iron. In abnormal uterine bleeding (AUB) a female can lose as much as one cup of blood (about 125 milligrams of iron) within a few months. Considering that humans normally absorb only about 1–2 milligrams of iron per day, prolonged bleeding can lead to iron deficiency within a short period of time.

Females as young as nine years of age can begin menstruating. Periods can often be irregular, skipping months, or a young female might have two or more periods within a month. This is due to the body trying to adjust to hormones that regulate ovulation and sexual development. Eventually the body will regulate itself and periods will become somewhat predictable. If within six months of onset periods are still irregular or abnormal, a physician should be consulted. A gynecologist, a specialist in female health, is one doctor that can be seen, but often family doctors and pediatricians can treat disorders of initial menses.

Blood loss in young males

Adolescent or teenage males do not typically have iron-deficiency anemia due to blood loss. If fecal or occult (not seen by the naked eye) blood is discovered in young males it is usually due to chronic use of aspirin-based pain relief medicine. Occult blood can also be due to prolonged periods of running (March hemoglobinuria), straining during bowel movements, bacterial or parasite infection, hemorrhoids, or more serious and rare causes such as polyp or tumor development or disease in the digestive system such as celiac disease, Crohn's, or ulcerative colitis. Another cause of anemia due to blood loss in youths is surprisingly due to alcohol abuse.

Alcohol abuse

Consumption of alcohol can damage the liver, causing it to become scarred (cirrhosis) or cancerous and to bleed significantly. This blood loss can result in anemia, but excessive and prolonged use of alcohol can also cause a B_6 (pyridoxine) deficiency, which not only results in anemia, but also in serious neurological and mental problems. Taking B_6 might help relieve some symptoms but the risk of liver damage and disease remains.

According to Hani Eshick of The CDM Group, a Maryland-based organization established to prevent alcohol use among children, "Excessive use of alcohol in youths is difficult to fathom, but alcohol use is known to occur as early as age nine and possibly even earlier." Statistically 3 million fourteen- to seventeen-year-olds are regular drinkers with confirmed alcohol-related problems. One in four eighth-graders has used alcohol in the past 30 days. These youths are at risk for numerous nutritional deficiencies, especially B_6 and zinc, which can not only lead to anemia, but can result in irreversible neurological and organ damage.

Other causes of anemia in youths

Lead poisoning is more common in younger children who live in low-income neighborhoods where lead-based paints are more prevalent. However, youths who work in environments where lead-based paint is present can inhale the metal and become poisoned if the exposure is prolonged.

Anemia accompanies inherited conditions such as thalassemia, sideroblastic anemia, sickle cell disease, and other forms of excessive red cell breakdown. Thalassemia is prominent in children of Greek or Italian heritage, although thalassemia, also called Cooley's anemia, is seen in Middle Eastern, African, Indian, and Southeastern Asian children. Sickle cell disease primarily affects children of African descent, but sickle cell disease can occur in Caucasians, Hispanics, and other ethnic populations.

The acquired form of sideroblastic anemia is rare in children but the inherited sex linked form of sideroblastic anemia can occur in male youths. Enlarged liver and spleen, liver disease, and increased skin pigmentation might be present in a youth with sideroblastic anemia. An autosomal (not sex linked) recessive form of sideroblastic anemia can occur in both males and females of affected families.

Diagnosing iron-deficiency anemia in juveniles

Diagnosing anemia in youths begins with a complete physical exam followed by routine blood work. According to the American Academy of Family Physicians, "When symptoms known to be associated with anemia are present, and hemoglobin values are below normal for age and gender, a complete blood cell count (CBC) with differential should be performed." When the complete blood count is abnormal an iron panel (fasting serum iron, total iron-binding capacity, and serum ferritin) may be ordered. Other tests that can be helpful include a reticulocyte (retic) count, and a fecal sample. During the physical examination, the physician will look for signs of anemia. A juvenile with anemia may have pallor (paleness), fatigue, and jaundice but may or may not be critically ill.

Findings that suggest chronic anemia include irritability, pallor (usually not seen until hemoglobin levels are less than 7 g/dL), glossitis (inflammation of the tongue), a heart murmur (occurs with the contraction of the heart muscle), blue sclera (bluish tint to whites of the eyes), growth delay, pica (eating nonfood items such as dirt, hair, coins, and paper) and spoon-shaped or indented fingernails. Children with acute anemia often present more dramatically with clinical findings, including rapid shallow breathing, rapid heartbeat, enlarged spleen, blood in the urine, and congestive heart failure.

Treating and preventing iron-deficiency anemia in youths

Because iron deficiency can have long-term consequences that are often irreversible, it is imperative that children get adequate iron in the early years of development. When a child has a hemoglobin level lower than the normal range for his age and has no known illnesses within the past two weeks, iron supplements, usually ferrous sulfate, are given to the child. The dose is based on the child's weight.

If the hemoglobin responds and increases by 1.0 g/dL within four weeks, the diagnosis of iron-deficiency anemia is made. Generally, the physician will advise continuation of supplements for two to three additional months to properly replenish iron stores. During this time, parents can become informed about diets that improve the absorption of iron. If the anemia returns after supplementation is discontinued, a work-up to identify the possibility of blood loss from the digestive tract is warranted.

The importance of a balanced diet cannot be stressed enough. Iron is absolutely essential to proper growth and development, but so are other nutrients and minerals such as copper and zinc, and vitamins A, B_6, B_{12}, folate, C, and E. These nutrients are involved in the absorption and utilization of iron and the making of red blood cells. Insufficiencies in any of these nutrients can result in a decrease in red blood cell production and anemia.

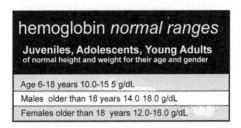

hemoglobin *normal ranges*

Juveniles, Adolescents, Young Adults
of normal height and weight for their age and gender

Age 6-18 years 10.0-15.5 g/dL	
Males older than 18 years 14.0 18.0 g/dL	
Females older than 18 years 12.0-16.0 g/dL	

ferritin	Normal Ranges

Juveniles, Adolescents, and Young Adults
of normal height and weight for their age and gender

Males ages 10-19	23-70 ng/mL
Females ages 10-19	6-40 ng/mL
Children ages 6-9	10-55 ng/mL
Children ages 1-5	6-24 ng/mL

In a 1997 study of food intakes of U.S. children and adolescents compared with recommendations, 3,307 U.S. children ages two to nineteen years were surveyed. Only 1 percent, that is about 33 children, met all recommendations for the Food Pyramid Guide. See chapter 35 for an illustration of the Food Pyramid Guide.

Changes in diet and behavior correspond with nutrition-related diseases such as obesity, deficiencies in vitamin A, C, and E. Though obesity does not directly cause anemia, food choices that lead to obesity can cause children to be under-nourished, increasing the risk for iron-deficiency anemia.

If youths consume sufficient meat, they will probably get adequate amounts of iron, zinc, copper, B_{12}, and B_6. However, trends indicate that youths are not eating enough fruits and vegetables, which are rich in folate, A, C, and K, and nutrients not found in meat (except liver) that can have an effect on blood cell production.

Statistics through 1996 indicate that anemia in older children, including teenagers, affects up to 20 percent of this population.

These numbers do not reflect the recent trends in behavior and diet for this group. Children are eating out more, choosing their own meals, and they are exposed to advertising and promotional gimmicks that encourage poor nutrition. As the results of these trends are taken into account, the incidence of anemia among youths in the United States might increase significantly.

Marion Nestle, New York University Professor of Nutrition and Food Studies, writes in her book *Food Politics: How the Food Industry Influences Nutrition and Health* a disturbing story of how the younger generation is being marketed into disease. Nestle calls for a "junk food" tax similar to the tax we pay on tobacco products. In her chapter "Pouring Rights" Dr. Nestle gives us a grim look at how the nutrition of our children is being altered by the power of the dollar.

According to The Prevention Institute, "In exchange for direct payments, school districts agree to sell only one company's products in vending machines and at all school events. Contract conditions frequently include the prominent display of advertising and marketing materials on school grounds and may include incentive payments for greater sales at the school sites. As many school districts struggle to pay for basic education, these contracts are an enticing extra source of funding to help pay for

---

According to a USDA Dietary-Intake Survey, twenty-five years ago teenagers drank almost twice as much milk as soft drinks. Today they drink twice as many soft drinks as milk.

---

sports equipment, computers, or furniture. Yet the promotion of high-sugar, high-caffeine beverages is in direct conflict with the mission of schools to promote the welfare of students."

Experts in nutrition agree that if these youngsters continue the habit of excessive consumption of high-sugar soft drinks, without adequate consumption of meats, fruits, vegetables, and grains, by the time they are in their early to mid-thirties, they will have developed any number of chronic illnesses. Among the diseases these youths may anticipate: diabetes, heart trouble, joint disease, depression, sexual dysfunction, impotence, hair loss, thyroid disorders, obesity, and cancers of the breast, bladder, prostate, and liver. Any one of these conditions can have anemia as a consequence.

According to a USDA dietary-intake survey, twenty-five years ago teenagers drank almost twice as much milk as soft drinks. Today teens drink twice as much soda as milk.

Taking action: prevention is key

- Watch for signs of anemia in your child: pallor; weakness or fatigue; eating or chewing on nonfood items such as ice, dirt, hair, coins, or paper; memory problems; irregular heartbeat; shortness of breath; spoon-shaped or indented fingernails; and unusual twitching in the legs.
- Talk to girls about normal and abnormal periods.
- Encourage your child to eat regular meals with variety, including some meat and lots of fresh fruits and vegetables rich in vitamin C and beta-carotene.
- Talk with your child about the health consequences of skipping meals, drinking too many soft drinks, and eating high-fat snacks and processed foods.
- If you smoke, try to stop, but at least protect your child from exposure to second-hand smoke, especially in closed areas such as a car or inside a home.
- Encourage your child not to smoke.
- Hinder your child's access to alcoholic beverages in the home.
- Know the signs of alcohol or drug use.

Resources

Numerous resources are available through the National Institutes of Health Library of Medicine, www.nlm.nih.gov; also, there are organizations that address specific disorders—look for them on the Internet. While compiling *Guide to Anemia*, the editors found these resources particularly helpful: American Academy of Pediatrics, www.aap.org; and the American Academy of Family Physicians magazine and their website www.aafp.org, as well as the following:

www.cdc.gov
www.nih.gov
www.kidshealth.org
www.nemours.org
www.menstuff.org/issues/byissue/teenhealth.html
www.youngwomenshealth.org/iron.html

7

Anemia in Adult Females

In the United States 7.8 million women are iron deficient; of these, 3.3 million women have iron-deficiency anemia.
—*National Center for Health Statistics, Centers for Disease Control and Prevention, Hyattsville, Maryland*

Before the birth of her son, Nancy was always on the go. She had her baby late in life; she was 36 when he was born. He had nursed well for seven months, then went onto solid foods. Nancy enjoyed the experience of breast-feeding and was disappointed when her son weaned himself. He was growing and healthy, keeping pace with other babies his age. He was always in the top 5 to 10 percent of the growth charts the pediatrician referred to at each visit.

The delivery had not been routine. Nancy had given birth by Cesarean section and needed two blood transfusions. She remained in the hospital for a week so that her recovery could be monitored. She felt great when she was discharged and looked forward to her new job as a mother.

Nancy had six weeks maternity leave from her job as a sales manager with a large financial company. The six weeks evaporated and she had to return to work. Lactation counselors had shown her how to express milk, bottle and freeze it for her son. In this way, she could continue nursing her son, providing the sitter with a bottle of breast milk. Nancy had read about the unique importance of breast milk and was dedicated to this task.

Her job became increasingly demanding; she continued to express milk but found she had less and less time to meet other obligations. She skipped checkups for herself, concentrating on getting her son to the doctor. Her periods had resumed and were heavy and irregular. It seemed she was always having a period.

At one checkup for her son, the pediatrician asked Nancy how she was managing. She remarked that Nancy looked a bit pale and asked if she was getting adequate rest. Nancy answered that things were great, even though they were not. Nancy did not want to confess that she had canceled appointments with her own doctor.

There just wasn't enough time to sit for hours in a doctor's office to be told that everything was normal, Nancy thought. Her initial checkups with the obstetrician had been good, and after all, she was not a smoker or drinker, except for an occasional glass of red wine; therefore, if she had any problems it would have to be due to stress, she rationalized.

Nancy noticed that she cried more easily lately, had developed an odd twitching sensation in her legs, and her heart sometimes felt like it was jumping or skipping a beat. She was terribly constipated, and she wasn't sleeping very well. She was often tired by mid-afternoon but felt the fatigue was due to her hectic schedule. Her weight hadn't gone down; in fact, she had gained some pounds and looked puffy in the face. At times, she had difficulty swallowing. Then there was her craving for ice. She had broken one tooth and had been warned by her dentist against this habit; he told her that this might be sign of a mineral deficiency and that she should see her doctor. Nancy made an appointment, but canceled it because of an emergency trip to Houston.

Weeks passed, her symptoms continued, but she ignored them. Nancy fought fatigue, participating in activities such as horseback riding and sailing when she really didn't have the energy to do so. On one weekend, while sailing, Nancy had an accident. She was knocked in the head with the boom of the sailboat she was manning. Her husband insisted that she go to the emergency room. Nancy agreed. Besides the expected X rays and scans, the physician did some blood work.

She did not have a concussion, but the physician told her that she was quite anemic. After discussing the symptoms she had been experiencing, the physician explained that some of the symptoms were associated with iron deficiency, but other symptoms needed to be investigated. Her doctor told her that her heavy periods were probably the cause of her anemia and that she needed to follow up with her family doctor because her anemia was fairly serious.

This time Nancy made the time to check with her ob-gyn. Her hemoglobin was 8.2 g/dL and her serum ferritin was 4 ng/mL. Her TSH (a test that measures thyroid function) was 43.28 (reference range of 0.3–3.0). Nancy revealed that she very rarely ate meat, especially avoiding red meat, and that she had stopped taking her daily vitamin, which had some iron in it. The physician put Nancy on birth control pills to regulate her periods, and 150 mcg of levothyroxine for an underactive thyroid. Additionally, she put Nancy back on her prenatal vitamins, which contained 60 milligrams of iron. She told Nancy to resume eating meat, take her thyroid meds and birth control pills at bedtime, and to take her prenatal vitamin midmorning with tomato or orange juice and not with the hormones because iron interfered with the absorption of thyroid medication.

Within six weeks, Nancy felt better. Her energy was back and she was sleeping through the night. At the eight-week checkup, her hemoglobin had improved greatly; it was 12.7 g/dL. Also, her TSH level had returned to a more acceptable range, closer to normal. Nancy was later diagnosed with Hashimoto's thyroiditis, an autoimmune disease (see chapter 12 for more details about this cause of anemia).

Iron deficiency is the greatest reason for anemia in women of childbearing age, but the causes vary. Blood loss, diet, and problems of absorption are key contributors to iron-deficiency anemia in females.

Blood loss

Heavy menstruation and blood loss from childbirth are common reasons for iron-deficiency anemia among females of childbearing age. Chronic blood loss can also be due to endometriosis or fibroids, which require a great amount of blood. Fibroids are usually benign, but can grow to the size of a baseball or grapefruit before they are detected. Fibroids of the uterus can interfere with delivery during childbirth, requiring Cesarean-section delivery. Von Willebrand disease is another overlooked cause of heavy menstrual bleeding in women (see chapter 28 for more about this disease).

The average menstrual period lasts anywhere from two to five days. Blood loss during this time is estimated to be as little as one ounce—a light or average period—to as much as one cup—a heavy period.

A unit of blood, taken during blood donation, is about 450–500 cc, or about one pint or two cups. A unit of blood contains about 200–250 milligrams of iron. A similar amount is lost during childbirth, about 500 cc (about a pint or approximately two cups) of blood. Thereby 200–250 milligrams of iron is lost. In addition, the newborn baby's blood and tissues contain another 500–800 milligrams of iron that originally came from the mother.

A woman's natural iron regulatory system takes care to increase absorption of iron from her diet during times of blood loss. Her normal absorption rate of 1 milligram is stepped up to 1.5–3 milligrams per day—the female body's natural response to blood loss.

Heavy blood loss during menstruation (menorrhagia) is called abnormal uterine bleeding (AUB). According to the National Women's Health Resource Center Hotline, AUB is one of the most common reasons women contact them.

Prolonged heavy bleeding (hypermenorrhea), where the duration might be as long as two weeks, or irregular bleeding (metrorrhagia) may eventually lead to anemia if the loss is not offset with increased iron intake.

Acute blood loss can also result from trauma or surgery or from taking aspirin or certain medications, especially those used to relieve arthritic pain, as well as from abusing alcohol. Another cause of blood loss is esophageal bleeding in a condition called Mallory-Weiss syndrome. In Mallory-Weiss, the lining of the esophagus is torn, usually from repeated vomiting, which can be seen in females who are bulimic.

Another menstrual problem that should be mentioned is amenorrhea, or the loss of a period. Women who experience amenorrhea can be at increased risk for iron overload, especially if menstruation is stopped for a prolonged period of time, and should ask their physician to check iron stores as well as functional iron in hemoglobin. Tissue iron rises significantly in females once they have reached menopause and stopped having a period. Women taking birth control pills or who have had hysterectomies are at increased risk for accumulating excessive amounts of body iron, which in time can lead to iron overload. Excessive body iron damages vital organs, causing them to fail. Outcomes of iron-related damaged organs include premature heart attack, diabetes, liver disease, osteoarthritis, osteoporosis, and hormone imbalances.

According to the U.S. Centers for Disease Control and Prevention, "Only one fourth of adolescent girls and women of childbearing age (twelve to forty-nine years) meet the recommended dietary allowance for iron through diet... 11 percent of nonpregnant women aged sixteen to forty-nine years had iron deficiency and 3 to 5 percent also had iron-deficiency anemia."

The most common anemia in females of childbearing age is iron deficiency due to blood loss, vitamin B deficiency, or because females typically do not eat much red meat. Also, females sometimes take supplements such as calcium with their iron-rich meals that inhibit the absorption of iron. Mineral deficiencies or imbalances in zinc, copper, vitamin A, B complex, and C can also lead to anemia in females because of their diets or because of impaired absorption.

Pregnancy and iron needs

"Among pregnant women, expansion of blood volume by approximately 35 percent and growth of the fetus, placenta, and other maternal tissues increase the demand for iron threefold in the second and third trimesters to approximately 5.0 milligrams of iron per day."[1]

Humans with normal iron metabolism have a natural regulatory mechanism that will assure adequate amounts of iron are absorbed to meet the demand, so long as sufficient amounts are consumed through diet. This mechanism has

---

1. U.S. Centers for Disease Control and Prevention, "Morbidity and Mortality Weekly Report (MMWR) Recommendations to Prevent and Control Iron Deficiency in the United States" (April 03, 1998, RR-3),1–36.

been observed in menstruating females who absorb up to 50 percent more iron during the days of menstruation than when not menstruating. In a British study of twelve pregnant women, iron absorbed from a normal diet was increased fivefold at twenty-four weeks of gestation and ninefold at thirty-six weeks as compared with the amount absorbed at the seventh week during the pregnancy.

For many decades, a large number of pregnant women have been advised to routinely take supplements of 25–65 milligrams of iron daily, even without laboratory evidence of subnormal hemoglobin values. The routine procedure, even though it may be unnecessary, often is considered to be harmless, and to have some unknown benefit. However, in 1993 a U.S. Prevention Service Task Force of the Office of Disease Prevention and Health Promotion, U.S. Public Health Service, carefully reviewed fifty published studies about iron supplementation. The task force concluded that controlled trials have failed to demonstrate that iron supplementation or changes in hematologic indexes actually improve clinical outcome for the mother or newborn. Additionally, the review found "no evidence that giving iron during pregnancy will reduce the incidence of childhood anemia or abnormal cognitive development."

There is agreement, however, that pregnant women who have subnormal hemoglobin values of 11.0 g/dL or less and whose ferritin is subnormal need supplemental iron. The American Academy of Family Physicians and the Institutes of Medicine recommend that pregnant females have serum ferritin measured along with hemoglobin values to assure moderately low normal hemoglobin values are in fact due to iron deficiency and not due to an undetected illness. Iron supplementation during this time is best monitored by a physician and discontinued once iron deficiency is corrected.

A few studies have examined the possibility that high as well as low hemoglobin values might be detrimental to the mother or fetus. In Wales, a study of 54,000 pregnancies demonstrated that prenatal mortality, low birth weight, and preterm birth were more common in women with hemoglobin values either less than 10.4 g/dL or greater than 13.2 g/dL than in women who had hemoglobin within the range of 10.5–13.1 g/dL.

Similarly, in the United States, a study of 22,000 pregnancies demonstrated that incidence of perinatal mortality was as much as twofold higher in women with hemoglobin values of 8.0 g/dL, and up to fivefold higher in women with hemoglobin values of 14.0 g/dL, than in women with hemoglobin ranges of 9.0 g/dL to 13.0 g/dL. In the same study, incidence of low birth weight and neonatal prematurity were greater in women whose hemoglobin was less than 8.0 g/dL or higher than 14 g/dL.

In a *Journal of American Medical Association* article entitled "Maternal Hemoglobin Concentration During Pregnancy and Risk of Stillbirth," Dr. Olof Stephansson and his colleagues report that stillbirths nearly doubled in women whose hemoglobin values were 14.5 g/dL or higher. The report went on to state that anemia, or hemoglobin values less than 11.0 g/dL, was not significantly associated with risk of stillbirth. It should be noted that hemoglobin will be elevated in women who are dehydrated or who smoke.

Supplemental iron for expectant mothers with normal iron metabolism does not significantly affect hemoglobin values for the mother or the fetus. Unneeded supplemental iron will be excreted or placed in ferritin, which is a containment vessel for iron.

Lactating and nursing females

Though lactating females can be iron deficient, the cause is probably due to blood loss as a result of childbirth, and not necessarily because they need extra iron to nourish a newborn. Another possible reason for iron deficiency, especially in the early weeks of lactation, is because during the third trimester, the mother sends a large quantity of iron to her developing offspring. If her diet is iron poor at this time, she will experience iron-deficiency anemia. Lactating mothers indeed require extra calories and adequate fluids to enable them to produce milk, but it is not necessarily true that they need supplemental iron. Nor is it true that supplemental iron taken by the mother will have an effect on her milk. Studies of breast milk of females with hemochromatosis, an inherited iron-loading disease, indicate that the excess iron stored in the tissues did not have an effect on the iron levels in the breast milk, suggesting that there is a complex iron regulatory system to assure that the proper balance of iron gets into human milk.

If a mother's hemoglobin is normal and ferritin adequate, an iron-rich diet that includes lean red meat, fresh fruits, and vegetables will likely provide sufficient amounts of iron for her and her newborn. For women who cannot afford meat, iron-fortified foods and supplemental iron may be essential. Regular checkups with a healthcare provider to monitor hemoglobin and ferritin are important.

Women are often prescribed daily calcium supplements in amounts greater than 500 milligrams per dose. Diminished iron absorption can result from a diet that includes foods or substances known to impair the bioavailability of iron. While heme iron absorption can be impaired by high doses of supplemental calcium, non-heme iron absorption can be impaired by numerous substances, such as tannin in coffee or tea, dairy products, or foods high in fiber. Women who are prescribed calcium supplements should take them at bedtime or mid-day and not with an iron-rich meal. Read about iron absorption in chapter 35.

Chemotherapy and radiation are among the cancer treatments that can result in anemia. Women anticipating cancer therapy who are anemic would benefit from improving hemoglobin and ferritin levels prior to cancer therapy. In one study of breast cancer patients, 61.9 percent developed moderate to severe anemia during chemotherapy treatment. Participants in the Austrian Breast and Colorectal Cancer Study Group were evaluated in a five-year follow-up. Those with breast cancer who developed anemia during chemotherapy were found to be three times more at risk of a recurrence of cancer in the same area of the affected breast as compared to the patients who did not become anemic during treatment. Restoring iron levels while facing chemotherapy can be difficult. Cancer patients are often tired and depressed and may not have much of an appetite. Liquid forms of supplements with iron added to fruit shakes or heme-based iron supplements may be better tolerated than other approaches to iron replenishment.

Anemia can also be a consequence of eating disorders such as bulimia. Blood loss from the digestive system may be due to laxative abuse or possible esophageal tearing due to repeat vomiting. Muscle wasting (catabolism) that generally accompanies an eating disorder increases serum ferritin concentrations, which may give a false impression that iron levels are adequate.

Exercise and anemia

March hemoglobinuria is a condition of blood loss from prolonged strenuous exercise. Female long-distance runners are at increased risk for this condition, which can lead to iron deficiency, sometimes without anemia.

Subclinical iron-deficiency anemia occurs when iron stores are depleted while hemoglobin levels remain within normal range. Females of childbearing age are more prone to subclinical iron-deficiency anemia than males.

According to a study conducted by Dr. Jere Haas, Professor and Director of the Division of Nutritional Sciences at Cornell, and his colleague Nancy Schlegel Meinig, Professor of Maternal and Child Nutrition, iron deficiency without anemia is a common problem among women of childbearing age. They report that "this condition affects about 16 percent of U.S. women and 40 to 80 percent of women in developing countries, most of whom are unaware of their iron deficiency."

Their study, published in *Journal of Applied Physiology* (2000), provides mounting evidence that iron depletion without anemia among women should be of greater concern. "These athletes have a much harder time sustaining exercise and adapting to training. But after a period of training, iron-deficient women who boost their body iron by taking supplements can improve their exercise endurance twice as much as iron-depleted women," reports Haas.

In a previous study published in 1998, Haas found that iron-depletion in nonanemic women results in lower capacity for physical work and impaired exercise performance. The present study by Haas and three other researchers shows that iron deficiency impairs the ability to increase aerobic endurance after a period of exercise training. "In other words, we now know that iron-deficient women don't benefit from training as much as women with higher iron status because of impaired metabolic responses to exercise, but that iron supplementation can compensate," Haas said.

In the latest study, 42 iron-depleted (but not anemic) women ages 18 to 33 participated in a randomized, double-blind trial. Half the group received an iron supplement (100 milligrams of ferrous sulfate per day) and half a placebo while training for four weeks, 30 minutes a day, five days a week at 75 to 85 percent of maximum heart rate.

Although all the women increased their endurance because of the training, those who improved their iron status cut 3.5 minutes off a 15-kilometer time trial on a stationary bike, compared with an average 1.5-minute improvement in the placebo group.

"That represents a 10 percent improvement in endurance performance after four weeks of training for the women who received iron," said Pamela Hinton, a postdoctoral research associate who is the first author of the study paper. "The study shows that women with moderate iron deficiency might not be getting all the fitness benefits of exercise training. They can improve aerobically but not optimally. Exercise for them is more difficult than for women with adequate iron."

Women who are physically active, dieting or vegetarians are particularly at high risk for iron depletion, the researchers point out. "In developing countries, iron depletion can have dramatic consequences on a woman's ability to do physical work and make a living," says Haas, who studies the functional consequences of mild to moderate forms of malnutrition worldwide.

Iron is an essential component of hemoglobin in the blood and plays an important role in oxygen transport and utilization. When people consume iron-deficient diets, the iron stores in ferritin are depleted first; at the final stage, they become anemic due to insufficient iron to produce new red blood cells. Haas and his coauthors focused on the first stage, while most medical practitioners are interested in the final stage.

"Because these women aren't anemic, we know they are getting enough oxygen to their muscles, but in iron-depleted, nonanemic women, the lack of iron has an effect at the muscle metabolism level," explains Hinton, with coauthors Christina Giordano and Thomas Brownlie.

To prevent iron depletion, the researchers recommend red

meat; for vegetarians, they recommend citrus fruit and juice (vitamin C) with meals to improve absorption from iron-rich foods, such as legumes, whole grains, and green vegetables. These women might also need supplemental B_{12}, especially those who are strict vegetarians.

Women can become iron deficient with or without anemia from causes other than childbirth related.

Diseases or conditions that can lead to iron deficiency with or without anemia or complicated iron balance in women of childbearing age are discussed in greater detail in specific chapters. These can include but not be limited to:

- eating disorders
- bariatric surgery
- problems of absorption
- cancer or cancer treatment
- hormone imbalances
- bone marrow failure
- autoimmune disease
- infection
- bleeding disorders
- alcohol abuse
- drug abuse
- drug interference
- long-distance running or intense exercise
- inherited or acquired diseases that interfere with blood cell formation or management
- anemia of inflammation or chronic disease

When determining iron deficiency with or without anemia in adult females, it is important to know that there are stages of iron deficiency. According to the World Health Organization, one in twelve reproductive-age women and teenage girls has a biochemical iron deficiency, but less than a quarter of these women are anemic. The stages begin when iron stores, as measured in serum ferritin, are low, 10–15 ng/mL, but not exhausted. There may be no symptoms present. The next stage is when iron stores are completely exhausted. Serum ferritin will be below 10 ng/mL. Symptoms of restless legs syndrome, increased infections, poor muscle coordination, shortness of breath upon exertion, fatigue, dizziness, sensitivity to cold, and decreased mental function may be present. In the final stage, no iron remains in the bone marrow stores, red blood cell production drops, and anemia is obvious in both lower than normal hemoglobin and ferritin less than 15 ng/mL. Symptoms can be severe in this stage.

Therapy

Females who are iron deficient may need to take supplemental iron for a period of time until symptoms are relieved, iron stores are replenished, and hemoglobin levels are back to normal range. Oral iron can be taken in a daily multivitamin if the iron deficiency is mild.

One good way to replenish iron stores is by eating meat, especially red meat at least three times per week. This approach may take a bit longer for iron stores to be replenished, but some added benefits to eating meat include getting the nutrients that are contained in meat and not dealing with side effects of some oral iron products. Vegetarians can get iron from foods, but many of these also contain fiber, which impairs the absorption of iron. While consuming either animal or plant iron-rich foods to replenish iron stores, a woman should avoid foods that inhibit the absorption of iron such as coffee, tea, grape juice or red wine, bran fiber, calcium supplements, eggs, or chocolate. These foods need not be eliminated from the diet; they can be eaten at other times of the day as snacks. Also, women trying to replenish iron stores can increase absorption of iron by consuming iron-rich meals with some form of vitamin C–rich juice or fresh fruit and vegetables that contain beta-carotene. Read more about dietary iron in chapter 35 on diet.

Taking action: prevention is key

- Know the signs of anemia: pallor; weakness or fatigue; eating or chewing on nonfood items such as ice, dirt, hair, coins, or paper; memory problems; irregular heartbeat; shortness of breath; spoon-shaped or indented fingernails; and unusual twitching in the legs.

- Report changes or concerns about your menstrual cycle (monthly period) to your doctor.
- Include red meat in your diet.
- Eat regular meals with variety, especially fresh fruits and vegetables rich in vitamin C and beta-carotene.
- Be aware of substances and foods that can impair the absorption of iron.
- If you smoke, try to stop.
- Get regular checkups and ask for an iron panel.

Resources

Numerous resources are available through the U.S. Centers for Disease Control and Prevention or National Institutes of Health Library of Medicine, www.nlm.nih.gov; also, there are organizations that address specific disorders—look for them on the Internet. While compiling *Guide to Anemia*, the editors found these resources particularly helpful:

www.nlm.nih.gov/medlineplus/druginformation.html
www.4woman.gov/
www.arborcom.com
www.nutritiouslygourmet.com
www.cdc.gov/Women/
www.aafp.org (American Academy of Family Physicians)
www.womenshealth.com/hotline.html
www.womenshealth.about.com
www.library.mcphu.edu/resources/womenres.htm

8

Anemia in Adult Males

"Less than 1 percent of men between the ages of twenty and fifty have iron-deficiency anemia."

—*U.S. Centers for Disease Control and Prevention MMWR, April 3, 1998*

Forty-five-year-old Jerold Townsend didn't feel well. He tired easily and seemed to run out of energy by mid-afternoon. He had noticed some blood in his stool but didn't think much of it. The blood was bright red and he attributed it to a recurring flare up of hemorrhoids. He also had mild cramping in the lower left portion of his abdomen, but he thought it was gas. Then one day at work he felt dizzy and short of breath; this alarmed him enough to go the doctor.

Blood work revealed a low hemoglobin (10.6 g/dL). The doctor pointed out that Jerold's hemoglobin (based on his medical file) normally ran around 15.5 g/dL and that the normal range for hemoglobin in males was 14.0–18.0 g/dL. His serum ferritin was 13 ng/mL. He did not have a fever, and his blood cells were normal size and normal color (normocytic/normochromic). His fecal sample was positive for the presence of blood. Jerold told the doctor about the bright red blood in his stool and how he hadn't been too concerned. He also reluctantly confessed that he liked beer and usually had about six before going to bed; he wondered if this could be the problem. The physician explained that the beer was probably not the cause of blood loss. Bright red blood can mean bleeding from the rectum or colon.

A diagnosis of iron-deficiency anemia was made and Jerold

was scheduled for a colonoscopy, which revealed a pocket in the colon that was bleeding. The physician told Jerold that he had diverticulosis, a condition where a weakness in the lining of the intestine leads to bleeding from tiny blood vessels in the colon. He also explained that these weaknesses or pockets can become impacted with fecal matter, causing pain, and that the impacted pockets can progress to diverticulitis (infection), which can be more serious.

> About 10 percent of Americans over the age of forty and about half of all people over the age of sixty have diverticulosis.

The physician treated Jerold and recommended that he take some iron supplements for a month. Upon recheck, Jerold's hemoglobin was improved. The physician talked with Jerold about increasing dietary fiber, eating more fruits and vegetables. He told Jerold to limit his beer to no more than four per day.

*   *   *

Iron-deficiency anemia is not as prominent in males as it is in females. This may be due primarily to the fact that males eat more meat, which contains the most easily absorbable form of iron. Also, males do not lose blood in the volumes that females do through menstruation or childbirth.

According to the U.S. Centers for Disease Control and Prevention, "Most men 20 to 50 years of age meet the recommended dietary allowance for iron through diet. Of the male adults studied who had iron-deficiency anemia, 62 percent had clinical evidence of internal blood loss that was determined to be caused by ulcers and tumors in the gastrointestinal tract. In the National Health and Nutrition Examination Survey (NHANES I), conducted during 1971–75, about two-thirds of anemia cases among men were attributable to chronic disease or inflammatory conditions."

Compare iron deficiency

	Iron deficiency	Iron deficiency anemia
Adult Males	1-4%	1-2%
Adult Females	5-11%	2-5%

Blood loss

Ulcers, colon polyps, bleeding hemorrhoids, liver disease, bleeding esophageal varices, tumors, cancer, celiac sprue, Crohn's or ulcerative colitis, chronic use of aspirin and aspirin-containing drugs, alcohol abuse, bacterial infection, overbleeding during treatment for hemochromatosis, intense exercise, and blood diseases are all possible sources of blood loss.

Bleeding disorders, such as hemophilia, or acute blood loss as a result of trauma or surgery can occur in males and result in anemia; however, chronic blood loss or severe problems of absorption that take place somewhere along the digestive tract are the most common reasons for iron-deficiency anemia in males.

When males, especially those between the ages of eighteen and sixty, are diagnosed as iron deficient—with or without anemia—one of the first areas a physician will investigate, given the patient's family history of disease, is blood loss from the digestive tract.

Causes of Bleeding in the Digestive Tract

Area	Condition
Esophagus	· inflammation (esophagitis) · enlarged veins (varices) · tears/rips (Mallory-Weiss syndrome) · cancer
Stomach	· ulcers · inflammation (gastritis) · cancer
Small Intestines	· duodenal ulcer · inflammation (irritable bowel disease)
Large Intestines & Rectum	· hemorrhoids · infections · inflammation (ulcerative colitis) · colorectal polyps · colorectal cancer · diverticular disease

Esophageal bleeding can be caused by inflammation, varices, tears in the lining of the esophagus, and from cancer. Esophagitis, or the inflammation of the esophagus, occurs when stomach acid is repeatedly pushed up into the esophagus. Constant irritation causes the tissues in the lower part of the esophagus to become inflamed, a condition known as Barrett's esophagus. If not corrected these inflamed tissues can bleed and in 5 to 10 percent of cases with Barrett's, cancer of the esophagus will develop.

Enlarged veins called varices can also cause blood loss from the esophagus. When engorged, these veins can rupture and bleed massively. Cirrhosis of the liver is the most common cause of esophageal varices. Cirrhosis is often seen in chronic alcoholics, patients with viral infections, or in persons with undetected and advanced hemochromatosis—iron overload disease. When iron overload disease is diagnosed in a person who has cirrhosis, the risk of liver cancer increases 200-fold.

Another cause of esophageal bleeding is from a condition called Mallory-Weiss syndrome. In Mallory-Weiss, the lining of the esophagus is torn, usually from repeated vomiting or uncontrolled and chronic coughing. Males who are heavy smokers or who have lung problems and who experience prolonged bouts of extreme coughing are most at risk for this syndrome.

The stomach is a frequent site of bleeding. Infections with *Helicobacter pylori* (*H. pylori*); alcohol abuse; and repeated consumption of aspirin, aspirin-containing medicines, and NSAIDS, particularly those used for arthritis, can cause stomach ulcers or inflammation (gastritis). Acute or chronic ulcers may enlarge and erode through a blood vessel, causing bleeding.

In the lower digestive tract, the large intestine and rectum are frequent sites of bleeding. Hemorrhoids are the most common cause of visible blood in the feces, especially blood that appears bright red. Hemorrhoids are enlarged veins in the anal area that can rupture and produce bright red blood, which can show up in the toilet or on toilet paper. If red blood is seen, however, it is essential to exclude other causes of bleeding since the anal area may also be the site of cuts (fissures), inflammation, or cancer.

Benign growths or polyps of the colon are very common and are thought to be forerunners of cancer. These growths can cause either bright red blood or occult bleeding. Colorectal cancer is the third most frequent of all cancers in the United States and often causes occult bleeding at some time, but not necessarily visible bleeding.

Different intestinal infections, such as salmonella, Campylobacter, *E. coli*, and Shigella (dysentery), which are bacteria, and G. lambda, a protozoan parasite responsible for giardiasis, can cause inflammation of the colon and bloody diarrhea. These infections are acquired from consuming water or foods contaminated with these pathogens. Swimming in lake waters, drinking water in some foreign countries, and eating in restaurants that have poor sanitary standards are ways people can become infected with these germs.

Diverticular disease can also have anemia as a consequence. Weaknesses in the colon wall allow pouches called diverticula to form. These pouches can remain without consequence or get filled with fecal matter and become inflamed (diverticulosis) or infected (diverticulitis). Diverticular disease typically occurs around the fourth or fifth decade of life. When onset is prior to the age of fifty, the incidence is three times more common in males than in females. When the onset is at age seventy or older, the reverse is true and incidence is three times more common in females. Symptoms range from mild cramping to pain in the lower left quadrant of the abdomen. Diarrhea, nausea, vomiting, and blood in the stool can accompany diverticulitis, whereas bloating and constipation are more common in diverticulosis. Blood may or may not be visible in the stool of patients with diverticulosis, although minute traces of occult blood (not visible to the naked eye) may be found upon medical examination.

Aspirin consumption and blood loss

Healthy adult males who are meat eaters will not likely become iron deficient due to aspirin ingestion; they may, in fact be helped by routinely taking a low-dose daily aspirin.

Many physicians recommend that patients take one 81 mg aspirin per day as a preventive measure against heart disease. The benefit may be due to the loss of blood and therefore the loss of iron that can build up undetected in organs such as the heart.

However, long-term use of aspirin, NSAIDs (non-steroidal anti-inflammatory drugs), or blood thinning medications can result in iron deficiency and anemia due to the chronic loss of blood. These males could lose a half-cup or more of blood per month, which is comparable to the blood loss of some menstruating females.

According to a New Zealand study of patients with

rheumatoid arthritis who were taking various types of pain medications, the amount of blood loss differed, depending upon the type of medication and frequency of use. Enteric-coated aspirin at a dose of one tablet (15 grains) three times a day produced an average fecal blood loss of 1.54 ml/day (one-third teaspoon). Uncoated aspirin at doses of three 5-grain tablets given three times a day resulted in an average fecal blood loss of 4.33 ml/day (nearly one teaspoon). Arthritis patients taking aspirin, fenoprofen calcium (an NSAID), or acetaminophen for pain averaged losses of 5.0 ml/day (one teaspoon) while taking aspirin, 2.2 ml/day while taking fenoprofen calcium, and 0.8 ml/day while taking acetaminophen.

Patients on these types of medications should be aware of their increased risk for iron deficiency and be checked periodically by their physician for anemia.

Alcohol abuse

Abusers of alcohol and some heavy drinkers have increased liver disease, frequent infections, and internal bleeding due to too few platelets. Abuse is defined as drinking in excess of one pint or more of 80- to 90-proof distilled spirits per day.

Inflamed livers (hepatomegaly), commonly seen in heavy drinkers, cannot function normally. These livers are unable to produce clotting factors, leading to an increased risk of bleeding, and anemia is the consequence.

Other causes of anemia in abusers of alcohol are folic acid and B_6 (pyridoxine) deficiency. Persons with deficiencies in these nutrients can have large red blood cells, a condition called macrocytic anemia. Eighty percent of males who abuse alcohol have macrocytic anemia.

One uncommonly known cause of iron deficiency is over-bleeding during therapeutic phlebotomy. Bloodletting, also called phlebotomy, is the therapy used for people with hemochromatosis, a leading cause of iron overload. Adult males are in the highest risk category for the classic type of this disease and therefore at higher risk for overbleeding. People with hemochromatosis have a metabolic disorder that causes them to absorb too much iron from their diet. In some cases they can absorb as much as four times what a person with normal iron metabolism absorbs. Iron cannot be excreted and over time these excesses build in vital organs such as the liver, heart, anterior pituitary, joints, and pancreas, resulting diseases, such as cirrhosis, diabetes, heart trouble, arthritis, depression, and impotence, or premature death generally from liver or heart failure. Excessive levels of iron must be reduced to avoid disease or premature death. Iron reduction is achieved with blood donation or therapeutic phlebotomy. It is not necessary to overbleed a hemochromatosis patient to lower excess levels of iron. "Overbleeding patients is a serious matter; we should not be trading one health problem for another," says William Dietz, MD, PhD, Director, Division of Nutrition and Physician Activity, U.S. Centers for Disease Control and Prevention, Atlanta.

Read more about hemochromatosis iron overload on our websites www.irondisorders.org or www.hemochromatosis.org.

Exercise-related anemia

Although the amount of iron lost through sweat or the gastrointestinal and urinary tract during exercise is negligible, over time, losses may be enough to deplete iron stores—especially in a nutritionally compromised athlete.

Heavy foot pounding during prolonged running or exercise can result in blood loss, which is detectable in the urine. March hemoglobinuria is a well-described intravascular hemolysis caused by exhaustive exercise. Such exercise has been associated with a fall in serum haptoglobin, the presence of free hemoglobin in the urine, a rise in plasma hemoglobin, and an increase in the number of younger red blood cells. The effect is magnified as the intensity of exercise increases. Hemolysis appears to be further influenced by running surface, resilience of shoe insoles, and running technique. In addition, red blood cell fragility may increase with exercise, a rise in body temperature, and the age of the red blood cells.

Exertional hematuria can be another cause of anemia and is found with some frequency in long-distance runners. Exercise-induced hematuria may have several causes. "Runner's bladder," which results in gross hematuria, is thought to be due to friction between the posterior bladder wall and the prostatic base. Another theory is that renal capillaries rupture in connection with increased vascular resistance that occurs during extreme physical exertion. Regardless of the cause, greater exercise duration and intensity raise the incidence of exercise-induced hematuria.

Gastrointestinal bleeding directly related to athletics has been described in marathon runners who reported bloody stools after running. A larger percentage of runners experienced occult blood loss after races. One cause for the blood loss is ischemic gastritis and colitis secondary to shunting of blood from the gastrointestinal tract to the exercising muscles. Stress-induced and NSAID-induced gastritis are also potential sources of gastrointestinal blood loss. Often, the pain associated with gastritis will be masked by the analgesic effect of the NSAID.

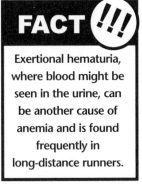

FACT

Exertional hematuria, where blood might be seen in the urine, can be another cause of anemia and is found frequently in long-distance runners.

According to Alabama sports medicine expert Raymond J. Browne, MD, MPH, "If an athlete has iron-deficiency anemia, it is typically caused by an inadequate diet or exercise-related occult blood loss. The diagnosis of sport- or exercise-related anemia should be a diagnosis of exclusion. Because bleeding is the primary cause of iron deficiency, many causes of gastrointestinal blood loss must be ruled out. That is why it's so important to do a thorough evaluation that includes medical history, family medical history, drug history, physical exam, and gastrointestinal referral if necessary."

Malabsorption and anemia

Impaired absorption is another common cause of iron-deficiency anemia. Insufficient hydrochloric acid (stomach acid), surgical removal of portions of the intestine, and gastrointestinal conditions such as celiac sprue and Crohn's disease can affect absorption. Malabsorption can also occur with *H. pylori* infection, excessive consumption of antacids, or calcium supplements.

Diseases or conditions that can lead to iron deficiency with or without anemia or complicated iron balance in men are discussed in greater detail in specific chapters. These can include but are not limited to:

- cancer or cancer treatment
- hormone imbalances
- bone marrow failure
- infection
- bleeding disorders
- alcohol abuse
- drug abuse
- drug interference
- inherited or acquired diseases that interfere with blood cell formation or management
- anemia of inflammation or chronic disease
- bariatric surgery

Diet

Males are rarely deficient in iron because of diet unless they are strict vegetarians. As vegetarians they are not only at risk of iron-deficiency anemia but for pernicious anemia, a B_{12} deficiency. B_{12} is contained in meat and meat products and to a small degree in brewer's yeast. As a precaution, these males can take a daily supplement that contains iron and B_{12}. Because B_{12} is not easily absorbed when swallowed, it must be placed sublingually (under the tongue) or given by injection.

Diagnosing and treating iron-deficiency anemia in males

Since males are rarely iron deficient because of diet, a moderately low hemoglobin, generally in the range of 9.5 g/dL, is suggestive of anemia of inflammation or chronic disease. When hemoglobin levels are below 9.5 g/dL, problems in the digestive tract are among the first causes to be suspected.

Additional tests such as a complete blood count with retic count, and an iron panel followed by an endoscope of the digestive system is likely the next step. If the scope procedure findings are negative, the next step might be a bone marrow aspiration.

Taking action: prevention is key

- Take aspirin or aspirin-based products in moderation.
- Take supplements only after knowing the upper tolerable limits and having a discussion with a nutrition expert.
- Eat regular meals with variety, especially fresh fruits and vegetables rich in vitamin C and beta-carotene.
- Be aware of substances and foods that can impair or increase the absorption of iron.
- If you smoke, try to stop or cut back.
- If you wish to drink, try to do so in moderation.
- Get regular checkups and ask for an iron panel.
- Have a periodic chest X ray and colonoscopy.
- Know the benefits of blood donation.

Resources

There are numerous resources available through the National Institutes of Health Library of Medicine, www.nlm.nih.gov; also, there are organizations that address specific disorders—look for them on the Internet. While compiling *Guide to Anemia*, the editors found these resources particularly helpful:

    http://arborcom.com
    www.cdc.gov
    www.aafp.org (American Academy of Family Physicians)

9

Anemia in the Elderly

"The prevalence of anemia in the elderly ranges from 8 to 44 percent, with the highest prevalence in men eighty-five years and older."

—*Douglas L. Smith, MD, "Anemia in the Elderly."*
The American Family Physician, 2000

At his regular checkup, eighty-year-old Arthur Nolan reported that except for a bit of lower back pain, he felt fine. The back pain, he told the doctor, was probably due to a pulled muscle caused by lifting some heavy books. All of his blood work was normal except for hemoglobin, which was 10.2 g/dL. The doctor asked Arthur if he had any symptoms of fatigue, dizziness, or irregular heartbeat. Arthur said that besides being a bit forgetful now and then, he felt great. He joked that he was getting older after all. The physician recommended that Arthur take ibuprofen for his pain, and iron pills, 325 milligrams, twice a day for anemia. He told Arthur to return for a recheck in one month to see if his hemoglobin value improved.

Five weeks later Arthur returned; his hemoglobin was 10.5 g/dL. The physician told him to continue taking the iron pills, but this time Arthur did not comply. He stopped taking the pills because he didn't think they were helping him. He had developed some stomach pain and concluded the iron pills were the cause. His back pain was now more persistent. He ignored the recommended one-tablet dose every four to six hours, and took two tablets every four hours. His neighbor had told him that over-the-counter medication was half-strength of prescription medication. Reasoning that if the physician gave him a prescription it would be twice the dose of his over-the-counter brand, he took the double dose each time without concern.

Arthur's son was visiting and noticed that his father looked exceptionally pale; his dad was weak, short of breath, and unsteady when he walked up the stairs. He also realized his father was repeating things and didn't seem to be as mentally sharp as usual. Additionally, he discovered that his dad wasn't eating well. Arthur agreed to see the doctor. His hemoglobin was 6.2 g/dL and he had a fever of 101 degrees. When the doctor told Arthur the test results, Arthur nearly fainted. His knees buckled as he tried to stand up. The doctor admitted him to the hospital immediately.

After hospitalization and six units of blood, Arthur felt better. He wanted to go home. The doctor explained that some of the tests indicated that there was blood loss, probably from the digestive tract. He had called in a specialist, a gastroenterologist, who ordered more blood tests, an endoscope, and an abdominal CAT scan.

Arthur's situation was complicated. His blood loss was attributed to a stomach ulcer that was bleeding significantly. He was positive for _Helicobacter pylori_ and the CAT scan revealed metastatic cancer in the lungs, liver, and pancreas. Arthur had a history of prostate cancer. Twenty years earlier, he had surgery to remove his prostate and after ten years his urologist told him his PSA (prostate specific antigen) was normal and he had no signs of cancer. The urologist did not check any other organs, run any other tests for cancer, or refer Arthur to a hematologist oncologist for follow-up.

After a lung aspiration, the tissue sample was examined to determine the primary cancer source. Arthur's final diagnosis was pancreatic cancer.

"Anemia should not be accepted as an inevitable consequence of aging."

—_Douglas L. Smith, MD, University of Wisconsin Medical School, Madison, Wisconsin_

Even though anemia is fairly prevalent among elderly persons, the underlying cause is not so easily revealed, especially during routine examinations. Symptoms of fatigue, pale skin,

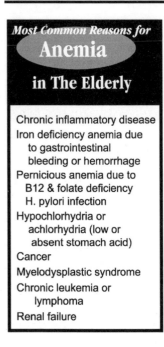

Most Common Reasons for

Anemia

in The Elderly

Chronic inflammatory disease
Iron deficiency anemia due
  to gastrointestinal
  bleeding or hemorrhage
Pernicious anemia due to
  B12 & folate deficiency
  H. pylori infection
Hypochlorhydria or
  achlorhydria (low or
  absent stomach acid)
Cancer
Myelodysplastic syndrome
Chronic leukemia or
  lymphoma
Renal failure

and decreased cognitive ability are easily attributed to getting older. Some physicians feel that mildly lowered hemoglobin is normal for an older patient. This may not always be the case. In healthy older persons, hemoglobin levels are generally normal. When anemia is present in older persons it is generally due to some underlying condition that requires further investigation or therapy.

Anemia of inflammation or chronic disease

Anemia of inflammation or chronic disease is the most common cause of anemia in the elderly. Numerous diseases have inflammation as a consequence; in the elderly some of the more common include acute or chronic infections, arthritis, or malignancy. Often in many older cases the underlying disease may not be identified right away. Physicians can mistake the transient condition of inflammation for iron-deficiency anemia and incorrectly prescribe iron pills.

Iron-deficiency anemia

Iron deficiency is the second most common cause of anemia in the elderly. The most common causes are blood loss, nutritional deficiencies, medications, cancer therapies, and poor absorption.

Long-term use of aspirin and nonsteroidal anti-inflammatory drugs (NSAIDs) can cause significant bleeding from the digestive tract. Many physicians recommend that patients take one baby aspirin per day as a preventive measure against heart disease. Usually the blood loss from this practice is minute. In cases where aspirin-based drugs are taken several times a day, a person can lose up to a half-cup or more of blood per month. Since a cup of blood contains about 100 to 125 milligrams of iron, an estimated 50 to 60 milligrams of iron can be lost per month in persons with prolonged use of these drugs.

Other causes of blood loss include esophageal varices, ulcers, tumor, colon cancer, diverticular bleeding, or intestinal lesions.

Without blood loss, iron-deficiency anemia takes several years to develop. Inadequate intake or inadequate absorption of iron can occur in older patients who have poor diets, do not eat much meat, or who have subnormal levels of stomach acid. Stomach acid is hydrochloric acid or HCl and is vital to absorption of iron. When HCl is low (hypochlorhydria) or absent (achlorhydria), in time the patient will develop iron-deficiency anemia or pernicious anemia due to B_{12} deficiency.

Blood Loss in the Elderly

Percentage Affected	Cause of blood loss
20-40%	Gastic ulcer Gastritis Esophagitis Gastric cancer
15-30%	Colon cancer Lesions Polyps Colitis Dialysis
10-40%	Cause not found

Iron deficiency is suspected when the serum ferritin is less than 15 ng/mL. Locating the source of bleeding is successful in many patients, but in as many as 40 percent of cases, the source of bleeding is not found.

Nutritional deficiencies

Elderly people who consume diets limited in variety are at risk for various nutritional deficiencies that can contribute to anemia. The two most common nutritional anemias seen in the elderly are the B vitamins, especially B_{12}, or folate; zinc and iron deficiencies are also frequently a cause.

Vitamin B_{12} (cobalamin) and folate deficiency (pernicious anemia)

Folate and vitamin B_{12} deficiencies are often present in the elderly but may be underdiagnosed. Symptoms of these deficiencies can include shortness of breath, fatigue, paleness, rapid heartbeat, loss of appetite, diarrhea, tingling or numbness of the hands and feet, unsteady gait, sore tongue, memory loss, depression, listlessness, confusion, irritability, and personality changes. Many of these symptoms are often attributed to aging. To further complicate the diagnosis, about 40 percent of patients with vitamin B_{12} deficiency have normal hemoglobin. Neurologic symptoms of B_{12} deficiency can develop before the patient's hemoglobin drops below normal. Anemia due to vitamin B_{12} or folate deficiency is usually macrocytic (abnormally large) but normocytic (normal size) or even microcytic (smaller than normal) cells can be seen in patients with these deficiencies when other diseases are present, causing iron deficiency or anemia of chronic disease.

Differentiating between folate and B_{12} deficiency is challenging because both deficiencies have nearly identical symptoms and specific tests are needed to differentiate between the two. Read more about testing for nutrient deficiencies in chapter 14.

The body can store only enough folate to provide for three to four months, whereas the liver stores enough B_{12} to provide for three years. Folate is found in leafy green vegetables, asparagus, broccoli, orange juice, liver, milk, and some grains. Meat and meat products such as dairy are good sources of B_{12}. Though older persons may not eat much meat, the likelihood of dietary insufficiency of B_{12} is not great unless the person is a strict vegetarian. More likely pernicious anemia due to lack of intrinsic factor, a hormone produced in the stomach that is vital to B_{12} absorption, is suspect in the older patient.

Lack of hydrochloric acid, surgical removal of portions of the stomach or small intestine, alcohol abuse, prolonged *Helicobacter pylori* infection, chemotherapy, medications such as anticonvulsants, bowel disease, poor kidney function, and hyperthyroidism can also contribute to B_{12} deficiency.

Zinc deficiency

Zinc is an essential mineral, which means that the body cannot produce zinc; it must be gotten from food. The elderly are at increased risk for zinc deficiency probably due to poor absorption, lead poisoning, or because they do not eat much red meat, an excellent source of zinc. Beef can contribute as much as 25 percent of the zinc in the diet. Many people who are iron deficient are also zinc deficient.

Lead poisoning

One cause of unexplained anemia can be lead poisoning, which is often overlooked as a reason for unexplained anemia in the elderly. The source of lead poisoning in older individuals can include the same exposures as children: beauty products (hair dyes, eyeliner), exposure to lead-based paints in ceramics or peeling paint in older homes, old water pipes, or ayurvedic medicines. These folk remedies are a traditional form of medicine practiced in India and other South Asian countries. Ayurvedic medications can contain herbs, minerals, metals such as lead, or animal products and are made in standardized and nonstandardized formulations. Blood lead levels and the erythrocyte protoporphyrin (EPP) blood test can determine lead levels or lead poisoning.

Diverticular disease can also have anemia as a consequence. Weaknesses in the colon wall allow pouches called diverticula to form. These pouches can remain without consequence, or get filled with fecal matter and become inflamed (diverticulosis) or infected (diverticulitis). Diverticular disease usually occurs around the fourth or fifth decade of life. When onset is prior to the age of fifty, the incidence is three times more common in males than in females. When onset age is seventy or older, the reverse is true and incidence is three times more common in females. Symptoms range from mild cramping to pain in the lower left quadrant of the abdomen. Diarrhea, nausea, vomiting, and blood in the stool can accompany diverticulitis, where bloating and constipation are more common in diverticulosis. Blood may or may not be visible in the stool of patients with diverticulosis, although minute traces of occult blood (not visible to the naked eye) may be found upon medical examination.

Diseases or conditions that can lead to iron deficiency—with or without anemia—or complicated iron balance in the elderly are discussed in greater detail in specific chapters. These causes can include but may not be limited to:

- myelodysplastic syndromes
- cancer or cancer treatment
- kidney disease
- hormone imbalances

101

- bone marrow failure
- autoimmune disease
- infection
- bleeding disorders
- alcohol abuse
- drug abuse
- drug interference
- inherited or acquired diseases that interfere with blood cell formation or management
- anemia of inflammation or chronic disease

Treatment

Treatment of anemia in the elderly patient might include diet changes, oral iron supplements, iron injections or infusions, blood transfusion, or an erythropoiesis-stimulating agent (ESA)*. Prompt treatment of anemia is necessary to avoid further complications, especially with the heart. Read about these therapies in chapters in part five.

Taking action: prevention is key

- Take aspirin-based products in moderation.
- Take supplements only after knowing the upper tolerable limits and consulting a nutrition expert.
- Eat regular meals with variety, especially fresh fruits and vegetables rich in vitamin C and beta-carotene.
- Be aware of substances and foods that can impair or increase the absorption of iron.
- If you smoke, try to stop or cut back.

---

*Erythropoiesis-stimulating agents (ESA) are genetically synthesized erythropoietin or recombinant human erythropoietin (rHuEPO) and available under the brand names Procrit® (Ortho Biotech), Epogen® (Amgen), and most recently Aranesp® or darbepoietin alfa (Amgen). These products are given primarily to kidney dialysis and chemotherapy patients who are not able to produce the hormone erythropoietin. Some physicians find that patients with anemia of chronic disease can benefit from short-term erythropoietin. Recent warnings about the use of ESAs issued by the FDA should be discussed with your physician.

- If you wish to drink, try to do so in moderation.
- Get regular checkups and ask for an iron panel.
- Have a periodic chest X ray and colonoscopy.

Resources

Numerous resources are available through the National Institutes of Health Library of Medicine, www.nlm.nih.gov; also, there are organizations that address specific disorders—look for them on the Internet. While compiling *Guide to Anemia*, the editors found these resources particularly helpful:

www.cdc.gov

www.aafp.org (American Academy of Family Physicians)

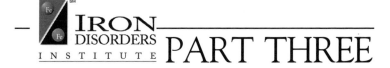

PART THREE

Common Causes—Sometimes Complicated Diagnosis

10

Anemia of Chronic Disease (ACD)

"ACD occurs commonly, but it is frequently misunderstood, underdiagnosed, or improperly treated. It is usually associated with infection, inflammation, malignancy, or trauma."

—Abramson & Abramson, "Common and Uncommon Anemias," American Family Physician, 1999

The gynecologist noted thirty-four-year-old Caron Whitfield's complaint of weakness and fatigue on her patient chart. Caron was having cramps but told the doctor that she often had menstrual cramps and fairly substantial periods. The doctor listened to Caron's lungs and heart, noting a slight arrhythmia, and measured Caron's hemoglobin, which was 10.2 g/dL.

Caron was given iron pills, 325 milligrams, and told to take them twice a day and return in one month. The pills seemed to make her sick, so she tried taking only one a day, which did not help. She bought a liquid form of iron from the health food store and mixed two to three drops in grape juice. This she could tolerate, but her symptoms did not improve. She called the doctor and spoke with a nurse who told her that she really needed to give the iron a chance to work. The nurse told Caron to keep up the supplementation for at least three weeks.

Later that afternoon her cramps got so bad that Caron took aspirin. Rather than helping, the aspirin seemed to make the pain worse. Caron noticed some blood in the stool and presumed that her period was about to start, but the following day, she had not begun her period.

Her pain was worse, now radiating into her back. She was

weak, nauseated, sweaty, cold, and had lost her appetite. She called the doctor again, but she was in such terrible pain she went to the Urgent Care Center. A urine sample was taken and a complete blood count was ordered. Her pulse rate was up, her breathing rapid and shallow, and she had a temperature of 100.7 degrees.

The physician told Caron that he suspected she had a urinary tract infection that may have spread to the kidneys. (The diagnosis would be confirmed the next day.) He prescribed Keflex, 250 milligrams every six hours per day for fourteen days, and Pyridium, 200 milligrams twice a day. He told Caron to drink plenty of fluids and rest as much as she could. He also told her she could stop taking the iron. He advised her to see her family doctor for a follow-up visit after the round of antibiotics was finished.

Within hours of taking the antibiotic Caron felt better and within days she had energy, no cramps or back pain and no fever. She returned to her gynecologist three weeks later for a follow-up visit. Her hemoglobin was a normal 12.4 g/dL.

Anemia of chronic disease (ACD) is also referred to as

"Iron supplementation provides no benefit in patients with anemia of chronic disease."

—*Douglas L. Smith, MD, "Anemia in the Elderly,"*
American Family Physician, *October 2000*

---

anemia of inflammatory disease. The latter term might better define this condition, because anemia of chronic disease suggests that a person has some terrible disease. Although ACD can accompany life-threatening illness, anemia of inflammatory or chronic disease is in fact a protective and natural phenomenon the human body employs to limit the amount of iron a person absorbs when potentially harmful agents such as bacteria have invaded the body. All living things, including bacteria and cancer cells, depend upon iron to sustain life just like humans and plants do.

For this reason, the human body will regulate how much iron it absorbs based on needs and the presence of any potential threat to life. If a person takes in too much iron he or she will actually absorb less and less as the supplemental amount is increased. When inflammation is present, the body will slow down absorption of iron so that just enough is available to make red blood cells but no surplus is left to nourish harmful pathogens. Depending on the underlying cause of disease, a modest drop in hemoglobin will occur; generally within the first three to four months of inflammation onset. Hemoglobin values will fall to around 9.5–10.5 g/dL and stabilize, remaining within this moderately low range until the underlying condition is cured.

The drop in hemoglobin often fools a physician into thinking the first stages of iron-deficiency anemia (IDA) are underway. Iron-deficiency anemia can also present with slightly lowered hemoglobin, but the hemoglobin is the last measure to drop in true iron-deficiency anemia. Iron stores in ferritin and iron in transport will get used up first in iron-deficiency anemia. IDA will be evidenced by a lowered serum ferritin and a lowered transferrin-iron saturation percentage with an elevated total iron binding capacity even before hemoglobin drops below normal. This is called subclinical iron-deficiency anemia, and clinical iron deficiency will follow if the underlying cause is not found and treated. In anemia of chronic disease total iron binding capacity will be lowered and transferrin iron saturation percentage will also be below normal but serum ferritin will be elevated. Taking iron pills for anemia of chronic disease could be harmful, even fatal.

The exact mechanism of ACD is not fully understood.

iron panel	IRON PANEL TESTS					
	Serum Iron	Serum Ferritin	Transferrin Iron Saturation Percentage	Total Iron Binding Capacity (TIBC)	Transferrin	Serum Transferrin Receptor
Anemia of Chronic Disease (ACD)	⬇	⬆	⬇	⬇	⬇	NORMAL
Iron Deficiency Anemia (IDA)	⬇	⬇	⬇	⬆	⬆	HIGH

Dr. Eugene Weinberg, Professor of Microbiology, Indiana University, and Iron Disorders Institute Medical & Scientific Advisory Board member, describes a natural defense mechanism, the Iron Withholding Defense System, which is activated as part of the inflammatory response. Since the mid-1950s Weinberg has been aware of the body's alteration of iron metabolism during disease. He first defined the iron with-holding defense system in the early 1980s when he described how the human body recognizes iron as a potential hazard to health. Iron is one metal that cannot be excreted by the body efficiently; so, extra precautions are taken by humans to avoid absorbing too much iron. When a harmful germ invades the body, the immune system team of white blood cells charges to the site to destroy the pathogen before it has time to multiply. Inflammation results as a part of this natural immune response. Inflammation triggers the release of chemicals that signal the iron regulation mechanism to adopt a defense mode.

What physicians see when the iron withholding defense system is activated is a mild drop in hemoglobin. However, what many physicians miss is that less iron is being absorbed and extra free iron is being collected by macrophages and stored in liver cells (hepatocytes). As a result serum ferritin rises. Anemia of chronic disease is not progressive. Hemoglobin values may remain in a slightly low range, but the levels can drop to as low as 7.0 g/dL depending on the severity of the inflammation and the length of time present. Other tests such as serum ferritin or C-reactive protein (CRP) can be performed to help differentiate between iron-deficiency anemia, where oral iron can be beneficial, and anemia of chronic disease, where oral iron should not be given.

In a U.S. Department of Agriculture study, investigators illustrate the iron withholding defense system at work. Drs. Fariba Roughead and Janet Hunt of the USDA Grand Forks Human Nutrition Research Center conducted a study of the effects of iron supplements on the body's control of iron absorption. In a randomized, placebo-controlled trial, heme and nonheme iron absorption by healthy men and women were measured from a test meal containing a hamburger, potatoes, and milkshake. These absorption measurements were made before and after a period of twelve weeks when the 57 participants were given 50 milligrams of supplemental iron or placebo daily while they consumed their usual diets.

Serum ferritin and fecal ferritin were measured during

supplementation and for a period of six months after supplementation was discontinued. Volunteers who took iron supplements, even those with initial ferritin less than 21 ng/mL, adapted to absorb less nonheme iron, but not less heme iron from meat.

Daily iron supplements caused these volunteers to absorb 36 percent less nonheme iron and 25 percent less total iron from food, and to have higher iron stores than those in the placebo group. The higher ferritin persisted for six months post supplementation, except in individuals who had low iron stores at the beginning of the study. Since iron stores were greater after iron supplementation, Drs. Roughead and Hunt's study demonstrated that adaptation in absorption did not completely prevent differences in body iron stores.

The adaptation to reduce iron absorption even in volunteers with low iron stores may indicate a localized control system to prevent excessive iron exposure of intestinal cells. The study is consistent with two systems at work, one that regulates how much iron we must absorb for normal function, and the iron withholding defense system, which protects us from nurturing harmful pathogens with excesses of iron we don't presently need.

In adults, anemia of chronic disease is likely due to some common ailment such as urinary tract infection, a head or chest cold, mononucleosis, tonsillitis or strep, stomach or intestinal flu, and bacterial infections such as *H. pylori*. ACD can also occur when an autoimmune disease is present. Most of these conditions are treatable and when the patient is cured, the anemia will be corrected. If the anemia persists once an illness is cured, the doctor will want to investigate further for a secondary underlying cause of anemia that may be more serious such as kidney disease, tumor, or cancer.

Anemia of chronic disease can be an indicator that a serious life-threatening condition is in the initial stages of development. However, when disease advances beyond this mild form of anemia, where treatment of the underlying condition cannot affect a cure, levels such as serum ferritin and transferrin iron saturation percentage change. For this reason, persons who have experienced anemia of chronic disease, where suspected underlying conditions have been addressed but the anemia persists, further investigation is needed. Blood loss, kidney function, bone marrow function, cancer, abnormal absorption, or chronic hemolysis could be pursued as causes.

Anemia of chronic disease can also be present even when tissues have excessive levels of iron. Tissue iron is different from functional iron in hemoglobin. Persons with hereditary hemochromatosis can have excessively high tissue iron but develop anemia because of iron damage to the kidney, anterior pituitary, or bone marrow. The damaged kidney produces less erythropoietin, a hormone vital to red blood cell production (erythropoiesis). An inflamed or damaged anterior pituitary can result in hypothyroidism, which causes diminished erythropoiesis and mild anemia. The bone marrow is the site of red blood cell formation.

Differentiating between anemia of chronic disease and iron-deficiency anemia

Patients with anemia of chronic disease do not generally have hemoglobin values below 9.5 g/dL, although on rare occasions levels can go much lower. Iron-deficiency anemia is often suspected in patients with anemia of chronic disease because the two conditions have many similarities. In both conditions, the serum iron level is low. Small or microcytic cells can be present in either disorder, though this type of cell is more indicative of true iron deficiency. Transferrin, a protein that transports iron, is elevated in iron-deficiency anemia, indicating that the body needs more iron. The total iron-binding capacity (TIBC), an indirect measurement of transferrin, is low in anemia of chronic disease because there is ample iron, but it is not easily available. TIBC tends to be increased when iron stores are diminished and decreased when they are elevated. In iron-deficiency anemia, the TIBC is higher than 400–450 mcg/dL because stores are low. In anemia of chronic disease, the TIBC is usually below normal because the iron stores are elevated.

In nearly two-thirds of the patients, the serum ferritin is one test that can be used to distinguish between anemia of chronic disease and iron-deficiency anemia. Ferritin is an acute-phase reactant, which means that it can be elevated in the presence

Comparing blood tests for anemia of chronic disease and iron-deficiency anemia	ACD	IDA
Hemoglobin (g/dL)	decreased*	decreased
Serum ferritin	increased	decreased
TIBC	decreased	increased
Serum iron	decreased	decreased
TS%	decreased	decreased
Erythropoietin	inadequate	adequate
MCV	normal to slightly decreased	decreased
White blood cell	variable	normal
Red blood cell	decreased	normal to slightly decreased
Serum transferrin receptor	normal	increased

*Hemoglobin can go as low as 7.0g/dL in some ACD patients.

of inflammation and this factor must be taken into consideration when examining the findings. Serum ferritin can be raised to normal levels even in the presence of iron deficiency. For this reason, difficulties arise in distinguishing iron deficiency in a patient with inflammation or infection from the anemia of chronic disease. Tests for inflammation like C-reactive protein (CRP) are not helpful in this case. For some cases in which both iron deficiency and anemia of chronic disease are possible, bone marrow aspiration with iron staining is the traditional means of determining that a person is iron deficient. However, the serum transferrin receptor test can be used to help differentiate between iron-deficiency anemia and anemia of chronic disease. The serum transferrin receptor is much less affected by inflammation than serum ferritin; results will be high in iron-deficiency anemia and usually low to low-normal in anemia of chronic disease. The ratio of the serum transferrin receptor to the logarithim of the serum ferritin concentration is better able to distinguish anemia of chronic disease from iron deficiency than is either test alone.

The greatest risk for harm is mistaking anemia of chronic

disease for iron-deficiency anemia and allowing the patient to take iron pills. This risk can be reduced or eliminated by differentiating between the two iron disorders with a serum ferritin test and by informing the patient about the differences between these two disorders.

Treatment

There is no treatment for anemia of chronic disease except to address the underlying condition. Iron supplementation is inappropriate in these patients because the added iron can become free to nourish bacteria and cancer cells.

Resources

Numerous resources are available through the National Institutes of Health Library of Medicine, www.nlm.nih.gov; also, there are organizations that address specific disorders—look for them on the Internet. While compiling *Guide to Anemia*, the editors found these resources particularly helpful:

    www.aafp.org (American Academy of Family Physicians)

    www.anemia.org (National Anemia Action Council (NAAC))

11

Endocrine System Disorders

"The status of the endocrine system must always be considered in evaluation of a normocytic, normochromic anaemia."

—Dr. J. K. Spivak, Johns Hopkins School of Medicine

Forty-year-old schoolteacher Sharon Parks described her symptoms to her doctor, who made notes. The chronic fatigue and weight gain were the worst of her symptoms, which included shortness of breath; constipation; difficulty sleeping; sensitivity to cold; coarse, dry hair; and cool, dry, pale skin. Sharon concluded that her libido was nonexistent. She had also gained forty pounds during the last ten years in spite of regular exercise. Sharon had been on estrogen hormone replacement therapy (HRT) and thyroid medication for more than ten years. Her medication had been changed several times, increasing or decreasing Synthroid®, estrogen, or progesterone, and on one occasion she was given testosterone. Prior to HRT, Sharon had always been on the slender side, and she was frustrated with the weight gain and the puffy look that accompanied the gain.

Her doctor told her that weight gain was a natural consequence of getting older. The physician explained that females often gained weight because they ate too much and their metabolism slows as they age. She recommended that Sharon increase her exercise and eat less. Her blood work, which included estrogen, testosterone, thyroid stimulating hormone, and a complete blood count, indicated that her thyroid medication was normal but her hemoglobin was a bit low, probably explaining the fatigue. The doctor renewed the prescription for Sharon's thyroid medication and recommended that she eat more red meat.

Wanting more energy, Sharon went to the health food store and stocked up on several items that were guaranteed to combat fatigue. Among her purchases were ginseng tea and iron pills. Without fail, Sharon took her thyroid medicine along with her iron pills every morning as soon as she got up.

Instead of improving, her symptoms got worse. She was having a terrible time with the heat; she was sweaty and her face was often flushed. Also, she had begun to stutter, couldn't remember simple things, and couldn't concentrate. She was having bouts of irritability followed by crying spells. Her skin was even drier and now itched. Her physician checked her thyroid levels and found the TSH (thyroid stimulating hormone) elevated. The doctor increased her thyroid medication from 125 to 150 mcg a day.

In time, Sharon ran out of the iron pills; she got busy and kept forgetting to run by the health food store to buy more. Time passed and then one day at school she realized she was talking almost incessantly. She was jittery; her heart was thumping hard and racing. She called her physician, who suspected the 150 mcg dose was too high. The dose was lowered back down to 125 mcg.

Within a week Sharon's symptoms improved and she actually felt good for the first time in a while. She remembered that she had been anemic and wanted to assure that she continued to feel good, so she picked up a bottle of iron pills at the health food store. Sharon resumed taking the iron in the morning along with her Synthroid®.

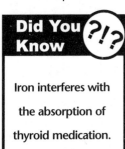

Did You Know

Her symptoms of hypothyroidism returned. This time the physician had Sharon come in for blood work. Her TSH was once again elevated. The doctor increased Sharon's dose back up to the 150 mcg. Within a few days, Sharon began to feel better.

Iron interferes with the absorption of thyroid medication.

Editor's Note: Sharon's story exemplifies how many of us associate the finding of "slightly low hemoglobin" with the need for iron pills. Sharon's physician did not perform a serum ferritin, which could have helped to determine if the slightly low hemoglobin level was in fact due to iron deficiency or inflammation. Here the patient assumes that iron pills will cure fatigue, when in reality, taking supplemental iron could have placed her health in serious jeopardy. The patient also contributed to her problems by not disclosing to her doctor that she was taking iron at the same time that she was taking her thyroid medication. Iron impairs the absorption of levothyroxin (generic); this patient was taking the brand name Synthyroid®.

The endocrine system

The endocrine system is a highly complex and interdependent network of ductless glands. Glands are organs of the body that manufacture substances called hormones. When the endocrine system is compromised, a wide range of conditions can result. It is the onset and progression of such conditions that result in anemia. Anemia of inflammation or chronic disease, iron-deficiency anemia, autoimmune hemolytic anemia, and pernicious anemia are among the types of anemia that can accompany endocrine disorders.

Organs of the endocrine system, called glands, discharge chemicals known as hormones directly into the bloodstream. Principal glands that make up the endocrine

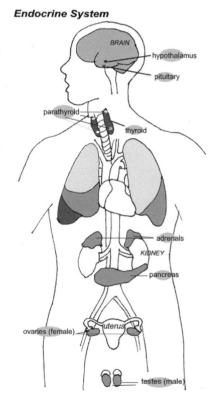

Endocrine System

Source: NIDDK

116

system include the hypothalamus, the pituitary, the adrenals, the pancreas, the parathyroids, the thyroid, and the testes and ovaries. The exocrine glands also discharge hormones or chemicals, but into ducts rather than directly into the bloodstream. Examples of the exocrine system include salivary glands, mucous glands in the lungs, sweat and tear glands, and mammary glands. The pancreas is part of both the exocrine and endocrine systems as it contains both types of glands. The thymus, brain, heart, lungs, skin, and placenta also produce and release hormones locally that act within those tissues, so they are not truly classified as endocrine glands.

The endocrine system affects the secretion of more than fifty different hormones.

Endocrine glands secrete hormones destined for a singular target organ or gland. Hormones are chemical messengers that carry instructions from one set of cells to another; they regulate specific functions such as metabolism, blood pressure, electrolyte and fluid balance, heart rate, mood, growth and sexual function development, tissue function, and the reproductive processes.

Once a hormone is secreted, it travels through the bloodstream to specific cells, which are called target cells. Many hormones bind with proteins that transport the hormone to its target cell. Each target cell has receptors either on its surface or within the cell for the specific hormone. This system is something like a lock and key—only a key designed for a certain lock will fit and function. Once locked in place, the cells receive the instructions carried by the hormone.

Receptors

Hormones   Target cell

Secreting gland

Not a target cell
No receptors

Source: NIAID

Hormone levels are regulated by a negative feedback system. When adequate amounts of a particular hormone are reached, the level activates a signal to the appropriate gland to stop production, much like when the level of water in a washing machine is high enough, a sensor sends a signal to a mechanism that controls the water and the water is shut off. Hormone levels can fluctuate depending upon factors such as infection, disease, stress, metabolic disorders, and nutritional imbalances. If these conditions are not corrected, eventually the gland affected works less efficiently and disorders such as hypothyroidism, diabetes, infertility, renal problems, or other illnesses can arise.

Because the system is so complex, one diseased or poorly functioning endocrine organ can have a profound impact on the function of other organs and systems. When organs of the endocrine system become inflamed or diseased, the body senses the presence of disease and a mild form of anemia is experienced. This condition is called anemia of inflammation or chronic disease. When the gland is atrophied (deteriorated), body function regulated by this gland slows down. Among some of the functions impaired is red cell production (erythropoiesis). In some cases, a diseased or dysfunctional gland can affect red blood cell destruction, resulting in hemolytic anemia, especially when the disease is autoimmune related.

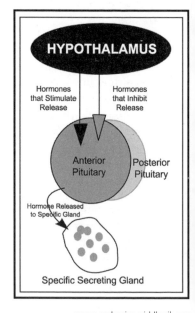

www.endocrine.niddk.nih.gov

Pituitary

The pituitary is often referred to as the master gland because of the numerous systems affected by its ability to function efficiently. The pituitary produces key hormones that not only stimulate the thyroid, adrenals, gonads (sex organs), uterus, and mammary glands but also promote growth of bones and muscles. This tiny gland is made up of anterior and posterior lobes; each lobe contains different hormones and regulates different functions.

When the glands relying upon adequate pituitary function are not properly stimulated, hormone secretion is decreased. As a result, these glands can deteriorate (atrophy), causing function to decrease. Anemias are often present in patients with abnormal pituitary function or other glands regulated by pituitary function. Pituitary overactivity can also lead to anemia, and it affects other endocrine functions as much as hypofunction.

Thyroid

The thyroid gland is located in the front of the neck and is shaped like a bow tie or butterfly. Thyrotropin, which is called thyroid stimulating hormone, or TSH, is secreted by the anterior pituitary and stimulates the thyroid gland to produce thyroxine, which is called T4. T4 is converted into triiodothyronine, or T3, which is the active form used by the body. In this form, the hormone affects metabolism or the rate at which the body expends energy. Proper thyroid function affects bone growth, brain development, and the nervous system in children; therefore, screening for hypothyroidism is performed at birth on every child born in the United States.

In an underactive thyroid (hypothyroidism), symptoms include chronic fatigue, loss of libido (sex drive), moodiness, low blood pressure, slow pulse, reduced temperature, cool dry skin, brittle nails, hair loss, weight gain, puffy face, dark circles under the eyes, ataxia (lack of coordination), aching muscles, joint stiffness and intolerance to cold, infertility, impotence, sterility, irregular menstrual periods, mild iron-deficiency anemia, and anemia of chronic disease.

When the thyroid is overactive (hyperthyroid), symptoms may include rapid weight loss, tremors, shakiness or nervousness, excessive sweating and sensitivity to heat, increased blood pressure, irregular heartbeat usually described as racing, and protruding eyes; also, the thyroid is often enlarged (goiter). B_{12} deficiency, anemia of inflammation, iron-deficiency anemia, and anemia with iron overload have been reported in patients with abnormal thyroid function.

Parathyroid

The parathyroids are four tiny glands attached to the four corners of the thyroid gland. They release parathyroid hormone that regulates the level of calcium in the blood. Parathyroid hormone also activates vitamin D, which is involved in absorption of calcium from the gut and deposition of calcium into the bones. Overproduction of parathyroid hormone causes hypercalcemia (high levels of calcium in the blood), which can lead to dehydration and trigger a sickling crisis in people with sickle cell disease. The chronic hemolysis associated with the sickling crisis can result in severe anemia.

Gonads (ovaries and testes)

The gonads are regulated by hormones secreted by the hypothalamus and the pituitary. The hypothalamus secretes gonadotropin-releasing hormone or GnRH that regulates the pituitary hormone LH and FSH, which, in turn, act upon the testes and the ovaries. In the testes, these hormones regulate testosterone production and sperm maturation. Testosterone regulates male characteristics, such as deepening of the voice, growth of facial and pubic hair, muscle growth and strength, sexual development including penile size, and the pubertal height-growth spurt. In the ovaries, these hormones regulate the menstrual cycle and control reproductive functions such as egg maturation. The female hormones estrogen and progesterone control female sexual features such as breast development and size, the pubertal height-growth spurt, and body fat distribution, especially on the hips and thighs. The sex hormones (testosterone and estrogen) also provide for the differences in sexual characteristics of males and females, such as voice, body hair distribution, and muscle formation. When the gonads do not function properly, early development of sex organs or menstrual onset (precocious puberty), loss of period, heavy and frequent periods, infertility, or sterility can result. Blood loss due to heavy menstruation is a leading cause of iron deficiency anemia in women of child-bearing age.

Adrenals

Adrenal glands are triangular in shape and are situated on

the top of each kidney. Adrenocorticotrophin, also called corticotropin or ACTH, is one of the hormones produced by the pituitary. This hormone stimulates the adrenals to make other hormones such as cortisol, aldosterone, and adrenal androgens. These hormones act on various organs of the body and influence metabolism, sodium and potassium balance, the body's response to stress, blood pressure, and heart rate. Cortisol serves as an anti-inflammatory agent in response to infection or bacteria. This inflammatory response can also trigger the iron withholding defense system, resulting in anemia of inflammatory or chronic disease. Since this is not a true anemia, where iron replenishment is needed, a person with abnormal adrenal function and lower than normal hemoglobin should be further evaluated with tests that can help distinguish the cause of anemia.

Diabetes mellitus

The pancreas produces two important hormones, insulin and glucagon. These two hormones work together to maintain a steady level of glucose, or sugar, in the blood and to keep the body supplied with fuel to produce and maintain stores of energy. When the pancreas fails to produce enough insulin, Type I diabetes, also called insulin dependent diabetes, occurs.

In Type II Diabetes the body produces insulin but is unable to respond to insulin. In fact, people with Type II diabetes usually have elevated insulin levels (hyperinsulinemia).

Diabetes often causes damage to the kidney, which affects production of erythropoietin, the hormone that stimulates the bone marrow to produce red blood cells. When chronic renal failure requires dialysis, vast amounts of iron and other nutrients are excreted. Chronic blood loss can be experienced as a result of kidney damage and lead to iron-deficiency anemia. About 50 percent of patients on dialysis develop iron-deficiency anemia. Infections associated with poorly controlled diabetes may lead to the anemia of chronic disease.

Endocrine disorders are pronounced in patients who are transfusion dependent. Although there are several conditions where blood transfusions are required therapeutically, patients with sickle cell disease or thalassemia must have regular blood

DIABETES	Type I	Type II
Age at onset	Early (before age 30)	Around age 40+
Symptoms	Frequent & abundant urination Thirst, weight loss Excessive hunger Ketoacidosis: abdominal pain Headache, rapid feeble pulse, Decreased blood pressure, Flushed, dry skin, irritability, Nausea, vomiting, air hunger/ Shortness of breath, double or Blurred vision	Frequent & abundant urination Thirst, weight change, itching Peripheral neuropathy
Therapy	Insulin & Diet	Diet, hypoglycemic drugs Possible insulin
Islet Cell Antibodies	Present at onset	Absent
Insulin in Blood	Little to none	Present
Body Weight	Normal/under	Obese (80%)
Blood Glucose	Elevated>200 mg/dL	Elevated>200 mg/dL
Symptoms of HYPOGLYCEMIA	Weakness, Tremor, Muscle twitching, Nausea, Vomiting, Pallor (paleness), Sweating, Confusion, Decreased blood pressure, Decreased heart rate, Palpitations, Air hunger (Shortness of breath, Sighing, Hiccups).	

transfusions to survive. Endocrine function is impaired in these patients because of iron-overload damage to the pituitary, resulting in impaired function of other endocrine glands, such as the thyroid, pancreas, gonads, and ovaries.

Treating anemia

Many family doctors recognize and know how to treat some endocrine problems; however, the family doctor is likely to refer the patient to a specialist such as an internist or an endocrinologist for a complete diagnosis and disease management.

Each endocrine gland has a specific test or diagnostic procedure to determine how well an organ is functioning. Besides these tests, ultrasound, computed tomography (CAT scan), and magnetic resonance imaging (MRI) treatment can be used to examine the specific organs for damage or the presence of cancer.

A patient's treatment varies depending upon the gland that is involved. The treatment for the anemia that accompanies endocrine disorders will also vary with the disease. The complete blood count, serum ferritin, and direct Coombs' test can help the physician to determine if the anemia is due to inflammation, iron-deficiency anemia, or autoimmune hemo-lytic anemia. A vitamin B_{12} and red cell folate can determine if the anemia is due to deficiencies of these nutrients.

Taking action

Anemia might be one of the first clues that an endocrine problem exists. Using the combined knowledge of symptoms, family history of disease, and the type of anemia present can help identify problems of the endocrine system early, when it is often easier to treat the underlying problem.

Resources

There are numerous resources available through the National Institutes of Health Library of Medicine, www.nlm.nih.gov; also, there are organizations that address specific disorders—look for them on the Internet. While compiling *Guide to Anemia*, the editors found these resources particularly helpful:

American Academy of Family Physicians
www.aafp.org

www.nlm.nih.gov/medlineplus/endocrinesystemhormones.html
www.endocrineweb.com

The American Thyroid Association

6066 Leesburg Pike, Suite 650
Falls Church, VA 22041
Tel: 703-998-8890
Fax: 703-998-8893
www.thyroid.org

National Institute of Diabetes and Digestive and Kidney Diseases (NIDDK)

www.niddk.nih.gov

12

Autoimmune Diseases

"Autoimmune diseases affect an estimated 8,511,845 persons in the United States or approximately 1 in 31 Americans."

—Jacobson, Gange, Rose, and Graham, "Epidemiology and Estimated Population Burden of Selected Autoimmune Diseases in the United States," Clinical Immunology & Immunopathology, 1997

Thirty-eight-year-old Tracy Lawrence went to her family doctor, an internist, because she had shortness of breath, severe fatigue, joint and muscle pain, headache, and an odd butterfly-shaped rash on her face. Her physician suspected systemic lupus erythematosus (SLE), which he confirmed with a test called antinuclear antibody (ANA). The doctor also performed other tests. Tracy's hemoglobin was quite low: 6.2 g/dL, her platelet count was elevated, her MCV (mean corpuscular volume) was low, and her RDW (red cell width) was elevated, suggesting iron-deficiency anemia. Tracy was given a corticosteroid called prednisone, oral iron pills (325 milligrams of ferrous sulfate), and ibuprofen for the joint and muscle pain.

For a while, she felt better, but then she began to get progressively worse. Within a year, Tracy's symptoms of fatigue, shortness of breath, and headache had returned; this time she also had a rapid heartbeat. The rapid heartbeat frightened her, so her neighbor took her to the emergency room. The emergency room doctor noted that Tracy was quite pale. He also noted that when resting her blood pressure and pulse were normal, but when he asked her to stand, her blood pressure dropped while her pulse increased. (This event is referred to as orthostatic and is seen in patients who have lost blood volume.)

An EKG and blood work were ordered. The EKG was normal, but the blood work showed that Tracy's white blood cell count was low, her platelet count was low, her hemoglobin was low, but her MCV (mean corpuscular value) was normal. A peripheral blood smear revealed spherocytes, which is suggestive of autoimmune hemolytic anemia (AIHA).

The doctor confirmed the diagnosis of AIHA with a direct Coombs' test. He referred Tracy back to her regular physician for follow-up. Tracy was taken off of iron, switched to acetaminophen for pain, and started on an immunosuppressive drug called Methotrexate. She continues to take all of these in addition to prednisone.

The word *auto* **is the Greek word for** *self.*

An autoimmune disease is a condition where the immune system mistakenly attacks the self, targeting the cells, tissues, and organs of a person's own body.

There are many different autoimmune diseases, and each can affect the body in different ways. For example, the autoimmune reaction is directed against the brain in multiple sclerosis and the gut in Crohn's disease. In other autoimmune diseases, such as systemic lupus erythematosus (lupus), affected tissues and organs may vary among individuals with the same disease. One person with lupus may have affected skin and joints whereas another may have affected skin, kidney, and lungs. In autoimmune hemolytic anemia, the attack is against the red blood cell. Because an autoimmune disease can affect so many systems of the body, anemia, especially autoimmune hemolytic anemia, is often a consequence. Iron deficiency anemia, anemia of chronic disease, and pernicious anemia are also among the possible findings of patients with an autoimmune disease.

From their incidence data investigators Jacobson, Gange, Rose, and Graham of the School of Hygiene and Public Health, Johns Hopkins University, Baltimore, Maryland, estimate "that approximately 1,186,015 new cases of… autoimmune diseases occur in the United States every 5 years…

Women are at 2.7 times greater risk than men to acquire an autoimmune disease."

The development of an autoimmune disease may be influenced by the genes a person inherits and the way the person's immune system responds to certain triggers or environmental influences. Some autoimmune diseases are known to begin or worsen with certain triggers such as viral infections.

Understanding the immune system

The immune system defends the body from attack by invaders recognized as foreign. It is an extraordinarily complex system that relies on an elaborate and dynamic communications network that exists among the many different kinds of immune system cells that patrol the body. At the heart of the system is the ability to recognize and respond to substances called antigens, whether they are part of the body (self-antigens) or infectious agents (nonself-antigens). Every system has its own antigens, which are proteins that the immune system is programmed to identify as self-antigens and not attack them.

Sometimes the immune system gets confused and attacks normal cell antigens. In a condition called genetic or molecular mimicry autoimmune disorder, some pathogens carry proteins on their surfaces that are indistinguishable from proteins on the host's cells. The immune system cannot distinguish between the normal cells and the germs that are invading them. For example, *H. pylori*, a common bacteria found in the stomach and small intestine, can "mimic" the cells of the stomach lining. As the immune system attacks cells in the lining of the stomach, gastrin production slows, intrinsic factor production slows, and over time the patient can develop pernicious anemia due to the lack of intrinsic factor.

Antibodies

The immune system is made up of nonspecific and specific immune mechanisms. Nonspecific types include white blood cells called neutrophils, monocytes, macrophages, and natural killer cells. Also, the nonspecific portion of the immune system includes sebum (for example, ear wax), mucus, enzymes, and hydrochloric acid. These may destroy pathogens but they are not activated for attack in the same way as the specific immune mechanisms. The specific types include white blood cells (lymphocytes) called T-lymphocytes or T-cells and B-lymphocytes or B-cells. These cells recognize specific pathogens and are mobilized when these pathogens have invaded the body.

B-lymphocytes and T-lymphocytes normally have the ability to differentiate between self-antigens and non-self antigens. B-cells do not attack pathogens directly themselves but instead produce antibodies that attack the pathogens or direct other cells, such as macrophages, to attack them. B-cells are classified as antibody-mediated-immunity. T-cells attack pathogens more directly, and are classified as cell-mediated-immunity. It is the T-cell that gets confused in cases of molecular mimicry, where the T-cell sends misinformation to the B-cell about the need for antibodies. The misinformed B-cell sends an antibody programmed to attack the self-antigen. This type of antibody is called autoantibodies and is the basis of autoimmune disease.

T Cell   Messenger Molecules   B Cell

Antibodies

Image courtesy of National Institutes of Allergies and Infectious Diseases.

Red blood cell surfaces have antigens just like any other cell. When the mistake in identity occurs and the attack is on the surface antigen of the red blood cell, the cell is destroyed. The bone marrow is then stimulated to produce more red blood cells and is reflected in an elevated reticulocyte count, which measures the rate of blood cell formation. As the new cells enter the blood stream, they are mistaken for invading pathogens, attacked, and destroyed. This continues the cycle of red cell production and early destruction (hemolysis) known as autoimmune hemolytic anemia (AIHA).

The direct Coombs' test is used to determine if a patient's red blood cells have been attacked by antibodies. If the red cells have antibodies on the surface, the cells will clump (agglutination) together.

Macrophages and neutrophils

Macrophages and neutrophils circulate in the blood and survey the body for foreign substances. When they find foreign antigens, such as bacteria, they engulf and destroy them. Macrophages and neutrophils destroy foreign antigens by making toxic molecules such as reactive oxygen intermediate. If production of these toxic molecules continues unchecked, not only are the foreign antigens destroyed, but tissues surrounding the macrophages and neutrophils are also destroyed. Macrophages also engulf old red blood cells or blood cells that have been destroyed by hemolysis. These cells release their iron back into the system for use in new red blood cells. When hemolysis is chronic, iron that is released by the macrophage can accumulate in the liver and other vital organs, leading to a condition of iron overload.

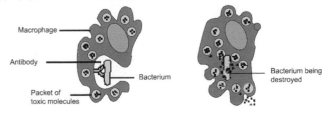

Image courtesy of National Institutes of Allergies and Infectious Diseases.

The inflammatory response

In rheumatoid arthritis, reactive oxygen intermediate molecules (free radicals) and other toxic molecules are made by overproductive macrophages and neutrophils invading the joints. The toxic molecules contribute to inflammation, which is observed as warmth and swelling, and participate in damage to the joint. Iron is a known oxygen reactant contributing to free radical activity throughout the body. When high levels of iron are present, which can occur with chronic hemolysis, the free-radical activity persists, as does the damage to the affected tissues. The body recognizes the destructive abilities of iron and when inflammation is present activates the iron-withholding defense system and slows release of iron from ferritin. A mild drop in hemoglobin and a rise in serum ferritin can be observed in the patient. This condition is called anemia of chronic disease, for which there is no cure except to correct the underlying cause of inflammation. The inflammatory response can be seen in autoimmune diseases such as sarcoidosis, Hashimoto's, Lupus, Graves' disease, or any condition known to be autoimmune related.

Detecting anemia in autoimmune diseases

Patients who have both Type 1 diabetes mellitus and autoimmune thyroid disease are at risk of developing pernicious anemia.

There are numerous autoimmune diseases in which anemia is present. It is crucial to find the underlying cause of the anemia, especially before self-medicating with over-the-counter supplements such as iron.

Inflammation associated with autoimmune diseases can often be mistaken for iron-deficiency anemia. Symptoms of many autoimmune diseases—such as fatigue—are nonspecific and usually associated with mild anemia, which can be mistakenly diagnosed as iron-deficiency anemia. Patients often associate the need for taking iron pills with the word *anemia*. In autoimmune diseases a serum ferritin or C-reactive protein (CRP) can help distinguish between the mild anemia that is caused by inflammation and iron-deficiency anemia. In iron deficiency, iron replenishment with iron pills can be appropriate. Taking iron for anemia due to inflammatory response can harm a person and even be fatal in rare situations.

Autoimmune hemolytic anemia (AIHA) is a group of disorders characterized by abnormal function of the immune system that produces antibodies, which attack red blood cells. AIHA is usually classified as either warm or cold type and in extremely rare situations "mixed"; each type is distinguished by testing for the specific antibodies. Individuals with AIHA experience early breakdown of red blood cells triggered by a rise or fall in the body temperature.

Iron-deficiency anemia generally results from blood loss due to medication used to treat the pain or inflammation associated with the autoimmune disease. Aspirin or aspirin-based products such as NSAIDs are among the most frequently used. Corticosteroids (prednisone) are also used in an attempt to stop inflammation.

Other medications used are intended to slow or suppress the immune system response involved in the autoimmune attack. These drugs are called immunosuppressive medications and include methotrexate, cyclophosphamide, azathioprine, and cyclosporin. Unfortunately, these medications also suppress the ability of the immune system to fight infection and have other potentially serious side effects.

Correcting anemia in patients with autoimmune disease will depend upon the type of anemia present. If the anemia is in response to the inflammation, treatment will center on medication specific to a cure or management of the underlying disease. Patients with autoimmune hemolytic anemia are treated with corticosteroids. Immunosuppressive drugs are sometimes used as well. Although some physicians may perform blood transfusions, these are done on a limited basis because the transfused cells may also be hemolysed rapidly and thus not very efficient. If the hemolytic anemia continues and the patient is not responsive to the steroid medications, the spleen may have to be removed (splenectomy).

If pernicious anemia is confirmed, injections of B_{12} (cobalamin) may be necessary. B_{12} injections may be given weekly initially and then once a month for the lifetime of the patient.

If the anemia is iron deficiency, oral iron or a combination of injected iron and erythropoietin may be considered. Some of these patients will also need supplemental folic acid.

Resources

There are numerous resources available through the National Institutes of Health Library of Medicine, www.nlm.nih.gov; also, there are organizations that address specific disorders—look for them on the Internet. While compiling *Guide to Anemia*, the editors found these resources particularly helpful:

NIAID Office of Communications & Public Liaison

Building 31, Room 7A-50
31 Center Drive MSC 2520
Bethesda, MD 20892-2520
Tel: 301-496-5717
www.niaid.nih.gov

Lupus Foundation of America, Inc.

1300 Piccard Drive, Suite 200
Rockville, MD 20850-4303
Tel: 301-670-9292
For medical questions select ext. #13
Fax: 301-670-9486
www.lupus.org

Arthritis Foundation

P.O. Box 7669
Atlanta, GA 30357-0669
Toll free: 800-283-7800
www.arthritis.org

American Autoimmune Related Diseases Association, Inc.

National Office
22100 Gratiot Ave.
E. Detroit, MI 48021
Tel: 586-776-3900
www.aarda.org

National Institute of Arthritis and Musculoskeletal and Skin Diseases (NIAMS)
1 AMS Circle
Bethesda, MD 20892-3675
Tel: 301-495-4484 or
877-22-NIAMS (226-4267) (free of charge)
TTY: 301-565-2966
Fax: 301-718-6366
www.niams.nih.gov

Foundation for Sarcoidosis Research
122 South Michigan Avenue
Suite 1700
Chicago, IL 60603
Tel: 312-341-0500
Fax: 312-322-9808
www.stopsarcoidosis.org/

13

Infection

"Infection and inflammation trigger an acute-phase response that can precipitate the development of mild to moderate anemia. In many cases, changes in hematological parameters may be the initial sign of an occult infectious or inflammatory disorder."

—N. Szymanski, Nephrology Nurse, 2001

Fifty-six-year-old Bess Tipton went to her doctor because of nausea, terrible stomach pain, and a burning sensation in her throat. Her temperature was normal, 98.4 degrees, and her blood work was unremarkable, except for a slightly lower than normal hemoglobin of 11.1 g/dL. Bess told the doctor that her hemoglobin often ran between 9.5 and 11.5, and this had never bothered her in the past. She also told the doctor that her body temperature was always sub, sometimes as low as 93 degrees. Her doctor ordered a barium swallow to examine the stomach. The doctor who read the X rays reported that there was no sign of an ulcer. Bess was given a prescription for Prilosec.

Bess's medical history included estrogen hormone replacement therapy, and hypothyroidism due to Hashimoto's disease, for which she took 112 mcg of Synthroid® daily. As a child she had numerous bouts of strep throat and scarlet fever. Her tonsils were removed when she was twenty-one. She had a mitral valve prolapse and often had heart arrhythmias.

Bess took the entire prescription of Prilosec and all of the pills in the sample packets, but the stomach pain and acid burning into her throat continued. Over the next few weeks Bess took Mylanta®, Pepto-Bismol® (liquid and chewable tablets), Tums®,

Pepsid-AC®, Maalox®, Rolaids®, Tagamet®, Zantac®, and Milk of Magnesia®. Besides these various medications Bess ate only white foods such as baked potatoes, rice, egg white omelets, yogurt, and milk.

None of the over-the-counter remedies or diet changes gave her any relief, except momentarily. Her doctor prescribed Prevacid and Cisapride suspension. Neither of these helped, but she took them anyway until her prescription ran out. Bess decided that because none of these medications worked that her stomach pain must be due to stress. She was under a great deal of pressure in her job and had lost two parents within six months.

While attending her mother's funeral Bess caught the flu, which developed into pneumonia. Because she was allergic to penicillin, she was given tetracycline and prednisone. She noticed after some time that her stomach pain had disappeared. She enjoyed nearly a year without stomach pain or burning in her throat. The only nagging symptom was halitosis. Bess saw her dentist, who recommended that she gargle twice a day.

Nearly a full year later the stomach pain returned with a vengeance. Bess doubled over, griping her midsection. Ironically, she had been researching for an article she was writing about *Helicobacter* (*H. pylori*). Many of the symptoms sounded familiar. She went directly to the Urgent Care Center and asked to be checked for *H. pylori*. The doctor told her that her blood work was normal and if she had *H. pylori* infection, she would have macrocytic (large) cells; hers were normocytic (normal). Bess lied to the doctor, telling him that her mother had *H. pylori* infection and she often shared her mother's food. This convinced the doctor to test her for the bacterium. The next day when Bess called for the results the doctor admitted his surprise that she was in fact positive for *Helicobacter*. He prescribed two week's worth of antibiotics (tetracycline), an antibacterial (flagyl), bismuth (Pepto-Bismol®), and a 30-day supply of Prilosec®—a proton pump inhibitor to reduce acid production and promote healing.

At the end of the two weeks Bess felt better; her stomach pain was gone and so was her bad breath.

Editor's Note: Generally people with a bacterial infection will run a fever. Because this patient also had hypothyroidism, which can cause low body temperature, the patient featured in this case example may in fact have had a fever with what appeared to be a normal temperature. It was also not determined if this patient was experiencing anemia of inflammatory response, pernicious anemia, which can be present with hypothyroidism, or if the patient experienced anemia due to iron deficiency. A serum ferritin could have helped to differentiate the cause of her mildly below normal hemoglobin.

Anemia can be present in a person as a direct consequence of an infection. Or some can be at greater risk for infection because of their anemia.

The onset of an infection takes place when a harmful germ invades the body through the skin or mucous membranes. These membranes are located in the lining of the mouth, eyes, nasal passages, lungs, gastrointestinal tract, vagina, and urethra. If the immune system is challenged in any way, the body cannot defend itself against some of the invading organisms and symptoms such as fever, vomiting, diarrhea, headache, nausea, joint pain, and heart problems, and anemia can result. Infection can be caused by viruses, protozoa, fungi, parasites (worms), or bacteria.

Anemia in individuals with infectious disease includes anemia of inflammatory response, also called anemia of chronic disease; iron-deficiency anemia usually due to blood loss; pernicious anemia due to the impairment of B_{12} absorption; and abnormal hemolysis (breakdown of red blood cells).

Bacteria and iron balance

Every surface of the human body is host to some type of bacteria. Mostly these bacteria are friendly; they are called normal flora. Normal body flora is part of our defense system that keeps harmful bacteria under control. These friendly bacteria assist immune system cells called B-cells, which secrete antibodies called immunoglobulin A. An Italian research team studied the effects of two "friendly bacteria," *Bifidobacterium bifidum* and *Lactobacillus acidophilus*, on the guts of twenty-five participants. The investigators found that "there were no significant changes in T-cell numbers or side effects as a result of receiving the bacteria. However, subjects given bacteria had statistically significant increases in the number of B-cells compared with others who received placebo. There were no changes in other types of blood cells. In subjects who had inflammation of their intestine, use of friendly bacteria decreased the inflammation by 50 percent compared with subjects on placebo who did not have a reduction in inflammation. Along with the reduction in inflammation, the numbers of white blood cells in those tissues were reduced in subjects given bacteria. This marked withdrawal of white blood cells (which were no longer needed) in those given bacteria compared to those given placebo was statistically significant."

Bacteria are single-cell organisms with a nucleus that is amorphic, meaning without specific shape. There are three different shapes of bacteria: spherical, spiral, or rod-shaped. Bacteria can divide, synthesize DNA and RNA, and adapt to hostile environments and grow resistant to antibiotics. *Helicobacter* is one of the best illustrations of the ability of bacteria to adapt.

Disease-producing bacteria can be transmitted sexually, by contaminated food or water, by insect bites, or by casual contact such as touching, kissing, drinking after, or breathing air exhaled by an infected person. Harmful pathogens are able to infiltrate the body by attaching directly onto the surface of cells of an organ or by secreting toxins, which can cause disease locally or systemically by getting into the bloodstream of the host.

Some virulent microorganisms can be harmful in one part of the body but not in other parts. To survive, regardless of where they are in the body, nearly all of these bacteria need iron and each obtains the metal in its own way. For example, the bacteria that cause tuberculosis can enter a macrophage, a cell that is intended to destroy the harmful germ. Macrophages, a type of white blood cell, engulf old red blood cells so that the iron in the hemoglobin of these cells can be recycled. When the bacteria enter the macrophage, they ingest the iron, which insures their survival. Other ways bacteria can get iron is from heme in hemoglobin or transferrin, an iron-transport protein found in the blood. Some bacteria can get iron directly from lactoferrin, a defense iron binding protein found in body fluids such as saliva, tears, breast milk, and vaginal and seminal (semen) secretions.

Helicobacter is an example of a pathogen that can get iron from lactoferrin. *Helicobacter* (*H. pylori*) is the leading cause of stomach ulcers and stomach cancers. This pathogen can be present in a person for decades before symptoms are noticed. Often symptoms of *H. pylori* infection will be attributed to stress or diet. When *H. pylori* was first discovered, clinicians did not believe that any bacterium could survive the highly acidic environment of the stomach. *H. pylori* is one exception; the bacterium burrows into the stomach lining escaping the acid.

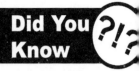

Did You Know

According to the U.S. Centers for Disease Control and Prevention, persons infected with *H. Pylori* have a two- to six-fold increased risk of developing gastric cancer and certain types of lymphoma.

Viruses

Structurally, viruses are less complex than bacteria. Unlike bacteria, viruses do not need iron to survive, but a virus will benefit from the presence of abundant iron in its host. A virus needs a specific host to survive and the infected host cells need iron to replicate the virus. The influenza virus, for example, can only proliferate in the cells of the respiratory system, which can contain great amounts of iron from inhaling tobacco smoke. Another example of a virus and its specific host is the herpes simplex virus, which survives in tissues of the mouth. Once inside a cell, viruses alter DNA or RNA. Here they are nurtured, multiply, and spread to other cells. Antibiotics, which work on bacterial infections, do not work on viral infections. Specific antiviral drugs are now available for many viral infections. Viruses are only vulnerable if a surface has been disinfected with some product, such as common household bleach. Some of the better known viruses include HIV; viral Hepatitis A, B, and C; poliovirus; and rubella, which causes German measles. Anemia associated with viral infections can be iron-deficiency anemia due to blood loss or hemolysis as a side effect of medications used as therapies for patients with viral infections. Anemia of inflammatory response can also be experienced by patients with viral infections.

Fungi

Yeasts and molds are types of fungi, whic can include benign or beneficial organisms as well as infection-causing organisms. Unlike plants, fungi cannot make chlorophyll; these organisms are nourished by organic matter such as feces, decaying animals, or foods. Characteristically fungi are similar to bacteria and originate in soils, in water, and on plants. The best-known fungi are mushrooms. A very familiar and troublesome fungus is the yeast Candida. Anyone who has had a yeast infection is familiar with this extremely common and virulent organism. Candida flourish anywhere in the body; they are nourished in body fluids such as saliva and tears by iron that has not been trapped by lactoferrin. Fungal infections may trigger an inflammatory response. Individuals who are anemic, have challenged bone marrow production, or are the recipients of transplants are at risk for increased fungal infection.

Protozoa

Protozoa are single-celled parasitic organisms with flexible membranes. They have the ability to move by means of pseudopods (false foot) or flagella (whip-like tentacles). Infections with protozoa are gotten from insect bites or from drinking or swimming in contaminated water or consuming food that has been handled by a person who has not washed his or her hands. Common protozoan infections include: trichomoniasis, vaginal infection due to the parasite Trichomonas; malaria, transmitted by an infected mosquito; amebic dysentery, generally from ingested contaminated water; and giardiasis from G. lamblia, which is contracted from ingesting contaminated water or by eating or drinking food or liquid contaminated by someone who is infected.

Some species of protozoa have the ability to survive hostile environments by secreting thick, protective capsules around themselves, or "encysting." As cysts, these harmful pathogens can remain dormant for weeks, or even months. Chlorine bleach can weaken the walls of these cysts but boiling water or food that might be contaminated with these cysts is necessary to kill the organism. Anemia that accompanies an infection with protozoa is generally caused by acute blood loss (iron deficiency) or anemia of chronic disease due to inflammation. In some cases of protozoan infection, hemolytic anemia can occur, leading to an inflamed or enlarged spleen.

Worms

There are several types of worms that humans can contract, but not all of them are accompanied by anemia. Hookworm and roundworm are two types of infestations that can lead to significant blood loss and anemia in infected humans. These worms are transmitted from animals that contaminate the soil with infected feces. A person can become infected with hookworm by direct contact with the contaminated soil, generally from walking barefoot, or accidentally swallowing contaminated soil.

Hookworms have a complex life cycle that begins and ends in the small intestine. Hookworm eggs require warm, moist, shaded soil to hatch into larvae. These barely visible larvae penetrate the skin, such as on the soles of the feet, are carried to the lungs, go through the respiratory tract to the mouth, are swallowed, and eventually reach the small intestine. This journey takes about a week. In the small intestine, the larvae develop into half-inch-long worms, attach themselves to the intestinal wall, and suck blood. The adult worms produce thousands of eggs. These eggs are passed in the feces (stool). If the eggs contaminate soil and conditions are right, they will hatch, molt, and develop into infective larvae again after five to ten days.

Round worms—human whipworm

Infestation with roundworm occurs in a similar way as hookworm. A person gets infected by swallowing the eggs by direct contact with contaminated soil (hands) or by ingesting food that is contaminated. The eggs hatch in the small intestine, and release larvae that mature and establish themselves as adults in the colon. The adult worms, which are approximately 4 cm in length (approximately 2 inches), live in the cecum and ascending colon. The adult worms are fixed in that location, with the anterior portions threaded into the mucosa. The females begin to oviposit sixty to seventy days after infection. Female worms in the cecum shed between 3,000 and 20,000 eggs per day.

The life span of the adults is about one year.

Infection is more frequent in areas with tropical weather and poor sanitation practices, and among children. It is estimated that worldwide, 800 million people are infected with worms. Anemia associated with this type of infection is generally iron-deficiency anemia due to blood loss and is seen mostly in children who are at the greatest risk for this type of infection.

At risk:

People at risk for anemia because of infection can include anyone at any age. People who are most at risk for infection because of their disease include individuals

- with compromised immune systems
- with weakened heart valve
- with abnormal bone marrow production: MDS, cancer, hypoplastic or aplastic anemias
- with enzyme deficiencies (G6PD, pyruvate kinase)
- with iron transport disorders (atransferrinemia, aceruloplasminemia)
- with inherited hemoglobin diseases (thalassemia, sickle cell disease)
- with bleeding and platelet disorders: von Willebrand's, hemophilia, paroxsymal nocturnal hemoglobinura (PNH)
- who are bone marrow transplant recipients
- with diabetes mellitus type I or II
- with kidney disease
- who have undergone surgery, especially to remove the spleen, generally to stop hemolysis

Enlarged spleen (splenomegaly) is seen in patients with acute or chronic hemolysis. In extreme cases, the spleen must be surgically removed to stop the continued breakdown of red blood cells. Once the spleen has been removed, the patient is more susceptible to infections with germs such as pneumococci, meningococci, H. influenzae, and some protozoan infections. Among other pathogens that thrive on the extra iron in the sera of splenectomized persons are strains of Hemophilus and of Capnocytophaga.

Detecting an infection

Infections can be acute (sudden onset) or chronic (lasting a long time), and symptoms are not always the same. Weakness and fatigue are two of the most common complaints of individuals with an infection, but numerous other symptoms can be displayed: fever, joint pain, muscle aches, vomiting, and diarrhea can mistakenly be attributed to the flu, and infections such as a tick bite can go undiagnosed for long periods of time. Diarrhea and vomiting can lead to dehydration very rapidly in a small child or frail adult. Anemia of inflammatory response or chronic disease present in people with infections can be mistaken for iron deficiency, and iron pills might be offered or taken by the patient who does not understand the differences between these two anemias. One is caused by blood loss and iron replenishment is needed; the other is a defense mechanism natural to the body to protect us against nourishing harmful germs. Regardless, iron should never be taken if a fever is present.

Infections can be isolated with specific tests that detect antibody reaction caused by the presence of a particular germ. This reaction triggers the release of immunoglobulins in the blood. IgG, IgA, and IgM are among the types of immunoglobulins associated in an antibody reaction. IgG detects about 75 percent of circulating blood antibodies for infections. IgA detects about 15 percent, and IgM is used more to detect chronic infections. Other tests confirm specific antibodies to bacterial or viral infections such as the heterophile antibody for infectious mononucleosis; viral hepatitis A, B, or C; or the *Helicobacter* antibody test.

Most tests to detect infections are done by obtaining blood from a vein in the arm. In some cases a fecal sample is needed, especially to examine for worms or to determine if an infection is cured, such as *Helicobacter pylori*.

Detecting anemia

A number of tests can confirm the type of anemia in a patient with infection. See chapters on the specific disease to learn more about detection of hemolysis or bone marrow failure. It is important for people with infections to determine if the anemia is due to iron deficiency or inflammatory response. With iron

142

deficiency anemia, serum ferritin will be low; with anemia of inflammatory response (our defense system), the serum ferritin will be elevated. Read more about this defense system in chapter 10.

Treatment
Treatment for infections varies and includes antibiotics, antivirals, and antifungals, sometimes in conjunction with other medications. Generally these drugs are taken for ten days to two weeks, followed by two weeks of probiotics, such as L. acidophilus. **Note:** Iron impairs the absorption of antibiotics.

Treatment for anemia will depend on the cause of anemia
Supplemental iron can be dangerous during the phase where the infection is being treated. Added iron at this time might cause the germ to proliferate and spread. Iron is best obtained from food sources such as red meat and not from supplements at this time. After the infection has been controlled, oral iron supplements can be used to replenish iron stores if they are still low. Regardless, iron replenishment in persons with infectious disease should not be done without proper medical supervision.

Taking action: prevention is key

- Wash hands frequently.
- Avoid spray from a cough or sneeze by an infected person.
- Do not share personal items such as a razor or toothbrush.
- Do not share other people's food, drink, or utensils.
- Do not take iron supplements if you have a fever or suspect an infection.

Resources

There are numerous resources available through the National Institutes of Health Library of Medicine, www.nlm.nih.gov; also, there are organizations that address specific disorders—look for them on the Internet. While compiling *Guide to Anemia*, the editors found these resources particularly helpful:

The Bad Bug Book
U.S. Food & Drug Administration
Center for Food Safety & Applied Nutrition
Foodborne Pathogenic Microorganisms and Natural Toxins Handbook
vm.cfsan.fda.gov/~mow/intro.html

www.cdc.gov (search by infectious disease)

National Institute of Allergy and Infectious Diseases (NIAID)
NIAID Office of Communications & Public Liaison
Building 31, Room 7A-50
31 Center Drive MSC 2520
Bethesda, MD 20892-2520
Tel: 301-496-5717
www.niaid.nih.gov

14

Nutrient Imbalances

"Learning about the possible side effects of over-the-counter nutritional supplements and products is just as important as knowing the side effects of any prescribed drug."

—John Beard, PhD, Professor of Nutrition, Penn State University, Iron Disorders Institute, Medical & Scientific Board Member

In the May 2000 issue of the *Journal of Pediatrics*, Dr. Timothy Porea and his colleagues Dr. John Belmont and Dr. Donald Mahoney Jr. describe the case of a seventeen-year-old male with zinc-induced anemia. The youth was referred to the Texas Children's Cancer Center and Hematology Service because he continued to have symptoms following the conclusion of treatment for an upper respiratory infection. At Texas Children's a complete blood count was among the first tests performed on the boy. His white cell count was low: 2.2 X 10⁹ (reference range 5 to 10 X 10⁹). His absolute neutrophil count (ANC) was 228 (reference range 1,800 to 2,000). An ANC below 1,000 is diagnostic of neutropenia (a condition of too few neutrophils). The boy's hemoglobin was 9.6 g/dL (normal for an adult male is 13.5 to 17.5 g/dL). A blood smear taken from the boy contained several abnormally shaped cells, some of which were suggestive of hemolytic anemia. His blood count when taken eight months earlier was normal.

In the months that followed, multiple tests were performed. Most of the test results were unremarkable except for the hemoglobin, which continued to remain low. His ANC, which varied in range from 220 to 860, was still below normal.

Immunoglobulins were normal, except for a mildly decreased IgM. He was negative for AIDS, Epstein-Barr, and human parvo-19 virus. A bone marrow biopsy was performed and findings were normal; so were folic acid, B$_{12}$, iron, and thyroid function.

The patient was referred to a neurologist because he was having headaches, fainting, and fatigued. An MRI of the brain was unremarkable; the neurologist started the boy on phenobarbital.

Some months later, a second bone marrow aspiration would lead to the boy's diagnosis. Findings with this sample included the presence of vacuoles in the marrow. Vacuoles are fluid- or air-filled precursor cells that will eventually become blood cells. This type of abnormality can be present in abusers of alcohol and individuals who are copper deficient. Prompted by these findings, the patient's serum copper and ceruloplasmin (protein that binds with and transports copper and is key to iron metabolism) were measured. His serum copper was 10 mg/dL; normal is 70–155 mg/dL. His ceruloplasmin was 2 mg/dL; normal is 23–49 mg/dL. His serum zinc was 199 mg/dL; normal range is 60–130 mg/dL.

After questioning the young man about over-the-counter nutrients, it was revealed that he had been self-medicating with 300 milligrams of zinc per day to treat acne. Once this was discovered the boy stopped taking the zinc supplements. Within one month his ceruloplasmin had risen to 9 mg/dL. Within two months his ANC was up to 2,640 and his hemoglobin was 14.6 g/dL. His chronic fatigue and headaches were gone. After nearly a year and half, his serum zinc was 71 mg/dL, copper 66 mg/dL, and ceruloplasmin 20 mg/dL. Excessive zinc causes low copper levels.

The recommended daily allowance (RDA) for zinc is 15 milligrams a day. Supplemental zinc can be used as treatment for the common cold and acne, but usually in doses of 30 milligrams or less. This youth had been taking up to 20 times the zinc RDA for nearly two years.

This case illustrates how excessive intake of a seemingly harmless nutrient can lead to a serious condition, not to mention the cost and time to perform the battery of tests and diagnostic procedures that can accumulate in trying to isolate the cause and reach a diagnosis. Nutrient imbalances can result in impaired red blood cell production, pernicious anemia, shortened red cell life span (hemolytic anemia), and iron-deficiency anemia. A number of possible side effects and symptoms can occur as a result of these imbalances. For this reason over-the-counter nutrients should not be taken without first investigating the consequences when doses exceed the recommended daily intake (RDI).

Healthcare providers need to know what supplements we are taking because of the potential to do harm to our health. Besides, today's healthcare providers are more receptive to using integrative strategies that include complementary, alternative, nonconventional, and nonpharmaceutical approaches to address health issues. Integrative medicine combines treatments from conventional medicine and complementary and alternative medicine for which there is some high-quality evidence of safety and effectiveness.

All nutrients contribute to healthy metabolism, but it is not fully known to what extent combinations of supplemental forms of nutrients interfere or promote metabolism. We know that deficiencies in vitamins A, B, C, D, E, and K and minerals iron, zinc, copper, manganese, and calcium can lead to abnormal formation and function of red blood cells. We also know that excesses in these same nutrients can result in the same type of abnormal formation or function.

The body is not made to handle high concentrations of nutrients found in many supplements. Some multivitamins are excessively loaded with thousands of times what is needed for balanced nutrition. Vitamin A, for example, is often found in quantities as high as 10,000 IU; amounts of this size can cause liver failure. Multivitamins can be beneficial but only if taken sensibly, otherwise these megadoses will put unnecessary strain on the liver, heart, and kidneys. Our bodies are equipped to manage whole foods, which are naturally in balance; whole foods, unless otherwise recommended by a healthcare provider, should be the main source of daily nutrients. In cases where certain nutrient levels are deficient, such as B_6, folate, B_{12}, zinc, or iron, one should not seek to remedy these shortages without seeking medical advice.

Balancing nutrients

Vitamin A is made in the liver from beta-carotene; it is important to the growth and differentiation of blood cells, especially in the early stages. Vitamin A helps to mobilize iron stores from tissues so that the iron can be used in hemoglobin. Deficiencies in vitamin A are somewhat uncommon in the United States, except among the very poor, whose diets may be limited by income. Vitamin A deficiencies can be related to the incidence of iron deficiency in developing countries, but this is not usually the case in developed countries. Vitamin A deficiencies usually result from poor dietary intake and a lack of beta-carotene. An imbalance of zinc and iron can cause changes in vitamin A absorption, transport, and production, so it is not unusual to observe alterations in all three nutrients simultaneously. Beta-carotene should be gotten from foods rather than from supplements as there is evidence that the supplemental form contributes to some cancers.

Vitamins C, E, and the mineral selenium are powerful antioxidants that protect against oxidative stress during the formation of the red blood cell structure and life span. Premature breakdown of red blood cells (hemolytic anemia) can occur with vitamin E deficiencies. But high doses of vitamin E can cause internal bleeding and result in iron-deficiency anemia. Vitamin C improves the absorption and utilization of iron. There is evidence that supplemental vitamin C can benefit patients who smoke or have suffered a stroke, but these reports come from controlled studies of patients who were under the care of trained investigators. The detrimental effects of excessive vitamin C are not well understood. One report from animal studies of high doses of ascorbic acid (vitamin C) resulted in increased esophageal (forestomach) cancers. More evidence exists to support the detriments of supplemental antioxidants when consumed in great excesses. Selenium, for example, can be fatal when taken in high doses. We get antioxidants from foods such as coffee, tea, nuts, fresh fruits, and vegetables.

Iron, zinc, and calcium are among the most frequently used over-the-counter supplements in the United States with their consumption second only to vitamin C as a supplement. These nutrients are often taken in amounts that far exceed a therapeutic dose, which results in imbalances too great for the body's ability to manage.

Iron, for example, is often taken in doses of 325 milligrams two to three times daily to treat anemia; in some cases the anemia is not due to iron deficiency. The person may be experiencing anemia of chronic disease (ACD), also known as anemia of inflammation. In this condition the body's natural defense is curtailing the amount of available iron by withholding it—placing the iron in ferritin (and elsewhere) until the danger of disease passes. Because the hemoglobin levels of people with anemia of inflammation can be lower than normal, they can mistakenly think that iron pills are appropriate. Iron pills could actually cause a fatality if taken in the presence of an infection. Read about anemia of chronic inflammatory disease in chapter 10.

As illustrated in the story at the beginning of this chapter, zinc taken in high doses interferes with copper absorption. Copper acts as a catalyst in the formation of hemoglobin, and the copper binding protein ceruloplasmin plays a major role in the distribution of iron throughout the body, especially in the brain, liver, and pancreas. According to copper metabolism experts Gitlan and Nittis, Washington University School of Medicine, St. Louis, Missouri, laboratory studies of patients with insufficient levels of this copper binding and iron shuttling protein demonstrate microcytic anemia (smaller than normal red blood cells) and elevated serum ferritin.

Zinc influences several aspects of vitamin A metabolism, including its absorption, transport, and utilization, while iron in supplemental doses greater than 25 milligrams can inhibit the absorption of zinc.

Calcium helps to regulate the timing of release or intake of iron into the red blood cell, which affects the life span of a red blood cell. Calcium competes for the same absorption pathways as iron, zinc, and copper. Deficiencies of these minerals can occur if one consumes great amounts of calcium, especially in amounts greater than 500 milligrams. When needed supplementally, calcium should be taken separately at bedtime.

B vitamins

B_{12} and folate deficiencies are commonly present in people with certain types of anemia, which are generally defined as a result of blood chemistries, a blood smear, or bone marrow aspiration. Folate and folic acid are forms of a water-soluble B vitamin. Folate is found in foods, where folic acid is the synthetic form found in supplements and fortified foods. Humans do not store great amounts of folate, and a deficiency can develop within a few months. Folate deficiency may occur in patients taking anticonvulsants, oral contraceptives, or drugs used to treat cancer, such as methotrexate, or in those who have liver disease, especially abusers of alcohol or patients who are on dialysis.

Vitamin B_6, also known as pyridoxine, helps in the formation of red blood cells. One form of sideroblastic anemia is pyridoxine-dependent and can be resolved with therapeutic doses of B_6, which must be supervised by a physician. B_6 can reach toxic levels in the body when taken in large doses for a prolonged period of time.

Vitamin B_2, also known as riboflavin, helps in the absorption of iron and iron utilization. Symptoms of anemia associated with a B_2 deficiency are very similar to vitamin B_{12}.

Vitamin B_{12} deficiency can result in pernicious anemia. A congenital form of pernicious anemia can be seen in children, but in otherwise healthy children, pernicious anemia is rare. The groups most at risk for this type of anemia are strict vegetarians and the elderly. Alcoholics generally have increased levels of B_{12} due to "gain of function" of the liver. When the liver is damaged for whatever reason, the damage can cause the liver function to increase. This can be dangerous, even life threatening, for anyone taking medications as the liver controls the amount of medication that gets into the bloodstream. Individuals with severe and prolonged hyperthyroidism such as Graves' disease have an increased demand for B_{12}, which is used up more rapidly because of the disease; therefore patients with Graves' are at an increased risk for pernicious anemia.

The terms "vitamin B_{12}" and "cobalamin" are used interchangeably. Cobalamin is a bright red crystalline compound that contains cobalt. It is essential for normal neurologic function, DNA synthesis, and blood cell formation. The most common form of cobalamin is cyanocobalamin, which must be converted before the body can absorb it. Cyanocobalamin can be changed

"Almost 800,000 elderly people in the United States have undiagnosed and untreated pernicious anemia..."

—R. Carmel, "Prevalence of Undiagnosed Pernicious Anemia in the Elderly," Archives of Internal Medicine, 1996

into hydroxycobalamin, methylcobalamin, and adenosylcobalamin, which are the active forms of B_{12} that the body can absorb.

Neither plants nor humans can make B_{12}, which is produced by bacteria found in the digestive tracts of grazing animals. The B_{12} is absorbed into the systems of these animals. Humans obtain B_{12} from eating the meat or dairy products that come from animals. Humans have these same B_{12}-producing bacteria in their colons, but B_{12} is absorbed in the small intestine

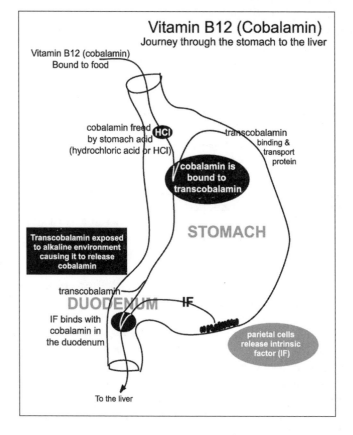

Vitamin B12 (Cobalamin)
Journey through the stomach to the liver

Vitamin B12 (cobalamin) Bound to food

cobalamin freed by stomach acid (hydrochloric acid or HCl) — **HCl**

transcobalamin binding & transport protein

cobalamin is bound to transcobalamin

STOMACH

Transcobalamin exposed to alkaline environment causing it to release cobalamin

transcobalamin

DUODENUM — **IF**

IF binds with cobalamin in the duodenum

parietal cells release intrinsic factor (IF)

To the liver

and only with sufficient amounts of stomach acid, transport proteins, and intrinsic factor—none of which is found in the large intestine.

Gastrin, a hormone produced by the lining of the stomach, stimulates the production of HCl, or stomach acid. HCl frees bound B_{12} from food so that it can be picked up by a transport protein, appropriately called Transcobalamin I. This protein transports B_{12} to the duodenum, the upper portion of the small intestine, where it is bound to intrinsic factor (IF). Pancreatic enzymes are released and B_{12} is eventually absorbed in the lower portion of the small intestine called the ileum. B_{12} is then transported by Transcobalamin II to the liver, where it is stored. Normally the liver maintains a three years' supply of B_{12}.

Deficiency in B_{12} can result in a form of anemia called megaloblastic anemia. A number of symptoms and findings are associated with megaloblastic anemia, including dementia, which can be mistaken for early Alzheimer's. Some refer to this state of dementia as "megaloblastic madness." Megaloblastic describes the large, nucleated, oval, or irregular shape of newly forming red blood cells seen in patients with pernicious anemia. Other symptoms and findings include fatigue, memory loss, optic nerve damage, loss of balance, stumbling or irregular gait, tingling and pain in the extremities, disease such as lesions in the spinal cord (myelin sheath), impotence, light-headedness, urinary incontinence, alternating diarrhea, constipation, and macrocytic anemia. Also present are elevated levels of homocysteine, a harmful compound in the blood that increases the risk of heart attack, blood clots, stroke, and elevated cholesterol.

Deficiencies in B_{12} due to lack of intrinsic factor in the stomach can result in pernicious anemia (PA). PA can be present in conditions of alcoholism, vegetarianism, poor nutrition or eating disorders, achlorhydria (lack of hydrochloric acid in the stomach), surgical removal of portions of the stomach or small intestine, *H. pylori* infection, celiac sprue disease, adrenal insufficiency, hyper- and hypothyroidism, diabetes, vitiligo, and myasthenia gravis. Additionally, pernicious anemia is observed in people with autism, Alzheimer's, Parkinson's, epilepsy, and Bell's palsy.

Diagnosing nutritional deficiencies

Nutrients can be measured directly in the tissue, blood, serum, or urine but some levels are not helpful.

The B_{12} level in serum, for example, is not an accurate indication of B_{12} deficiency. Normal ranges for B_{12} vary from lab to lab. Some set the normal low level of B_{12} at 100 ng/L; some use higher levels such as 200 ng/L up to 295 ng/L. For many patients, by the time the B_{12} level reaches 200 ng/L permanent neurological damage may have occurred.

Blood cell parameters such as mean corpuscular volume (MCV) can be helpful in the diagnosis of B_{12} deficiencies. The normal range for MCV is 82–98 fL. Below normal MCV is considered microcytic anemia, which is seen in iron-deficiency anemia. Above normal value is macrocytic anemia, which occurs with pernicious anemia. An MCV greater than 130 fL is associated with B_{12} or folate deficiency in nearly 100 percent of patients. Elevated MCV can

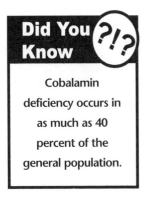

Did You Know ?!?

Cobalamin deficiency occurs in as much as 40 percent of the general population.

also be seen in patients with acquired sideroblastic anemia.

The Shilling test is one way to diagnosis pernicious anemia. The test involves swallowing a dose of radioactive B_{12} to evaluate absorption by measuring the levels of B_{12} in the urine. The Shilling test can be done with or without intrinsic factor. This two-step method helps to clarify whether absorption is the cause of the anemia. A bone marrow aspiration and serum B_{12} levels might be done prior to the Shilling test.

Urine methylmalonic acid (UMMA) and homocysteine are sensitive for the diagnosis of B_{12} deficiency. Abnormal UMMA

iron panel	IRON PANEL TESTS						
	Serum Iron	Serum Ferritin	Transferrin Iron Saturation Percentage	Total Iron Binding Capacity (TIBC)	Transferrin	Serum Transferrin Receptor	Hemoglobin
Vitamin B12 Deficiency (pernicious anemia)	⬆ or Normal	⬆ or Normal	⬆ or Normal	⬇ or Normal	⬇ or Normal	Normal to HIGH	⬇
Iron Deficiency Anemia	⬇	⬇	⬇	⬆	⬆	HIGH	⬇

levels usually precede abnormal blood counts or below normal serum vitamin B_{12} levels. Measurement with UMMA is especially useful for patients whose serum B_{12} levels are in the range of 200–350 ng/L.

High levels of folate can mask a B_{12} deficiency. Folate can correct anemia associated with a B_{12} deficiency but it will not correct the neurological damage often associated with the B_{12} deficiency. Therefore it is important to examine both B_{12} and folate levels when pernicious anemia is suspect.

MMA and homocysteine will both be elevated in B_{12} deficiencies. In folate deficiencies homocysteine levels will be elevated but MMA will not. According to *The Mayo Clinic Proceedings*, urine methylmalonic acid (uMMA) test is preferred because of convenience and sensitivity. It is not necessary to order the homocystine test for detecting vitamin B_{12} deficiency. The uMMA test reflects both tissue and cellular vitamin B_{12} deficiency.

Though vitamin B_{12} is stored in the liver, it is a water-soluble vitamin and not likely to reach toxic levels in the body of even persons with normal B_{12} levels. MRIs of patients with lesions of the spinal column substantiate the fact that neurologic damage caused by B_{12} deficiency can be reversed, if it is found and treated early. Since there is not evidence that B_{12} is harmful, some physicians will administer doses of B_{12} in high risk patients who have symptoms of mild dementia even when their hematological values are within the "normal" range.

B_{12} can be administered by injection or in oral supplementation sublingually (under the tongue). According to the American Academy of Family Physicians, injection doses are usually 1,000 micrograms, often given daily for one week to build up stores, then weekly for one month, and then monthly thereafter. Oral

B12/Folate panel	VITAMIN B-12 AND FOLATE TESTS					
	Hemoglobin	MCV	UMMA	Homocysteine	Red Blood Cell Size	Red Blood Cell Color
Vitamin B12 Deficiency (pernicious anemia)	⬇ or Normal	⬆	⬆	⬆	MACRO CYTIC	NORMO-CHROMIC
Folate Deficiency	⬇ or Normal	⬆	Normal	⬆	MICRO CYTIC	HYPO CHROMIC

MCV=mean corpuscular volume UMMA=urine methylmalonic acid

doses range from 1,000 to 2,000 micrograms daily. Previously oral vitamin B_{12} supplementation was not thought to be effective. Recent studies indicate that the oral doses can be as effective as injected doses. The oral doses are generally higher than injected doses.

B_{12} deficiency takes about two decades to develop. When deficiency in B_{12} is found in youths, it is generally due to some compounding factor, such as long-term antiseizure medication, chemotherapy, problems of absorption, and intestinal diseases such as Crohn's, colitis, or celiac sprue. B_{12} deficiencies are often seen in autistic children, though the exact mechanism is not known.

Achieving nutrient balances

Eating a balanced diet that includes some meat, grains, vegetables, and fruits will assure adequate intake of nutrients for the majority. Everyone should inform his or her healthcare provider of any supplements being taken. Those requiring therapeutic doses of a supplement should do so only with medical supervision. People with exceptional conditions that might need therapeutic doses of supplements might include but is not limited to individuals with Graves' disease or Hashimoto's thyroiditis, AIDS, disease of the small intestine, multiple sclerosis, stomach surgery, or diabetes; individuals who have a history of acid reflux, especially those who have taken "proton pump inhibitors" or long-term antacid products that might inhibit absorption are also candidates.

Bariatric surgery is more frequently becoming an approach used in controlling obesity, especially in morbidly obese people. There are four types of operations that are commonly offered in the United States: adjustable gastric band (AGB), Roux-en-Y gastric bypass (RYGB), gastric sleeve (GS), and biliopancreatic bypass with a duodenal switch (BPD). Some of these procedures can result in life-threatening nutrient deficiencies that must be met with strict medical supervision. Each bariatric procedure has its own benefits and risks and should be discussed fully with physicians who specialize in these types of procedures. The National Institutes of Health provides excellent educational information about these procedures.

Content in this publication is not intended to be a substitute for professional medical advice, nor is it intended to replace the services of a medical professional or impair the patient–healthcare provider or caregiver relationship. Content in this publication should be used as information only and be discussed with a medical professional who is qualified to diagnose and treat your condition. Iron Disorders Institute, all contributors, and the publisher of this book are not responsible for the content on websites listed in the resources, nor do we endorse products promoted on such sites. We advise you to always seek the advice of a qualified health provider before making any changes to diet, supplementation, or starting any new treatment. Any application of the information or recommendations in this book is made at the reader's discretion.

Resources

There are numerous resources available through the National Institutes of Health Library of Medicine, www.nlm.nih.gov; also, there are organizations that address specific disorders—look for them on the Internet. While compiling *Guide to Anemia*, the editors found these resources particularly informative:

USDA Food Composition Nutrient Data Laboratory
www.nal.usda.gov/fnic/foodcomp/Data

Bariatric surgery information:
National Institutes of Health Weight Control Information Network
www.win.niddk.nih.gov

Center for Science in the Public Interest
Nutrition Action Newsletter, June 2008 (This issue features multicomplex vitamins.)
www.cspinet.org/

National Center for Complementary and Alternative Medicine
nccam.nih.gov/

Patients may order the uMMA test kit from Norman Clinical Laboratories. Call 513-521-TEST (8378), or see the website for fees and insurance coverage details. www.b12.com

15

Alcohol Abuse

"Alcohol has numerous adverse effects on the various types of blood cells and their functions."

—Harold S. Ballard, MD, Associate Chief of Hematology and Oncology, New York Department of Veterans Affairs Medical Center, New York, New York

The emergency medical attendants rushed forty-seven-year-old Larry Bonner to the hospital. His wife Sarah had called them when Larry passed out and fell down the front steps. He was moving slightly, groaning and trying to say something, but his words were slurred. He was very drunk. He had lost his balance at the top of steps, toppling backward and falling the full length of the concrete stairs and onto the sidewalk. Sarah knew that her husband was a heavy drinker. On this day she knew for a fact that he had consumed more than two pints of whiskey.

In the emergency room, the physician noted that Larry was very thin, except for a paunch; his skin was jaundiced (yellow color). His eyes were bloodshot and yellow; his tongue was smooth, swollen, and dry. He had a slight fever and normal blood pressure, but rapid pulse. Upon physician examination, the ER physician suspected that Larry's abdomen was filled with fluid (ascites). The liver was enlarged and edema was present on Larry's legs and feet. The physician also noted abrasions on Larry's left ankle, arm, and wrist. He ordered a set of X rays, an IV of fluids, and waited for the laboratory findings.

The radiologist confirmed that the left ankle was broken; the wrist had a hairline fracture. The lab work provided that Larry's hemoglobin was 10.2 g/dL, his mean corpuscular volume (MCV) and red cell distribution width were elevated. His liver enzymes were elevated, and he was hypoglycemic (low blood sugar). There was no blood in the stool but his urine was positive for bilirubin. His red cell folate was seriously low but his B_{12} was quite high.

Larry spent two days in the hospital where he was given fluids and therapeutic doses of folic acid. The physician discussed therapy with Larry's wife, who seemed frustrated, embarrassed, and saddened by the event. She told the doctor that Larry would rather have "booze" than a meal. The doctor provided her with the contact information for several support organizations.

Editor's note: This family eventually did seek counseling and further medical attention, and was helped.

People who abuse alcohol are at risk for numerous alcohol-related medical complications, including those affecting the blood (i.e., the blood cells as well as proteins present in the blood plasma) and the bone marrow, where the blood cells are produced. Alcohol's adverse effects on the blood building, or hematopoietic, system are both direct and indirect. The direct consequences of excessive alcohol consumption include: toxic effects on the bone marrow; the blood cell precursors; and the mature red blood cells (RBCs), white blood cells (WBCs), and platelets. Alcohol's indirect effects include nutritional deficiencies that impair the production and function of various blood cells.

These direct and indirect effects of alcohol can result in serious medical problems for the drinker. For example, anemia resulting from diminished RBC production and impaired RBC metabolism and function can cause fatigue, shortness of breath, lightheadedness, and even reduced mental capacity and abnormal heartbeats. A decrease in the number and function of WBCs increases the drinker's risk of serious infection, and impaired platelet production and function interfere with blood clotting, leading to symptoms ranging from a simple nosebleed to bleeding in the brain (i.e., hemorrhagic stroke). Finally, alcohol-induced abnormalities in the plasma proteins that are required for blood clotting can lead to the formation of blood clots (i.e., thrombosis).

In this chapter, the terms "chronic alcohol abuse" or "chronic excessive alcohol consumption" refer to the ingestion of one pint or more of 80- to 90-proof alcohol (i.e., about eleven drinks) per day. However, alcohol-related hematological problems can occur at much lower consumption levels. The drinker's risk for developing these problems grows with increasing alcohol consumption.

Alcohol's effects on iron metabolism

In addition to interfering with the proper absorption of iron into the hemoglobin molecules of red blood cells (RBCs), alcohol use can lead to either iron deficiency or excessively high levels of iron in the body. Because iron is essential to RBC functioning, iron deficiency, which is commonly caused by excessive blood loss, can result in anemia. In many alcoholic patients, blood loss and subsequent iron deficiency are caused by gastrointestinal bleeding. Iron deficiency in alcoholics often is difficult to diagnose, however, because it may be masked by symptoms of other nutritional deficiencies (e.g., folic acid deficiency) or by coexisting liver disease and other alcohol-related inflammatory conditions. For an accurate diagnosis, the physician must therefore exclude folic acid deficiency and evaluate the patient's iron stores in the bone marrow.

Conversely, alcohol abuse can increase iron levels in the body. For example, iron absorption from the food in the gastrointestinal tract may be elevated in alcoholics. Iron levels also can rise from excessive ingestion of iron-containing alcoholic beverages, such as red wine.

The increased iron levels can cause hemochromatosis, a condition characterized by the formation of iron deposits throughout the body (e.g., in the liver, pancreas, heart, joints,

Approximately 20 to 30 percent of alcohol misusers acquire up to twice the amount of dietary iron as normal persons. These iron-loaded individuals are at increased risk for the same pathogens as those persons with hemochromatosis.

—"Alcohol: How Much Is Safe?" idInsight Magazine, *Third Quarter, 2000* anterior pituitary, and gonads). Moreover, patients whose chronic alcohol consumption and hemochromatosis have led to liver cirrhosis are at increased risk for liver cancer.

"If cirrhosis is present at the time of diagnosis of hemochromatosis, the chance of developing liver cancer is increased 50–200-fold."

—Herbert L. Bonkovsky, MD, Chair, Iron Disorders Institute
Medical & Scientific Advisory Board; Vice President for Research,
Director of Research, the Liver Center, Carolinas Health Care System;
Professor, University of North Carolina; Professor, University of Connecticut

Alcohol's effects on the bone marrow and on RBC production

Alcohol is the most commonly used drug whose consequences include the suppression of blood cell production, or hematopoiesis. Because its toxic effects are dose dependent, however, significantly impaired hematopoiesis usually occurs only in people with severe alcoholism, who also may suffer from nutritional deficiencies of folic acid and other vitamins that play a role in blood cell development. Chronic excessive alcohol ingestion reduces the number of blood cell precursors in the bone marrow and causes characteristic structural abnormalities in these cells, resulting in fewer-than-normal or nonfunctional mature blood cells. As a result, alcoholics may suffer from moderate anemia, characterized by enlarged, structurally abnormal RBCs; mildly reduced numbers of WBCs, especially of neutrophils; and moderately to severely reduced numbers of platelets. Although this generalized reduction in blood cell numbers (i.e., pancytopenia) usually is not progressive or fatal and is reversible with abstinence, complex aberrations of hematopoiesis can develop over time that may cause death.

Many bone marrow abnormalities occurring in severe alcoholics affect the RBC precursor cells. These abnormalities most prominently include precursors containing fluid-filled cavities (i.e., vacuoles) or characteristic iron deposits.

Development of vacuoles in RBC precursors

The most striking indication of alcohol's toxic effects on bone marrow cells is the appearance of numerous large vacuoles in early RBC precursor cells. It is unknown whether these vacuoles affect the cell's function and thus the drinker's health; however, their appearance generally is considered an indicator of excessive alcohol consumption. The vacuoles usually appear in the pronormoblasts five to seven days following the initiation of heavy alcohol consumption. Moreover, the vacuoles on average disappear after three to seven days of abstinence, although in some patients they persist for up to two weeks.

To a lesser extent, vacuoles also develop in the granulocyte precursors of alcoholics. This finding is not specifically alcohol-related, however, because other events that interfere with WBC production (e.g., infections) may induce similar structural changes in the granulocyte precursors.

The precise mechanism underlying vacuole development in blood cell precursors currently is unknown. Microscopic analyses of early blood cell precursors grown in tissue culture suggest that when the cells are exposed to a wide range of alcohol concentrations, the membrane surrounding each cell is damaged. These alterations in membrane structure may play an influential role in vacuole formation.

Less commonly, vacuole development in pronormoblasts also can occur after treatment with the antibiotic chloramphenicol. The two conditions can easily be distinguished, however, because in contrast to the alcohol-induced vacuolation, chloramphenicol-induced vacuolation is accompanied by the disappearance of virtually all later RBC precursors.

Sideroblastic anemia

One component of RBCs is hemoglobin, an iron-containing substance that is essential for oxygen transport. Sometimes, however, the iron is not incorporated properly into the hemoglobin molecules. Instead, it is converted into a storage form called ferritin, which can accumulate in RBC precursors, often forming granules that encircle the cell's nucleus. These ferritin-containing cells, which are called ringed sideroblasts, cannot mature further into functional RBCs. As a result, the number of RBCs in the blood declines and patients develop anemia. Many patients also have some circulating RBCs that contain ferritin granules called Pappenheimer bodies. The presence of these cells in the blood serves as an indicator of sideroblastic anemia and can prompt the physician to perform a bone marrow examination to confirm the diagnosis.

Sideroblastic anemia is a common complication in severe alcoholics: Approximately one-third of these patients contain ringed sideroblasts in their bone marrow. Alcohol may cause sideroblastic anemia by interfering with the activity of an enzyme that mediates a critical step in hemoglobin synthesis. Abstinence can reverse this effect. The ringed sideroblasts generally disappear from the bone marrow within five to ten days, and RBC production resumes. In fact, excess numbers of young RBCs called reticulocytes can accumulate temporarily in the blood, indicating higher-than-normal RBC production.

Megaloblastic anemia

Blood cell precursors require folic acid and other B vitamins for their continued production. Under conditions of folic acid deficiency, precursor cells cannot divide properly and large immature and nonfunctional cells (i.e., megaloblasts) accumulate in the bone marrow as well as in the bloodstream. This impaired hematopoiesis affects mainly RBCs, but also WBCs and platelets. The resulting deficiency in RBCs, WBCs, and platelets (i.e., pancytopenia) has numerous adverse consequences for the patient, including weakness and pallor from anemia, infections resulting from reduced neutrophil numbers, and bleeding as a result of the lack of platelets.

Megaloblasts occur frequently in the bone marrow of alcoholics; they are particularly common among alcoholics with symptoms of anemia, affecting up to one-third of these patients. These alcoholics generally also have reduced folic acid levels in their RBCs. The most common cause of this deficiency is a diet poor in folic acid, a frequent complication in alcoholics, who often have poor nutritional habits. In addition, alcohol ingestion itself may accelerate the development of folic acid deficiency by altering the absorption of folic acid from food.

Alcohol-related RBC disorders

Alcohol-related abnormalities in RBC production manifest themselves not only in the bone marrow but also through the presence of defective RBCs in the blood. For example, grossly enlarged RBCs can occur in the blood, a condition called macrocytosis, as well as oddly shaped RBCs that are subject to premature or accelerated destruction (i.e., hemolysis) because of their structural abnormalities. As a result, alcoholics frequently are diagnosed with anemia.

Macrocytosis

The routine examination of blood samples from alcoholic and nonalcoholic patients using automated blood cell counters has resulted in the identification of many people in whom the average size of individual RBCs, the mean corpuscular volume (MCV), is significantly larger than normal. However, an increased MCV does not automatically lead to a diagnosis of macrocytosis. For example, cells with an increased MCV can be found in patients with folic acid or vitamin B_{12} deficiency (as in the case of megaloblastic anemia) or with chronic liver disease. Moreover, the presence of enlarged RBCs in the blood can be indicative of a variety of disorders in addition to alcoholism, including different kinds of anemia and a dysfunction of the thyroid gland. To establish a diagnosis of macrocytosis, the physician must examine the blood cells under a microscope to identify structural features characteristic for each disorder. Thus, the enlarged RBCs in patients with macrocytosis generally are uniformly round, in contrast to the more oval cells characteristic of megaloblastic anemia. In addition, a diagnosis of macrocytosis resulting from alcohol requires that the physician investigate all potential causes of RBC enlargement, including the patient's alcohol-consumption history.

People who drink excessive amounts of alcohol can develop macrocytosis even in the absence of other factors associated with RBC enlargement, such as alcoholic liver disease or folic acid deficiency. In fact, alcohol abuse is the disorder most commonly associated with macrocytosis. Up to 80 percent of men and 46 percent of women with macrocytosis are alcoholics. The precise mechanism underlying macrocytosis still is unknown. However, alcohol appears to interfere directly with RBC development, because the macrocytes disappear within two to four months of abstinence.

Hemolytic anemia

Hemolysis can be an underlying cause of anemia, and several types of hemolytic anemia may be caused by chronic heavy alcohol consumption. Two of these disorders are characterized by the presence of malformed RBCs—stomatocytes and spur cells, whereas one alcohol-related hemolytic anemia is caused by reduced phosphate levels in the blood (i.e., hypophosphatemia).

Diagnosing hemolysis in alcoholic patients is not easy because these patients frequently exhibit confounding conditions, such as alcohol withdrawal, abnormal folic acid levels, bleeding, or an enlarged spleen.

Stomatocyte hemolysis

Stomatocytes are RBCs with a defect in their membranes that causes the cells to assume a mouthlike—or stoma—shape when examined under a microscope. Stomatocytes have a shortened life span because they become trapped in the small capillaries of the spleen and are subsequently destroyed. In healthy people, stomatocytes account for less than 5 percent of the RBCs, whereas their number can be significantly higher in alcoholics. In fact, more than 25 percent of alcoholics exhibit an increased proportion of stomatocytes in the blood (i.e., stomatocytosis).

The exact mechanism by which alcohol causes the formation of stomatocytes still is unclear. Alcohol-related liver disease may play a role in the development of stomatocyte hemolysis, because all four of the binge-drinking alcoholics in whom stomatocytosis originally was iden-

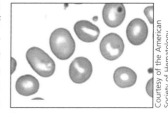

Stomatocytes

Courtesy of the American
Society of Hematology

tified also had some evidence of liver dysfunction. Alternatively, alcohol may directly affect the RBCs. This hypothesis is supported by the observation that in the four original patients, the stomatocytes disappeared during abstinence, but reappeared when alcohol consumption was resumed.

Spur-cell hemolysis

Spur cells are distorted RBCs that are characterized by spike-like protrusions of their cell membrane. These spurs are caused by the incorporation of excess amounts of cholesterol into the cell membrane, resulting in an increase of the cell's surface area without a corresponding increase in cell volume. Modestly elevated membrane cholesterol levels result in a flattened RBC shape, whereas larger increments of cholesterol cause the membrane to be thrown up into spikes. Spur cells may be prematurely eliminated in the spleen.

Spur-cell hemolysis occurs in about 3 percent of alcoholics with advanced liver disease, causing anemia that progresses relentlessly and is eventually fatal. Clinicians have tried unsuccessfully to treat the disorder using various agents with choles-

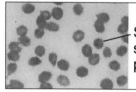

Spur cells have spike-like protrusions

Courtesy of the American Society of Hematology

terol-lowering properties. Consequently, surgical removal of the spleen is the only treatment capable of slowing the hemolytic process. However, most alcoholic patients with spur-cell hemolysis are not acceptable candidates for major abdominal surgery, because their coexisting advanced liver disease increases their risk of bleeding. Moreover, the procedure may precipitate liver failure.

Hypophosphatemia

Although hypophosphatemia-induced hemolysis is rare, its most common cause is alcoholism, especially during the withdrawal phase. Phosphate is an essential component of adenosine triphosphate (ATP), a compound that provides energy for many cellular processes. Alcohol causes phosphate to be excreted with the urine. Profound hypophosphatemia may cause the phosphate and ATP levels in the RBCs to decline substantially. This depletion of the store of ATP in the RBCs leads to increased rigidity of the RBC membranes, eventually damaging the cells. These damaged cells are prematurely destroyed in the spleen, and the patient may develop acute hemolytic anemia.

Alcohol's effects on WBCs

Since the 1920s, clinicians have noted an association between excessive alcohol ingestion and the development of infections. These observations suggest that alcohol interferes with the normal production and/or function of WBCs, which form the body's defense against microorganisms and other foreign substances. Because alcoholics commonly develop bacterial infections, much research has focused on alcohol's effects on neutrophils, the primary cell of defense against bacterial invasion. However, alcohol also impairs the function of monocytes and macrophages, which attack bacteria and other microorganisms, and of lymphocytes, which mediate the immune response. Alcohol-induced impairment of neutrophils and monocytes is discussed in the following sections.

Neutrophils

When a severe bacterial infection occurs, the body's response usually includes an increase in the number of WBCs—especially neutrophils—in the blood, a condition called leukocytosis. In contrast, alcoholics suffering from bacterial infections often exhibit a reduced number of neutrophils in the blood (neutropenia). For example, in a study of ten alcoholics with severe bacterial pneumonia or other bacterial infections, neutropenia was present in five patients when they were admitted to the hospital and developed in the other five patients within twenty-four to forty-eight hours (McFarland and Libre, 1963). The neutropenia was transient, however, and in several patients a rebound leukocytosis occurred between five and ten days after hospital admission.

The observed neutropenia may be related to impaired neutrophil development in the bone marrow. Thus, bone marrow analysis of alcoholic patients during the neutropenic stage demonstrated that virtually none of the neutrophil precursors had matured beyond an early developmental stage. Moreover, the neutrophil stores that are maintained in the bone marrow to allow a quick response to a bacterial infection were depleted more rapidly in active alcoholics than in healthy control subjects.

Alcohol consumption also interferes with the neutrophils'

ability to reach the site of an infection or inflammation (i.e., neutrophil delivery). When traveling to such a site, the neutrophils adhere to the walls of the blood vessels before migrating out of the blood vessels into the affected tissue. In tissue-culture experiments using nylon fibers to mimic this adherence, neutrophils could not adhere to the fibers if the blood samples were incubated with alcohol. This effect was more pronounced the higher the alcohol doses were. Neutrophils obtained from intoxicated volunteers had the same defect. The degree and duration of this adherence defect correlated with the inhibition of neutrophil delivery observed in the body. Moreover, drugs that corrected the adherence defect in tissue-culture experiments also improved neutrophil delivery in humans.

The function of neutrophils, including their adhesion ability, is regulated by hormonelike substances called leukotrienes. Thus, the impaired neutrophil functioning observed after alcohol treatment could be attributable to reduced leukotriene production or to the neutrophils' inability to respond to the leukotrienes. Some research results indicate that alcohol can interfere with leukotriene production.

In an effort to overcome or prevent the alcohol-induced impairment of the body's antibacterial defense, researchers have studied the effects of a growth factor called granulocyte-colony stimulating factor (G-CSF) in animal experiments. During normal neutrophil production in the bone marrow, G-CSF promotes the multiplication and functional activity of neutrophils. The studies found that G-CSF stimulated neutrophil recruitment specifically to the site of an infection and ameliorated the alcohol-induced impairment in the defense against bacterial infections.

Monocytes and macrophages
The monocyte-macrophage system, like neutrophils, constitutes an important line of defense against infections. Monocytes and macrophages clear invading microorganisms as well as foreign or defective proteins from the blood by engulfing and subsequently destroying them. Alcohol interferes with the function of the monocyte-macrophage system, with clinically significant consequences. For example, compared with healthy people,

alcoholics are less resistant to infections by microorganisms that normally are eradicated by monocytes and macrophages, such as the bacteria that cause tuberculosis and various forms of pneumonia. Similarly, studies of intoxicated laboratory animals demonstrated reduced elimination of bacteria by the monocyte-macrophage system. These effects generally appear to be temporary. Thus, in alcoholic patients whose monocyte-dependent elimination of a defective form of albumin (a protein normally present in the blood) is reduced at admission to a hospital, monocyte function generally returns to normal within one week of abstinence from alcohol. Further studies indicate that alcohol impairs monocyte-macrophage function rather than production. Thus, the cells frequently remain at their normal locations in the tissues rather than migrate to the sites of infections. In addition, alcohol inhibits the monocytes' adhesion abilities.

Alcohol's effects on the blood–clotting system

Blood clotting, or coagulation, an important physiological process that ensures the integrity of the vascular system, involves the platelets, or thrombocytes, as well as several proteins dissolved in the plasma. When a blood vessel is injured, platelets are attracted to the site of the injury, where they aggregate to form a temporary plug. The platelets secrete several proteins (i.e., clotting factors) that, together with other proteins either secreted by surrounding tissue cells or present in the blood, initiate a chain of events that results in the formation of fibrin. Fibrin is a stringy protein that forms a tight mesh in the injured vessel; blood cells become trapped in this mesh, thereby plugging the wound. Fibrin clots, in turn, can be dissolved by a process that helps prevent the development of thrombosis (i.e., fibrinolysis).

Alcohol can interfere with these processes at several levels, causing, for example, abnormally low platelet numbers in the blood (i.e., thrombocytopenia), impaired platelet function (i.e., thrombocytopathy), and diminished fibrinolysis. These effects can have serious medical consequences, such as an increased risk for strokes.

Platelets actually are not intact cells but disc-shaped cell fragments without nuclei that are released from giant precursor cells in the bone marrow called megakaryocytes.

Thrombocytopenia

Thrombocytopenia, an abnormal decrease in platelet count, is a frequent complication of alcoholism, affecting 3 to 43 percent of non–acutely ill, well-nourished alcoholics, and 14 to 81 percent of acutely ill, hospitalized alcoholics. Thus, apart from acquired immune deficiency syndrome (AIDS), alcoholism probably is the leading cause of thrombocytopenia. Except for the most severe cases, however, the patients generally do not exhibit manifestations of excessive bleeding. Moreover, alcohol-related thrombocytopenia generally is transient, and platelet counts usually return to normal within one week of abstinence. Therefore, patients generally require no therapeutic intervention other than that needed to ease alcohol withdrawal. Only in patients whose thrombocytopenia is severe and associated with excessive bleeding are platelet transfusions indicated.

In many patients with thrombocytopenia, rebounding platelet numbers even exceed normal values. This rebound thrombocytosis after cessation of alcohol consumption also occurs in the majority of patients whose platelet counts are normal at the time of hospitalization. In these patients, the extent of the excess in circulating platelets usually is higher than in patients presenting with thrombocytopenia.

The exact mechanisms underlying alcohol-related thrombocytopenia remain unknown. Some researchers have suggested that alcohol intoxication itself, rather than alcohol-related nutritional deficiencies, causes the decrease in platelet numbers. This view is supported by findings that thrombocytopenia developed in healthy subjects who received a diet containing adequate protein and vitamin levels (including large doses of folic acid) and consumed the equivalent of 1.5 pints (745 milliliters) of 86-proof whiskey for at least ten days (Lindenbaum, 1987). The subjects' platelet levels returned to normal when alcohol consumption was discontinued. Similarly, platelet counts can be reduced in well-nourished alcoholics who do not suffer from folic acid deficiency. The available data also suggest that alcohol can interfere with a late stage of platelet production as well as shorten the life span of existing platelets.

Failure of the platelet counts to rise after five to seven days of abstinence usually indicates the presence of another underlying disorder affecting the platelets. Individual drinkers appear to differ in their susceptibility to alcohol-induced thrombocytopenia. Thus, clinicians have noted that some people who consume alcohol in excess repeatedly develop thrombocytopenia (often severely), whereas other drinkers maintain normal platelet levels.

In addition to differences in the quantity of alcohol consumed, inherited or acquired variations in an individual drinker's biochemistry may account for these differences in susceptibility.

Thrombocytopathy

Alcohol affects not only platelet production but also platelet function. Thus, patients who consume excessive amounts of alcohol can exhibit a wide spectrum of platelet abnormalities when admitted to a hospital. These abnormalities include impaired platelet aggregation, decreased secretion or activity of platelet-derived proteins involved in blood clotting, and prolongation of bleeding in the absence of thrombocytopenia.

Because alcohol impairs the function of the normal blood-clotting system, it also can adversely interact with over-the-counter and prescription medications that prolong bleeding or prevent coagulation. For example, alcohol can potentiate the prolongation of bleeding time caused by aspirin and other nonsteroidal anti-inflammatory drugs (NSAIDs) (e.g., ibuprofen or indomethacin), particularly when alcohol ingestion equivalent to about four drinks occurs simultaneously with or following ingestion of normal doses of these medications. As a result, the concomitant use of alcohol and aspirin or NSAIDs greatly increases the patient's risk for gastrointestinal bleeding. Similarly, alcohol can enhance aspirin-induced fecal blood loss.

To prevent such adverse reactions, healthcare professionals should proactively counsel patients who regularly consume alcohol about the proper choice and safe use of aspirin and other over-the-counter NSAIDs. Alcohol also can interact with anticoagulants, prescription medications that prevent blood clotting and which are used to treat patients who are at increased risk of developing thrombosis or an embolism in the lung. One commonly used anticoagulant is warfarin. However, warfarin treatment is not indicated for alcoholic patients, because alcohol ingestion can significantly interfere with the proper management of warfarin maintenance therapy.

Fibrinolysis

The body's ability to prevent excessive bleeding using the coagulation system is balanced by the fibrinolytic system, which helps ensure blood flow in peripheral organs and tissues by dissolving inappropriate fibrin clots. Alcohol's effect on fibrinolysis is controversial. Whereas some older studies reported an increase in fibrinolytic activity after alcohol consumption, more recent, better controlled studies have demonstrated that alcohol diminishes fibrinolysis the day after alcohol ingestion or during prolonged alcohol consumption. These observations suggest that alcoholics may be at increased risk for thrombosis.

Fibrinolysis is controlled in part by the presence in the blood of two proteins: tissue plasminogen activator (TPA) and plasminogen activator inhibitor 1 (PAI-1). TPA promotes fibrinolysis, whereas PAI-1 reduces fibrinolytic activity. The activities of both proteins must be well balanced to maintain an adequate level of fibrinolysis. Alcohol can alter the activities of both TPA and PAI-1. Thus, moderate alcohol consumption stimulates TPA activity. Because increased TPA activity reduces the risk of inappropriate blood-clot formation, this alteration may have a beneficial, cardioprotective effect. Conversely, recent studies also have indicated that high levels of alcohol or its degradation product, acetaldehyde, could stimulate PAI-1 production and thereby suppress fibrinolysis.

Stroke

Alcohol-induced impairment of the blood-clotting and/or fibrinolytic systems can have serious medical consequences. Most significantly, clinical epidemiological data suggest that a recent bout of heavy drinking increases the drinker's risk of suffering a hemorrhagic or ischemic stroke. During a hemorrhagic stroke, the blood flow to a brain area is impaired due to a ruptured blood vessel that results in bleeding in the brain. If the blood flow is interrupted because a blood vessel is blocked by a blood clot, the condition is called an ischemic stroke. Alcohol conceivably can contribute to both conditions by interfering with the normal coagulation system and by reducing fibrinolysis, respectively.

Hematogical markers of alcoholism

An important focus of alcohol research is the search for biological markers that could be used in simple screening tests to identify people who are at risk for alcoholism or who already are chronic heavy drinkers. Two categories of biological markers exist: state markers, which reflect a person's alcohol consumption, and trait markers, which indicate a predisposition for alcoholism.

State markers fall into two main groups: screening markers and relapse markers. Screening markers, which detect chronic alcohol consumption, could complement information obtained from patients in the course of taking their medical history. This physical information could provide important diagnostic clues because, as clinical observations suggest, many people do not accurately report their level of alcohol consumption. Thus, screening markers could be useful in the early identification of alcoholism, especially in patients who consume alcohol in amounts that do not lead to acute medical problems but that could have long-term behavioral or medical consequences. In contrast, relapse markers, which are sensitive to acute alcohol consumption, could play an important role in monitoring recovering alcoholics and other heavy drinkers. State markers that would permit the identification of heavy drinkers even when alcohol is no longer present in the blood would be particularly valuable diagnostic tools.

Trait markers could help identify people at risk for alcoholism who could benefit most from early, targeted prevention and intervention approaches. These high-risk populations most prominently include first-degree relatives of alcoholics. Trait markers also could provide important research tools for evaluating the genetic and environmental factors that may pre-dispose a person to alcoholism.

State markers

Chronic ingestion of large quantities of alcohol alters many physiological and biological processes and compounds, includ-ing several blood-related (i.e., hematological) variables. Because blood samples are relatively easy to obtain, structural and func-tional changes in circulating blood cells and plasma proteins potentially can form the basis of laboratory tests for screening, diagnosing, and monitoring alcoholism. Two hematological state markers commonly used for these purposes are the pres-ence of carbohydrate-deficient transferrin (CDT) in the blood and an increase in the size of red blood cells (RBCs), as mea-sured by the mean corpuscular volume (MCV).

Carbohydrate-deficient transferrin (CDT)

CDT is one of the newest, and perhaps the most promising, of the hematological state markers. Transferrin is an iron-containing protein in the plasma that transports iron, which is stored at various sites in the body, to the developing RBCs in the bone marrow for incorporation into hemoglobin. Transferrin molecules in the blood usually contain several car-bohydrate components. In chronic heavy drinkers, however, the number of carbohydrate components in each transferrin molecule is reduced, resulting in CDT. The mechanism underly-ing this alteration still is unclear.

Because elevated CDT levels in the blood appear to be a spe-cific consequence of excessive alcohol consumption, a recent study investigated the utility of repeatedly monitoring serum CDT to detect relapse among recovering alcoholics. The study found that in most of the subjects who relapsed, the elevation of CDT levels preceded self-reported alcohol consumption by at least 28 days. These findings suggest that repeated testing of alcoholic patients for CDT permits early relapse detection and thus may lead to early intervention. Early intervention, in turn, may decrease the need to rehospitalize patients for alcohol withdrawal and prevent some of the complications associated with sustained excessive drinking.

Mean corpuscular volume (MCV)

The MCV is elevated in approximately 50 to 60 percent of people who chronically ingest excessive alcohol quantities. With the advent of automated instruments that determine the MCV during routine blood counts, physicians and other healthcare providers frequently detect elevated MCVs in patients who are well nourished and who have no obvious disorders to explain this finding. In these patients, a moderately increased MCV may be a clue to unsuspected alcoholism. Analysis of blood smears can support this diagnosis: In patients with an alcohol-related increase in MCV, the enlarged RBCs are round and of uniform size. Conversely, in patients with certain types of anemia that result in an increased MCV, the RBCs typically are oval and of variable size. Because the MCV usually returns to normal within two to four months of abstinence, the increase in RBC size apparently is a direct effect of alcohol on RBC production.

Trait markers

Researchers have proposed numerous genetic and genetically determined biochemical characteristics that might potentially serve as trait markers of alcoholism. Because of the easy availability of blood samples, many research efforts have focused on biochemical markers that can be found in circulating blood platelets. These studies have identified two enzymes that appear to be viable markers of alcoholism and whose activities can be measured in isolated platelets: monoamine oxidase (MAO) and adenylyl cyclase (AC).

Monoamine oxidase

MAO is an enzyme that breaks down certain neurotransmitters (e.g., dopamine and serotonin) that have been implicated in mediating various phenomena related to the risk of developing alcoholism (e.g., tolerance to alcohol's effects). Although MAO acts primarily in the brain, platelets also contain the enzyme. MAO activity levels are genetically determined, and many studies have demonstrated that people with a certain alcoholism subtype or with particular psychiatric disorders (e.g., schizophrenia and mood disorders) exhibit abnormally low MAO activity levels. In fact, low MAO activity in the platelets and other tissues of certain alcoholics is the most replicated biological finding in genetic alcoholism research. The available data also suggest that low MAO activity in the platelets predicts a risk for alcoholism in relatives of a certain type of alcoholic. This alcoholism subtype is characterized by an early age of onset of alcohol-related problems, frequent social and legal consequences of drinking, and a strong genetic predisposition.

Adenylyl cyclase (AC)

AC is an enzyme that plays a role in the transmission of signals from a cell's exterior to its interior; the enzyme's levels in the body are genetically determined. Several studies have found that AC levels in the platelets as well as in some white blood cells are frequently reduced in alcoholics compared with nonalcoholics, even after long periods of abstinence. Because a single gene appears to determine the level of platelet AC activity, it is likely that low platelet AC activity is an inherited trait in many alcoholics and therefore could be used as a trait marker. Recent studies indicate, however, that the gene responsible for low AC levels does not actually cause alcoholism, but may increase the risk of developing the disease.

Numerous clinical observations support the notion that alcohol adversely affects the production and function of virtually all types of blood cells. Thus, alcohol is directly toxic to the bone marrow, which contains the precursors of all blood cells, as well as to the mature cells circulating in the bloodstream. Moreover, long-term excessive alcohol consumption can interfere with various physiological, biochemical, and metabolic processes involving the blood cells. The medical consequences of these adverse effects can be severe. They include anemia, which in severe cases can have debilitating effects; an increased risk of serious bacterial infections; and impaired blood clotting and fibrinolysis, which can cause excessive bleeding and place the drinker at increased risk of strokes. These direct effects may be exacerbated by the presence of other alcohol-related disorders, such as liver disease and nutritional deficiencies. Abstinence can reverse many of alcohol's effects on hematopoiesis and blood cell functioning.

Treatment for alcohol-related anemia

Treatment for anemia associated with alcohol abuse will vary depending upon the extent of organ damage, iron levels, and whether or not the individual has stopped consuming alcohol. The attending physician may use a combination of iron replacement therapies.

Content in this publication is not intended to be a substitute for professional medical advice, nor is it intended to replace the services of a medical professional or impair the patient– healthcare provider or caregiver relationship. Content in this publication should be used as information only and be discussed with a medical professional who is qualified to diagnose and treat your condition. Iron Disorders Institute, all contributors, and the publisher of this book are not responsible for the content on websites listed in the resources, nor do we endorse products promoted on such sites. We advise you to always seek the advice of a qualified health provider before making any changes to diet, supplementation, or starting any new treatment. Any application of the information or recommendations in this book is made at the reader's discretion.

We appreciate the contribution of this important chapter, extracted with permission from Alcohol Health & Research, *a NIAAA publication. Dr. H. S. Ballard, author of the article, is the associate chief of hematology and oncology at the New York Department of Veterans Affairs Medical Center, New York, New York. Susanne Hiller-Sturmhofel is a science editor of* Alcohol Health & Research.

Resources

We encourage physicians to request *The Physicians' Guide to Helping Patients with Alcohol Problems*, a free publication published by The National Institute on Alcohol Abuse and Alcoholism. A copy may be obtained by writing to:

The National Institute on Alcohol Abuse and Alcoholism
Publication Distribution Center
P.O. Box 10686
Rockville, MD 20849-0686
Fax a request to: 202-842-0418
Also, the full text is available online: www.niaaa.nih.gov

16

Cancer

"Anemia may be a major factor in cancer-related fatigue and quality of life in cancer patients."

—*Vogelzang et al., "Fatigue Coalition,"* Seminars in Hematology, *1997*

In 1997, Edward "Eddie" Leigh went to his doctor because of abdominal pains, diarrhea, and mild fatigue. He thought he had a case of the stomach flu. He certainly didn't think he had something as serious as cancer, since most of his relatives with cancer were diagnosed in their seventies. Eddie was only thirty-nine and the epitome of good health. He ate nutritiously, didn't drink, didn't smoke, exercised regularly, and had a positive attitude. His family doctor dismissed him without a single test. The diagnosis was "too much stress," which Eddie found ironic since he helps people cope with stress through his work as a motivational speaker.

Months passed; the abdominal pain intensified. This time the physician recommended a sigmoidoscopy, which was normal. What was not known at the time was that Eddie had a serious tumor growing in the right (ascending) portion of his colon—a section that a sigmoidoscopy cannot reach. A colonoscopy, which views the entire colon, would have found the tumor. He was diagnosed with irritable bowel syndrome.

Eddie continued to work, coping with the pain until he experienced rectal bleeding so severe that he was admitted to the hospital. This time the focus of attention centered on a coincidental discovery of food poisoning and rested there—no further tests were done to investigate the rectal bleeding.

Two months later the rectal bleeding recurred. Symptoms of diarrhea, nausea, abdominal pain, and fatigue persisted. The diagnosis this time was hemorrhoids. No tests were done. Six months later the rectal bleeding was so severe that Eddie passed out; when he became conscious, he was lying in a pool of his own blood. The doctor recommended another sigmoidoscopy.

Eddie never had the second sigmoidoscopy, since he was in the process of switching insurance companies. An additional sigmoidoscopy would have been normal once again, since the cancer was on the right side of the colon. Incidentally, he was switching insurance carriers to get a better coverage, not because of the family doctor. Eddie felt confident that the doctor was giving him accurate information about his condition.

One month after the change in insurance, and nearly two years since his initial doctor visit Eddie saw a new physician. The abdominal pain had become excruciating and the symptoms of diarrhea, nausea, and fatigue were still present. This doctor performed a simple blood test, a CBC (complete blood count) and found that Eddie was anemic (his hemoglobin was 10.2 g/dL—a normal hemoglobin range for a healthy male is 13.8–17.2 g/dL). An immediate colonoscopy was performed. Eddie still did not consider cancer a possibility; he thought he had a bleeding ulcer.

The colonoscopy revealed a large tumor on the right portion of the colon. Soon after, Eddie had surgery to remove one-third of his colon. The pathology report revealed two of seventeen lymph nodes removed were malignant, which classified his colon cancer as stage III.

Eddie began chemotherapy within a month of surgery, and continued chemo for a year. During this treatment he battled side effects, which included nausea, fatigue, anemia, low white blood cell counts, loss of appetite, and "the runs." His oncologist watched his numbers carefully and discussed with Eddie a conservative treatment to address the anemia, which persisted because of the chemotherapy. She suggested that a daily multivitamin with iron and iron-rich foods be the first line of therapy. Eddie agreed, appreciating her conservative approach.

Three years post diagnosis, Eddie has no sign of cancer. He has an abdominal scan every six months, and a CBC and liver panel every three months along with a physical to check his weight, blood pressure, heart rate, and lungs. He also has a colonoscopy every year.

Eddie shares his message of survival, hope, joy, and optimism with others. On the *Today Show*, known colon cancer prevention advocate Katie Couric asked Eddie what advice he would give the viewers. Eddie replied, "Having a sigmoidoscopy is like having a mammogram and examining only one breast." His comment has had a powerful impact on millions of people who can now relate to the importance of examining the entire colon, which the colonoscopy provides.

Eddie's cancer may have been caught at an earlier stage (before the lymph metastases) if years earlier a simple blood test and full scope had been done. Still, he maintains his positive attitude; instead of using his energy to blame the first doctor, he uses his experiences to help others. Today he will tell you that anemia saved his life; he credits his present physician with the wisdom to perform a simple blood test, the CBC, and to follow up with a colonoscopy.

Edward Leigh has a master's degree in health education; he is a motivational speaker who travels throughout the world sharing his message of prevention, hope, and humor. He even has been able to find humor in his struggle with cancer. Since he had one-third of his colon removed, he refers to himself as a "semicolon." If you would like more information about Edward Leigh, go to www.EdwardLeigh.com or call him at 800-677-3256. Update as of 2008: Eddie has campaigned heavily to promote disease prevention. Most recently Montel Williams featured Eddie on his show. A clip of the show is available through Internet sites such as YouTube®.

Cancer explained

The word *cancer* is derived from the Latin word for "crab." A tumor is a cluster of cancer cells, and it grows in planes of least resistance in the silhouette of a crab. Nearly every type of living cell in the human body may be susceptible to uncontrolled growth or cancer, such that approximately 200 distinct varieties of cancers are known. The biggest risk factor for developing cancer is aging. The longer one lives the more likely one is to develop some form of cancer. In the United States it is expected that one of every two men and one of every three women will develop some form of cancer. Although most of the 200 varieties of cancer are rare, deaths due to cancer are attributable to only a few common cancers such as lung, breast, colon, skin, and blood cancers. Some types of cancer are preventable. Some types of cancer are

Cancer Cancer Cancer		
TYPES	**Organ affected**	
Carcinomas	Liver	Breast
	Skin	Uterus
	Lung	Ovary
	Glands	Testes
	Bladder	Colon
	Kidney	Brain
Sarcoma	Bone	Fibrous tissue
	Muscle	Fat
	Cartilage	
Lymphomas	Lymphatic System	
Leukemia	Blood or Blood forming organs	

caused by environmental factors and some are caused by genetic factors. Early detection combined with a healthy lifestyle, limited sun exposure, and cessation from smoking are several ways to reduce the chances of developing cancer.

Several factors determine how cancer is defined, diagnosed, and treated, including where the cancer originates and how the cancer cells appear under the microscope. All cancers, however, fall into one of four broad categories: carcinoma, sarcoma, leukemia, and lymphomas. When cancers affect the blood or blood-forming organs, they are called myeloid; when the cancer involves other tissues that do not directly affect the formation of blood cells, they are referred to as nonmyeloid. These distinctions are critical to therapy and the treatment of anemia that accompanies the various forms of cancer.

Cancers are defined by the tissue where the abnormal cell growth originates. For example, a person might have breast cancer because the disease is believed to have begun in the tissues of the breast, even though the cancer may have spread to other organs such as the lung. This patient would be diagnosed with primary breast cancer with lung metastases.

Different types of cancers are defined by the organ of the body involved. Carcinomas originate in the liver, lungs, glands (i.e., prostate or thyroid glands), bladder, kidney, breast, ovary, uterus, testes, colon, skin, and brain. Sarcomas originate in bone, muscle, cartilage, and fibrous tissue (i.e., connective tissue or fat). Leukemia originates in the bone marrow; myeloma is a subset of leukemia and is a cancer of plasma cells (i.e., type of B cell responsible for producing antibodies). Lymphomas originate in the lymphatic system.

Approximately 80 percent of all cancer cases are carcinomas. Sarcomas are rare, representing only about 1 percent of all cancers and are usually seen in the pediatric population. Most cancers are considered sporadic, meaning that no clear cause can be attributed. Congenital or hereditary cancers can be passed from a parent to a child, but this does not mean that the child will develop the cancer. The presence of the gene variation responsible for several cancers, breast or ovarian cancer and other suspect gene variations, place the individual who inherits them at increased risk for that type of cancer. Screening family members can provide the benefit of early detection, where preventive measures can be taken to reduce the risk of cancer development.

Leukemia, lymphoma, and myeloma are from an acquired (not inherited) genetic injury to the DNA of a single cell, which becomes abnormal (malignant) and multiplies continuously. The accumulation of malignant cells interferes with the body's production of healthy blood cells and makes the body unable to protect itself against infections.

Diagnosis of cancer

Cancers are diagnosed in various ways, again depending upon the primary source of the cancer. Often used is the biopsy, which involves surgically obtaining a small tissue sample that is examined under a microscope. A biopsy can be done of all tissues, including the bone marrow. The biopsy helps to identify the primary cancer. Another diagnostic tool is the endoscope, which can examine major organs and the entire digestive system. Radiographs (i.e., X rays), ultrasound, computed axial tomography (CAT) scan, positron-emission tomography (PET) scan, and magnetic resonance imaging (MRI) are other ways that tumors can be detected. Additionally, blood tests may help to diagnose the cancers. Some tumors release substances called tumor markers, which can be detected in the blood. For example, a blood test for prostate cancer measures the amount of prostate specific antigen (PSA). Higher-than-normal concentrations of PSA may indicate cancer. Recently, a blood test for ovarian cancer, known as CA-125, has become available. Blood tests by themselves, however, are inconclusive. Use of simple screening aids such as an occult blood test or chest radiograph with a patient's family history of disease or symptoms adds to the overall picture that may assist in the prompt detection and diagnosis of cancer.

Early detection can lead to a better cure rate whereby the person can be expected to have a normal life expectancy as if he or she had never had cancer. Once cancer has become metastatic and the disease has spread to other organs, the cure rate can be dramatically less optimistic.

"In addition to the mechanisms associated with the anemia of chronic disorders, anemia in cancer patients may result from marrow replacement by tumor or tumor-induced fibrosis, or from the effects of therapy, which include marrow toxicity, renal toxicity (impairing erythropoietin production), and poor nutrition."

—*Robert T. Means, Jr., MD; University of Kentucky College of Medicine, Department of Internal Medicine, Hematology/Oncology; Member, Iron Disorders Institute Medical & Scientific Advisory Board*

Symptoms of cancer

Symptoms can be silent, particularly in the early stages of development. Some symptoms are specific to certain types of cancer, such as difficult urination for prostate cancer, or flu-like symptoms and easy bruising for acute leukemias. Sudden weight loss, a thickening or lump, unexplained bleeding, coughing, or a wound that will not heal are some of the many symptoms related to cancer. Many times symptoms are non-specific, that is, common to many other conditions. Anemia is a good example; often, the discovery of anemia can prompt the early diagnosis of cancer.

Anemia in cancer patients can be due to blood loss, hemolysis, bone marrow suppression due to chemotherapy, renal toxicity resulting in reduced production of erythropoietin, infiltration of the bone marrow by the malignancy itself, or inflammation, otherwise called anemia of chronic disease.

Anemia of chronic disease (ACD)

ACD is one of the most common syndromes in clinical medicine. Patients with ACD have anemia characterized by inadequate iron concentration in the blood, although they have adequate iron stores in the body. Typically, ACD occurs in patients with chronic infectious, inflammatory, or neoplastic diseases, although 40 percent of patients have no known cause for their anemia. The pathogenesis of ACD is characterized by both a blunting of the native erythropoietin response to anemia, and a relative resistance to therapeutic erythropoietin (i.e., Epogen® or Procrit®). Although most patients with ACD have only a moderate degree of anemia, approximately 25 percent of patients are sufficiently anemic to potentially require transfusion.

Anemia due to blood loss or surgery

Iron, folate, B_{12}, and zinc are nutrients that are essential to red blood cell production. Patients with cancer may be deficient in stores of these nutrients because of malnutrition, surgery, or bleeding. Tumors, whether malignant or benign, require a great deal of blood to grow. In some cases the tumors can be growing significantly but no sign of blood loss is detected in fecal samples. The anemia is confirmed with blood tests such as hemoglobin and serum ferritin, but the confirmation of the tumor requires more extensive investigation with endoscopy, radiograph, CAT scan, or MRI. Significant blood loss can occur in the advanced stage of the disease, especially in cancers of the lung, esophagus, stomach, colon, rectum, ovaries or uterus, liver, kidney, or bladder, as the tumor invades and destroys healthy tissues and blood vessels.

Patients who have had surgery to treat cancers of the stomach and small intestine are especially at risk for nutritional deficiencies. The stomach produces HCl, which is an acid that helps digest food, particularly proteins. When stomach acid is inadequate (hypochlorhydria), food is not well digested and is excreted. Surgical removal of large portions of the stomach can result in hypochlorhydria. Nutrients released by stomach acid are then absorbed in the upper portion of the small intestine called the duodenum. Vitamin B_{12} continues to be absorbed in the ileum, which is the lower end of the small intestine. Some investigators believe that there is a secondary site for the absorption of iron and other nutrients lower in the small intestine in the jejunum and the ileum. Therefore the surgical removal of other sections of the small intestine may also contribute to poor absorption.

When the nutrient deficiencies are due to blood loss, the source of blood loss must be identified and corrected. Blood transfusion may be required short term. Thereafter, when hemoglobin concentrations improve, diets that include red meat, which is rich in iron, zinc, and vitamin B_{12}, and other foods that are high in folate, vitamins C, A, and E, and beta-carotene may improve hemoglobin concentrations within a few weeks, if other causes of anemia also are eliminated. Some physicians will recommend oral supplements of iron and folic acid (synthetic form of folate). When the nutrient deficiency is due to surgical removal of absorption sites, replacement of these nutrients can be achieved by intravenous iron, B_{12} injection, or total parenteral nutrition (TPN). TPN is a technique used to feed a person intravenously, replacing the normal eating and digestion process.

Anemia due to hemolysis

Hemolysis is the destruction of red blood cells and is a normal part of the blood cell cycle. Premature hemolysis is not normal and can occur when red blood cells are damaged or an immune response is mounted against red blood cells. Hemolytic anemia can be caused by chemotherapy drugs, an immune response to infection, transfused blood, or bone marrow transplantation.

Anemia due to invasion or suppression of bone marrow

Red blood cells are formed in the bone marrow. When cancer invades the bone marrow, blood cell production is diminished or stopped completely. Marrow activity can also be affected by chemotherapy. Chemotherapy drugs cannot differentiate between cancer cells and the cells of healthy tissue, including bone marrow. With too few red blood cells to circulate in the blood, inadequate oxygen concentrations may cause the patient to feel weak and fatigued.

Managing anemia

The management of anemia in cancer patients will depend upon the cause of anemia and the type of cancer. For example, anemia of chronic disease or inflammatory response (ACD) may be corrected when the underlying cause of inflammation or infection is cured. Iron-deficiency anemia can often be corrected with diet or oral supplementation. Anemia due to acute blood loss can be corrected with blood transfusion while investigation to determine the source of blood loss is pursued.

Further need for transfusions depends on the type of blood disease in question and the type of drugs used in the chemotherapy. For example, almost all patients with leukemia (a disease primarily affecting the bone marrow and blood) require some transfusions during their care. Many patients with Hodgkin's or non-Hodgkin's lymphoma (diseases primarily affecting the lymph nodes and spleen) may not require transfusions unless they require a marrow or blood stem cell transplant or if the lymphoma involves the marrow.

Anemia due to bone marrow failure or chemotherapy can be improved with products such as epoetin alfa. Epoetin alfa is sold under the brand names of Epogen® brand marketed by Amgen; and Procrit® marketed by Ortho Biotech (Raritan, NJ). Darbepoetin alfa, trade name Aranesp® (manufactured by Amgen), is another product that is approved for use in patients with chemotherapy-induced anemia. Darbepoetin alfa, like epoetin alfa, stimulates the production of red blood cells and can be administered either as a subcutaneous injection or an intravenous infusion. Darbepoetin alfa has a threefold longer half-life in the blood than epoetin alfa, which means that it does not need to be injected as often as epoetin alfa.

For leukemia patients, products such as Procrit®, Epogen®, and Aranesp® are of benefit if the anemia is due to chemotherapy, although some researchers believe that ACD associated with cancer in general may benefit from these products.

There has recently (2006–2008) been controversy about how best to use erythropoietin agents in patients with cancer. This resulted from studies suggesting that certain groups of cancer patients receiving rHuEPO products had shorter survival than comparable patients not receiving these products. Interpretation of these studies is complicated by a variety of factors, such as the degree to which anemia was to be corrected, the point at which rHuEPO therapy was started, and specific patient characteristics. Physicians considering rHuEPO therapy for their patients should review the most current guidelines, and discuss the risks and benefits with the patient.

Chemotherapy–induced neutropenia and thrombocytopenia

Chemotherapy not only destroys red blood cells and the bone marrow's ability to make more; it also destroys white blood cells and platelets. Granulocyte-colony stimulating factor (G-CSF) and granulocyte macrophage-colony stimulating factor (GM-CSF) are two endogenous proteins that act on bone marrow to produce white blood cells. White blood cells are necessary to help prevent infections. Recombinant human G-CSF is marketed in the United States as Neupogen® or as the extended-release form Neulasta® (both manufactured and distributed by Amgen). Recombinant human GM-CSF is marketed in the United States as Leukine® (Immunex).

Platelets are important blood cells that aid in the clotting of blood, and these cells and their progenitors may be destroyed by some forms of chemotherapy. One product, a recombinant human interleukin, Neumega® (Wyeth) is approved for use in patients with chemotherapy-induced thrombocytopenia (low platelet count).

Taking action: prevention is key

Early detection of cancer is key to survival. With the major advances in cancer and cancer treatment, many cancers are treatable if detected early. Routine physical exams and screening procedures such as the colonoscopy, mammogram, pap smear, and lung X ray along with specific blood tests are among the ways cancer can be detected before disease advances. Not smoking, cutting back on fatty, processed, and high-sugar foods, and drinking only in moderation are choices that not only lower one's risk for cancer but may provide other health benefits as well.

Knowing one's iron levels can also be beneficial in the prevention of cancer. Serum ferritin will rise in the presence of tumor development and might be a helpful test to add during an annual physical for adults.

Finally, reading and becoming knowledgeable about one's condition is also very important. Most physicians today appreciate a well-informed patient and often can benefit from the efforts of such patients.

Resources
For more information about myeloid cancers, such as leukemia, lymphoma, and myeloma, regarding incidence and treatment, including bone marrow transplantation, contact:

The Leukemia & Lymphoma Society
1311 Mamaroneck Ave.
White Plains, NY 10605
Information Resource Center: 800-955-4572
www.leukemia-lymphoma.org

There are a number of excellent cancer treatment facilities. The following centers were helpful in compiling this particular chapter:

The University of Texas M. D. Anderson Cancer Center

1515 Holcombe Blvd, Houston, TX 77030
800-392-1611 (USA) / 713-792-6161
www.mdanderson.org

The Hollings Cancer Center

Medical University of South Carolina, Charleston
86 Jonathan Lucas St.
Charleston, SC 29425
Tel: 843-792-9300
Fax: 843-792-1407
http://hcc.musc.edu

The following websites provide hundreds of links to various Web-based cancer-information sites:

Colon Cancer Network

www.colorectal-cancer.net

The Cancer Research and Prevention Foundation

www.preventcancer.org

Association of Cancer Online Resources

www.acor.org

Colon Cancer Alliance

www.ccalliance.org

For more information about familial adenomatous polyposis (FAP):

IMPACC (Intestinal Multiple Polyposis and Colorectal Cancer)

P.O. Box 11
Conyngham, PA 18219
Contact: Mrs. Ann Fagan, Administrator
Tel: 570-788-1818
Fax: 570-788-4046

The National Cancer Institute
NCI Public Inquiries Office
Suite 3036A
6116 Executive Boulevard, MSC8322
Bethesda, MD 20892-8322
In the United States and its territories, call 800-4-CANCER
(800-422-6237)

17

Celiac Sprue

"Iron-deficiency anemia is the most common clinical presentation in adults with celiac sprue."

—R. J. Farrell and C. P. Kelly, New England Journal of Medicine, 2002

At a blood drive where she worked, forty-nine-year-old Lucile Parker had been turned away from donating blood because she was anemic. She had been diagnosed with anemia before and periodically took iron pills except when bouts of diarrhea would flare up. Additionally, each day she took a daily vitamin and an extra 400 milligrams of calcium with magnesium and vitamin D. She had been told by her gynecologist that she needed calcium for a bone condition, but she could not remember what it was called, "osteo-something."

Her family doctor confirmed that she had iron-deficiency anemia with blood work. Her hemoglobin was 9.7 g/dL and her serum ferritin was 11.0 ng/mL. During the examination Lucile talked about her fatigue, especially in the late afternoons and evenings and bouts of diarrhea, grumbling noises in her gut and her "paunch," which was how she described her bloated abdomen. The doctor noted that her abdomen was slightly distended. He referred Lucile to a gastroenterologist and told her to continue taking the iron pills and her calcium supplement.

Lucile decided not to see the gastroenterologist. She assumed her diagnosis was iron-deficiency anemia and that the iron pills would take care of her problem. Two months later she was hit with a terrible bout of diarrhea. The problem persisted for four days and was so severe that she had to call in sick to work.

After a week at home alone, she called her older brother who came by to check on her. He thought she looked terribly pale and thin. Since she refused food, he urged her to take some Pedialyte and a teaspoon of liquid trace minerals in a glass of juice. She was embarrassed to talk about the diarrhea, but because her brother stayed for several hours he was able to figure out what was happening.

He reminded Lucile that as a baby she was hospitalized for severe feeding problems and diarrhea; he told her that she almost died. After nearly two months in the hospital and a special diet, she had been allowed to go home. He remembered that she'd had to remain on the special diet, which was wheat-free, he thought, for several years. He reminded his sister of how excited she had been when the doctor told her that she could go off the special diet, when she was about seven. It was cause for celebration, because the diet had been a real pain— she hadn't been allowed to eat pizza, breads, and cereals like the rest of the family.

Her brother's story triggered a memory for Lucile of a trip to the doctor as a teenager. Her mom had taken her to the doctor because of the severe cramps, diarrhea, and weight loss. The doctor suspected that Lucile was bulimic or anorexic, but this was not the case. She was anemic according to her blood work. Her mother told the doctor that Lucile had often been anemic; she also told him about Lucile being hospitalized as a child and the gluten-free diet that seemed to help.

Lucile recalled that the doctor seemed unimpressed by her mother's remark about the diet, possibly convinced that Lucile had an unconfessed eating disorder. At home, her mother put her back on the diet and after a while, the diarrhea, cramping, and bloating all disappeared.

After reliving her history of bowel problems and anemia by talking with her brother, Lucile agreed to see the gastroenterologist. Upon physical examination, Lucile had pallor, dark circles under the eyes and a mildly distended and tympanitic (drum-like sound when tapped) abdomen. At this point she was very weak and had difficulty getting up and down from the examination table. Her muscle strength was good despite her weakened state, and she had no signs of neurological problems. The gastroenterologist listened to Lucile's history of illnesses, making notes as she spoke.

Lucile underwent numerous tests including blood and urine, abdominal CAT scan, upper and lower endoscope, and a bone biopsy. Her hemoglobin, serum ferritin, and red cell folate were low; her red cells were microcytic (small) and hypochromic (not much color) with elliptocytosis (oval shaped). Her B_{12}, platelet, SED rate, and white blood count were normal. She was positive for IgA endomysial antibodies. Her bone biopsy provided that she had osteoporosis (thinning of the bones) and osteomalacia (softening of the bones). Her endoscope revealed abnormalities in the small intestine consistent with celiac disease: "villous atrophy, crypt hyperplasia, and intraepithelial lymphocytosis."

Lucile was prescribed Fosamax, 5 milligrams once daily on an empty stomach for her bone loss. It was recommended that she take iron supplements, 325 milligrams per day, and she was instructed to follow a gluten-free diet.

"Celiac disease (CD) is not rare in the United States and may be as common as in Europe... According to a large multicenter study... in at-risk groups, the prevalence of CD was 1:22 in first-degree relatives, 1:39 in second-degree relatives, and 1:56 in symptomatic patients. The overall prevalence of CD in not-at-risk groups was 1:133."

—*Alessio Fasano, MD, University of Maryland*

Celiac disease, also called sprue, celiac sprue, non-tropical sprue, and gluten-sensitive enteropathy, is a condition of sensitivity to gluten grains containing glidian protein found in wheat, oats, barley, and rye. These grains are often used as fillers in many products. Celiac sprue should not be confused with tropical sprue, a different condition with symptoms similar to celiac. Celiac disease is classified both as a malabsorption disorder because the absorption of nutrients is impaired, and as an autoimmune disease. Villi, fingerlike projections along the lining of the small intestine, become damaged in the presence of gluten. Inflammation occurs that activates the immune response. T-cells of the immune system that are sent to destroy an invading germ instead initiate an attack on the villi.

When villi are damaged, the patient loses the ability of normal absorption of nutrients from food. As the nutrients pass unabsorbed into the large intestine, gas, cramping, bloating, and fatty diarrhea can be experienced. Chronic malabsorption can lead to malnutrition, with weight loss, retarded growth in children, and vitamin and mineral deficiency disorders such as folate and iron-deficiency anemia.

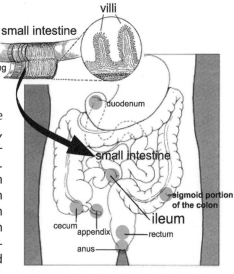

Image adapted from National Cancer Institutes and the National Institutes of Diabetes & Digestive & Kidney Diseases

Celiac disease occurs mostly in people of northern European descent and is frequently seen in children. Celiac disease is believed to be underdiagnosed in the United States because of the strong European heritage of Americans. We do not screen for the condition in the United States, where the diagnosis can take on average ten years to obtain.

In European countries where children are screened for celiac disease, the disease is identified early and prevention with a gluten-free diet employed. Children who are screened in infancy for the antibodies to gluten are protected from the developmental delays that can result from iron-deficiency anemia, a consequence of celiac disease. About 10 percent of an affected person's first-degree relatives (parents, siblings, or children) will also have the disease.

Symptoms are not always reliable; some people have several symptoms, some only a few symptoms, and others have no symptoms but still present with mild deficiencies such as iron and folate. Symptoms and findings known to be associated with celiac disease include:

- Recurring abdominal bloating and pain
- Chronic diarrhea
- Weight loss
- Pale, foul-smelling stool
- Iron-deficiency anemia
- Folic acid deficiency
- Calcium deficiency
- Gas
- Bone pain
- Bone loss or softening
- Behavior changes
- Muscle cramps
- Fatigue
- Delayed growth
- Failure to thrive in infants
- Pain in the joints
- Seizures
- Tingling numbness in the legs (from nerve damage)
- Pale sores inside the mouth, called aphthus ulcers
- Painful skin rash that itches, called dermatitis herpetiformis
- Hives
- Tooth discoloration or loss of enamel
- Missed menstrual periods (often because of excessive weight loss)

In a rare finding by Mayo Clinic's celiac disease expert Joseph Murray, MD, an obese woman with constipation, two symptoms not usually associated with CD, presented with active celiac disease. Another finding not usually associated with celiac is suspect iron overload.

Variation C282Y of HFE, the gene for hereditary hemochromatosis, the leading cause of iron overload disease, has been noted in some patients with celiac. These patients may exhibit an elevated serum ferritin in spite of the absorption difficulties associated with CD. Although no known studies to date substantiate the prevalence of HFE in celiac patients, experts such as Murray suspect the incidence might be significant at least in some populations. Investigators Butterworth, Cooper, and Rosenberg reported in *Gastroenterology* 2002 that carrying the gene for hemochromatosis could explain why some celiac disease patients do not become iron deficient.

Serum ferritin, which can be indicative of iron overload disease, can also be elevated by inflammation, a condition called anemia of chronic disease (ACD). In ACD, the serum ferritin is elevated but the transferrin saturation percentage is normal and usually accompanied by a normal to low-normal hemoglobin.

In severe prolonged cases of celiac disease the patient can develop pernicious anemia, a vitamin B_{12} deficiency. B_{12} is absorbed in the ileum portion of the small intestine where the majority of damage occurs in celiac disease. When pernicious anemia is found in a patient with celiac, investigation for cancer should be considered.

Other consequences of celiac disease can include lymphoma and adenocarcinoma in the intestine, osteoporosis or osteomalacia, and miscarriage. Congenital malformation of a developing fetus, such as neural tube defects, is a risk for untreated pregnant women with celiac disease because of malabsorption of nutrients such as folic acid.

In undiagnosed children, short stature results when celiac disease prevents nutrient absorption during the years when nutrition is critical to a child's normal growth and development. Children who are diagnosed and treated before their growth stops may have a catch-up period. Seizures, or convulsions, result from inadequate absorption of folic acid. Lack of folic acid causes calcium deposits, called calcifications, to form in the brain, which in turn cause seizures.

Celiac disease is often seen in children with insulin-dependent diabetes. A group of Medical College of Wisconsin researchers, Lee, Parton, Werlin, Wyatt, Aktay, and Kumar, tested diabetic patients at Children's Hospital of Wisconsin for signs and symptoms of celiac disease and found that at least 4.6 percent of the children who participated in the study suffered from celiac disease, while even more had indicators that could be early signs of the disease. These researchers recommend that children with insulin-dependent diabetes mellitus (IDDM) be tested for celiac disease.

In one study at Mayo Clinic, William Hu, MD, PhD, a neurology resident, reported cognitive impairment or decline in celiac patients. This decline improved in some patients on gluten-free diets. This reversal or stabilization of the cognitive symptoms provides a good argument against chance as an explanation of the link between celiac disease and cognitive decline. Dr. Joseph Murray offers some possible theories to explain the connection between celiac disease and cognitive decline as nutritional deficiencies, immune attack on the brain, or inflammatory cytokines (chemical messengers).

Diagnosing celiac sprue

Diagnosing celiac disease can be delayed because some of its symptoms are similar to those of other diseases, including irritable bowel syndrome, Crohn's disease, ulcerative colitis, diverticulosis, intestinal infections, chronic fatigue syndrome, and depression.

To differentiate between these conditions, physicians test the patient's blood to measure levels of antibodies to gluten. These antibodies are antigliadin, anti-endomysium, and antireticulin. If a patient tests positive for these antibodies, the next procedure is an endoscopy to obtain a biopsy of the small intestine. Biopsy of the small intestine is the best way to diagnose celiac disease, but when a person responds to the gluten-free diet, the physician will know for certain that the diagnosis of celiac disease is correct.

Treatment

The only treatment for celiac disease is to follow a gluten-free diet, that is, to avoid all foods that contain gluten. For most people, following this diet will stop symptoms, heal existing intestinal damage, and prevent further damage. Improvements begin within days of starting the diet.

The gluten-free diet is a lifetime requirement. Eating any gluten, no matter how small an amount, can damage the intestine. This is true for anyone with the disease, including people who do not have noticeable symptoms. Depending on a

Diet for celiac disease

Not okay to eat	Foods that contain wheat (including spelt, triticale, semolina, and kamut), rye, barley, and possibly oats—in other words, most grain, pasta, cereal, and many processed foods, which can contain fillers made of gluten.
Okay to eat	Flours made of potato, rice, soy, or bean. Plain meat, fish, rice, corn, tapioca, poi, fruits, and vegetables do not contain gluten, so people with celiac disease can eat as much of these foods as they like.

person's age at diagnosis, some problems, such as delayed growth and tooth discoloration, may not improve.

A small percentage of people with celiac disease are not responsive to therapy. These people may not be strictly adhering to the diet or they may have severely damaged intestines that cannot heal even after eliminating gluten from the diet. These individuals can become gravely ill and require intravenous nutrition supplements.

For the anemia that accompanies celiac disease, lean red meat, if it can be tolerated, is a good source of iron. Oral iron supplements may be used; low doses are best and iron should be taken with a rich source of vitamin C for improved absorption. Key foods and substances that impair iron absorption include coffee, tea, chocolate, and calcium and should be avoided. Since many celiac patients are given calcium supplements, these are best taken at bedtime and not with the iron.

Taking action
Read more about celiac disease by visiting the websites of organizations listed at the end of this chapter. These sites contain excellent resources and diet information. Portions of this chapter are from the NIDDK section on celiac disease. If you think you

may have this condition, please discuss it with your doctor so testing can be done before you start a new diet, because changing your diet can make it very hard to make the diagnosis.

Resources
American Celiac Society
PO Box 23455
New Orleans, LA 70183
Tel: 504-737-3293
Email: americanceliacsociety@yahoo.com
www.americanceliacsociety.org

Celiac Disease Foundation
13251 Ventura Blvd. #1
Studio City, CA 91604
Tel: 818-990-2354
Fax: 818-990-2379
Email: cdf@celiac.org
www.celiac.org

Celiac Sprue Association of the USA, Inc.
P.O. Box 31700
Omaha, NE 68131-0700
Tel: 402-558-0600
Toll Free: 877-CSA-4CSA
Email: celiacs@csaceliacs.org
www.csaceliacs.org

GIG (Gluten Intolerance Group)

15110 10th Ave. SW, Suite A
Seattle, WA 98166
Tel: 206-246-6652
Fax: 206-246-6531
www.gluten.net

National Institute of Diabetes and Digestive and Kidney Diseases (NIDDK)

2 Information Way
Bethesda, MD 20892-3570
www.niddk.nih.gov/
Use the search feature with words *celiac disease*

National Center for Nutrition and Dietetics

American Dietetic Association
216 West Jackson Boulevard, Suite 800
Chicago, IL 60606-6995
Tel: 1-800-366-1655
Email: hotline@eatright.org
Internet: www.eatright.org

Find recipes, gluten-free products, and upcoming events on the Celiac Disease & Gluten-Free Diet Support website: www.celiac.com.

18

Crohn's and Ulcerative Colitis

"Some 1,000,000 Americans suffer from these inflammatory bowel diseases."

—*The Crohn's and Colitis Foundation, New York, New York*

Her first recollection of any intestinal distress was in 1972. At that time twenty-eight-year-old Carol Rooney became very ill with pains in her stomach. She was unable to keep anything down, not even a glass of water. She called her physician, who made a telephone diagnosis of colitis and sent her to the hospital to have an IV inserted and fluids for twenty-four hours. After the fluids and the stay in the hospital Carol began to feel better and returned home. She never gave her "colitis" diagnosis a second thought because she didn't know what colitis was; besides, she did not have another episode for nearly sixteen years.

When Carol's second bout of intestinal distress occurred, it seemed much more severe and lasted longer. Still, she never related the two incidents until many years later, when she became ill from eating undercooked chicken. The symptoms ranged from nausea, vomiting, and stomach pains to running a very high fever. The nausea, vomiting, and stomach pains lasted only twenty-four hours and she assumed whatever she had was over. The spiking fevers, however, continued for months.

Carol finally ended up in the hospital where her primary care physician diagnosed the problem as appendicitis and told her she would need surgery. Fortunately, another physician who examined her felt it was something other than appendicitis and ordered an upper GI series, which confirmed Crohn's disease.

Crohn's disease! Carol had no idea what this condition was. She started asking her doctor questions, "What do I do to get rid of it? How did I get it, and will it lead to anything else?" His reply was typical for that period in time: "It is an incurable disease, and we don't know how you got it, but the good news is it isn't fatal."

Shortly thereafter her husband's employer transferred them to another state, which meant she would have to find new doctors. This turned out to be a blessing in disguise because Carol found an excellent gastroenterologist who was knowledgeable about Crohn's disease. Every question she posed for which he had no answers, he checked with other gastroenterologists and hospitals for answers. This was the beginning of a journey of learning about the disease, its symptoms, the medications, their side effects, the long-term effects of the drugs, surgeries, and so on.

Carol continued to suffer many flare-ups with Crohn's disease, and had many hospitalizations for total parenteral nutrition (TPN). TPN is a technique where all life-sustaining nutrients are fed through a large vein in the chest in order to give the bowels total rest in the hopes they might begin to heal on their own. Many times Carol was put on an elemental diet, a specially prepared liquid meal that contains all necessary nutrients. She suffered with severe intestinal pains, diarrhea, spiking fevers, chills, joint pain, vomiting, fatigue, and anemia off and on for five years before finally agreeing to surgery. A bowel resection to take out as much of the infected area of her small bowel as possible would restore her to good health for nearly eighteen months. Carol was grateful for every single day that she was free of symptoms. She points out that she cannot say that she was free of the disease because even if the diseased part of the small bowel was removed, the Crohn's disease still remained. It would almost certainly come back and for Carol, it did. Her second surgery was exactly twenty-three months after the first. This time the surgeon removed even more of the small bowel, which left her very close to having short bowel syndrome.

One big concern for Carol has been anemia, though currently it is not a problem. Her physician ordered large doses of iron and vitamin C to be taken three times a day until the anemia was under control. Additionally, Carol underwent a battery of tests to determine the cause of the occult blood loss and the anemia. Carol used her experience to help others with Crohn's disease. "I have found over the years that a positive attitude, coupled with as much knowledge of Crohn's disease as I can get, gives me the tools I need to combat this debilitating disease," says Carol Rooney, former president of the Crohn's and Colitis Foundation, Carolinas chapter and former Development Director for the chapter.

Inflammatory bowel disease

An inflammatory bowel disease (IBD) is described as any condition that causes inflammation in the small or large bowel, including appendix, rectum, and colon, or organs leading to the bowel including the mouth, esophagus, and stomach. Most such diseases are acute and short-lived and are due to bacterial, protozoal, or vital infections, such as salmonella, shigella enteritis, giardiasis, or rotavirus. The most important forms of chronic idiopathic (unknown cause) inflammatory bowel disease are Crohn's disease and ulcerative colitis. They may have similar symptoms, which makes distinguishing between these conditions a challenge. Anemia is a common complication of IBD.

Anemia of chronic disease can be present due to the inflammation; iron-deficiency anemia is generally due to blood loss. Pernicious anemia, a vitamin B_{12} deficiency, is due to decreased absorption. B_{12} absorption depends upon a well-functioning stomach and ileum (lower portion of the small intestine). Therefore, patients who have inflammation in these areas or who have had surgery involving these organs frequently develop a B_{12} deficiency.

Crohn's disease typically manifests itself as inflammation of the lower part of the small intestine, the colon, and other parts of the digestive tract such as the esophagus, stomach, rectum, appendix, and anus. Crohn's usually involves all layers of the intestinal wall. Ulcerative colitis is not found in the small intestine. Colitis is a condition that results in inflammation and superficial ulcers in the colon (large intestine) and the rectum.

Crohn's disease affects males and females alike and onset

is usually before the age of thirty during the mid-teens to early twenties. The most prominent symptoms include persistent diarrhea, abdominal pain in the lower right quadrant, rectal bleeding, fever, loss of appetite, weight loss, skin or eye irritations, delayed growth and sexual maturation in children, and anemia. There are multiple genetic factors that predispose people to develop Crohn's disease. Thus it tends to run in families.

Comparing Bowel Diseases

Condition	Symptoms		Most at Risk

Crohn's	- Persistent diarrhea
	- Abdominal pain
	- Rectal bleeding
	- Fever
	- Loss of appetite
	- Weight loss
		- Skin or eye irritations
		- Delayed growth and
		  sexual maturation in
		  children
		-Nutritional deficiencies
		-ACD, IDA, PA
			Men and women generally at age 30 but onset can occur in mid teens

Ulcerative Colitis	- Bloody diarrhea - Visible pus or mucus in stool - Abdominal pain - Loss of appetite - Weight loss	- Arthritis - Osteoporosis - Liver & Kidney Disease - Skin rashes -Nutritional deficiencies -ACD, IDA, PA	Men and women generally ages 15 to 40
Diverticulosis	- Mild cramps - Bloating	- Constipation - ACD	Age 40+ Incidence: Onset <age 50

Diverticulitis	-Diarrhea
	-Nausea
	-Vomiting
		-Blood in stool
		-Pain in lower left
		  portion of the
		  abdomen
		- ACD, IDA
			Males are 3X
			  more affected
			Onset 70+
			Females are 3X
			  more affected

Celiac Disease	· Recurring abdominal gas, bloating, and pain · Chronic diarrhea · Weight loss · Pale, foul-smelling stool -Nutritional deficiencies	· Bone pain · Bone loss or softening · Behavior changes · Muscle cramps · Delayed growth · Failure to thrive in infants -ACD, IDA, PA	All ages, including infants

ACD=Anemia of Chronic Disease IDA=Iron Deficiency Anemia PA=Pernicious Anemia

Ulcerative colitis occurs most often in people ages fifteen to forty, although children and older people sometimes develop the disease. Ulcerative colitis affects men and women equally and appears to run in some families. About half of patients have mild symptoms. Others suffer frequent fever, bloody diarrhea with visible pus or mucus in the stool, nausea, and severe abdominal cramps. Ulcerative colitis may also cause problems outside the large intestines, such as arthritis, inflammation of the eye, liver disease (fatty liver, hepatitis, cirrhosis, and primary sclerosing cholangitis), osteoporosis, skin rashes, anemia, and kidney stones. No one knows for sure why problems occur outside the colon. Scientists think these complications may occur when the immune system triggers inflammation in other parts of the body. These problems are usually mild and go away when the colitis is treated.

Inflammatory bowel disease is medically incurable. Its cause is unknown. Some suspect that a bacterial or viral infection can initiate the disease process, but this theory remains unproven. Emotional stress does not cause inflammatory bowel disease, although life stresses may trigger or worsen GI symptoms in virtually all of us, whether we have underlying IBD or not. Diet does not cause IBD, but dietary modifications may reduce symptoms. Deficiencies of essential nutrients may occur in IBD disease depending on the location and extent of the disease. The major essential nutrients are: carbohydrates, fats, protein; vitamins A, B_{12}, and folic acid; C, D, calcium, iron; copper, magnesium, and zinc. Some fats and proteins are considered "essential" because our bodies are unable to make them from other building blocks. There also are micronutrients such as selenium, manganese, and others, which are essential for optimal health but for which the amount needed is low. The best protection is to eat a variety of foods from the four basic food groups, choosing sources that are rich in the nutrients you need and that conform to any dietary modifications that you may require. Most people who eat a well-balanced, mixed American diet do not require vitamin or mineral supplements. In fact, taking too much vitamin A, D, or E may actually cause serious disease. Still, modest doses (recommended daily allowance) are unlikely to do harm beyond that caused by the expense of paying for unneeded medication. Some patients with increased metabolic demand (e.g., pregnant or lactating women; patients with malabsorption or maldigestion syndromes) may require vitamin and/or mineral supplementation.

Diagnosing inflammatory bowel disease (IBD)

Inflammatory bowel disease can be extremely difficult to diagnose. Because it shares the symptoms of so many other intestinal illnesses, it sometimes takes years before a correct diagnosis is made. Physicians rely on the patient's history, physical examination, a variety of procedures, and laboratory tests to reach a correct diagnosis and to differentiate between Crohn's disease and ulcerative colitis. Some of these tests also are used to monitor patients' progress. These tests can be categorized as follows:

Blood and urine tests. Blood chemistries provide information about specific antibodies, nutritional status and general health, electrolyte balance, and liver and kidney function. Urinalysis is used to look for bacteria or blood cells in the urine.

Stool examinations. Stool tests are important in differentiating between IBDs and infections, which may produce similar symptoms.

Radiological procedures such as magnetic resonance imaging (MRI) and computed tomography imaging (CAT scan), barium enemas, and GI series with small bowel follow through aid in diagnosis of IBD, and in monitoring illness activity and progression.

Endoscopic procedures examine the insides of hollow organs such as the esophagus, stomach, small intestine, and large intestine. Flexible tubes, called endoscopes, can be passed through the rectum or the mouth, and aid physicians in the examination of the GI tract. They allow for removal of biopsies, polyps, and other abnormalities. Capsule endoscopy can also be performed. In this procedure, patients swallow a capsule that contains a miniature camera and transmitter. As it passes through the GI tract from the mouth to the anus it transmits images of the inside of the tract. These images can be displayed on video viewers. Because of the relatively higher costs of capsule endoscopy compared to conventional endoscopy and because polyps or other abnormalities seen cannot be removed or biopsied, capsule endoscopy is usually used only when conventional endoscopy has failed to yield a diagnosis in a patient in whom the clinical suspicion of organic bowel disease is high.

Differentiation between Crohn's and ulcerative colitis depends in part upon the portion of the digestive tract involved. Although Crohn's disease can affect any and all parts of the GI tract , from the mouth to the anus, it usually occurs in the terminal part of the small intestine called the ileum, or the colon (large intestine), or both. About 35 percent of Crohn's cases involve only the ileum, about 20 percent involve only the colon, and about 45 percent involve both the ileum and colon. In contrast, ulcerative colitis involves the rectum and colon. Usually, it involves the lower parts of the colon, the rectum and sigmoid colon, but it may march up to involve all portions of the colon and occasionally with total colonic involvement, may even involve the terminal ileum ("backwash ileitis").

Diagnosing Bowel Diseases

Condition	Area of the bowel involved	Key test used for diagnosis
Crohn's	Primarily small intestine & colon Can be present in mouth, esophagus, stomach, duodenum, large intestine, appendix, and anus.	Small bowel biopsy with endoscope
Ulcerative Colitis	Colon & rectum	Large bowel biopsy with endoscope
Diverticulosis	Colon	Colonoscopy
Diverticulitis	Colon	Colonoscopy
Celiac Disease	Small intestine	Blood test for antibodies to gluten

Treatment for IBD

Medications help control IBD. Unfortunately, none of the current medications used to treat IBD provides a cure. However, most people respond favorably to careful, well-directed, long-term medical management. Current therapies can help control disease by:

- Suppressing the abnormal and destructive immune response
- Promoting healing of intestinal tissue
- Relieving symptoms of diarrhea, abdominal pain, and fever

Surgery may be needed if drugs do not control symptoms or if complications arise. Approximately two-thirds to three-quarters of individuals with Crohn's disease undergo at least one surgical procedure during the course of their illness. Unfortunately, although surgery can alleviate complications and help to manage the symptoms of Crohn's disease, it is not a cure. In fact, 40 to 50 percent of people with Crohn's disease who have had surgery for it later require a second, third, or fourth operation. Because of this, physicians try to avoid surgery if possible.

Some patients with chronic, idiopathic ulcerative colitis must eventually have their colons removed because of massive bleeding, severe unrelenting inflammation, severe distention or rupture of the colon, or development of cancer, or precancerous changes (intestinal dysplasia). Sometimes the doctor will recommend removing the colon if medical treatment fails or if the side effects of corticosteroids or other drugs threaten the patient's health. Although cancer is not a universal sequela of ulcerative colitis, about 5 percent of these patients go on to develop cancer of the colon. Risks of cancer development are higher in those with more extensive disease (most of colon involved) and those with disease for a longer time. Because of the risk of cancer development, patients with ulcerative colitis should undergo regular screening colonoscopies. The frequency of screening depends upon the clinical features of the patient.

In celiac disease the diet is the cure. In Crohn's or ulcerative colitis, the diet is not a cure but can help relieve symptoms and replace lost nutrients. When IBD is active, it is not unusual for eating to cause cramping and intestinal discomfort. This is especially true when the small intestine is inflamed. Since there are several reasons why this occurs, it is important to observe any association between specific foods or types of food and the onset of gastrointestinal symptoms. Any of the following foods can cause discomfort:

- Milk and milk products
- High fiber foods
- Fried or greasy foods
- Large meals

Keeping in shape is important for everyone, but it can be especially helpful for people with inflammatory bowel disease. The long-term benefits of exercise—even if the routine is periodically interrupted—can include faster recovery from abdominal surgery, reversal of muscle weakness and wasting, and prevention of calcium and protein loss from the bones.

Anemia in those suffering from inflammatory bowel disease often occurs as a complication of IBD, with reported frequencies ranging widely (20 to 70 percent). Its onset is usually gradual, sometimes taking years to develop, and many patients may not immediately realize the effect on their daily performance. Occasionally, a low red blood cell count is the initial clue to the diagnosis of IBD, but in general, anemia occurs well after intestinal symptoms have begun.

The main manifestations produced by anemia are weakness and fatigue. Shortness of breath, especially with physical activity, is also common. Patients often find they just can't do things with as much energy as they used to. Lightheadedness and nausea are also frequently noticed. In older patients or those with coronary artery disease, anemia can lead to chest pain (angina) because of the decrease in oxygen supply to the heart. Headaches and other neurological symptoms also may occur due to the diminished oxygen level in the brain.

The causes of anemia in IBD are generally due to many

factors, anemia of chronic disease and iron deficiency being the most common. Anemia of chronic disease is in response to the inflammation. Iron-deficiency anemia develops from blood loss, which is either obvious to the patient, or occurs in such small amounts as not to be noticed (occult blood loss).

Correcting anemia

For anemia of chronic disease, treating the underlying condition is the only therapy. Once the inflammation is under control, the anemia of chronic disease will disappear. If the anemia is due to iron deficiency, it is usually successfully treated with replacement of iron taken orally. Iron injections or infusions may be needed if the anemia is severe and the patient is not responding to oral supplements. Treatment with recombinant human erythropoietin (rHuEPO)—brand names Procrit®, Epogen®, Aranesp®—might be used to stimulate the bone marrow to produce more red blood cells.

Because vitamin B_{12} is absorbed only in the terminal ileum, patients with disease in this part of the bowel or those who have required surgical removal of the terminal ileum require lifelong regular injections of B_{12}. The usual dose is 100 mcg intramuscularly once each month.

Resources

Anyone interested in learning more about inflammatory bowel diseases is encouraged to visit the websites listed below and to contact the Crohn's & Colitis Foundation of America (CCFA) for further information.

Crohn's & Colitis Foundation of America, Inc. (CCFA)

386 Park Avenue South, 17th floor
New York, NY 10016-8804
Tel: 212-685-3440, 800-932-2423
Email: info@ccfa.org to get information or to locate the address and telephone number of your local chapter. Each chapter can provide the location and contact number of local support groups, as well as information on how to become a volunteer in the fight against IBD.
www.ccfa.org

National Institute of Diabetes and Digestive and Kidney Diseases (NIDDK)

2 Information Way
Bethesda, MD 20892-3570
www.niddk.nih.gov
Use the search feature with the words *Crohn's, ulcerative colitis*

The New People Not Patients: A Source Book for Living with Inflammatory Bowel Disease by David B. Sachar, MD, Chief, Division of Gastroenterology, Mount Sinai Medical Center, and David S. Kaminstein, MD, FACG, Philadelphia, PA. Published by the Crohn's and Colitis Foundation of America.

19

Renal Disease

"Anemia continues to cause serious health consequences for patients with chronic kidney disease... Even though the anemia can be managed by available therapies, anemia associated with chronic kidney disease often goes under-recognized and under-treated."

—*Allen R. Nissenson, MD, FACP, Associate Dean, Department of Medicine, Division of Nephrology, David Geffen School of Medicine at UCLA; and Director, Dialysis Program, DaVita Dialysis Center, Los Angeles, California*

Health problems for Terry Cox all started with a diagnosis of bladder cancer. His physician thought that the cancer was contained and had not spread and could be removed surgically. Following surgery, Terry became progressively more tired. When he tried to work in the yard he found that he had to sit down frequently to rest. His wife Louise took him back to the doctor, where it was discovered that Terry's hemoglobin was 6.0 g/dL—dangerously low. He was admitted to the hospital and given 5 units of blood. This improved his hemoglobin and energy level but soon the fatigue returned. Terry went back to his doctor who ran more tests and performed various procedures including endoscopy of the upper and lower gastrointestinal system, scope of his bladder, and a spinal tap. It seemed that his body was not making new red blood cells but his storage iron (ferritin) was quite elevated.

While monitoring his red cell count, the physician ran some tests to check Terry's kidney function. The findings indicated that Terry's kidneys were not functioning properly. This was another surprise for Terry as he thought his kidneys were just fine; in fact, he often got up two or three times during the night to use the bathroom. An image of his kidneys showed that one of his kidneys was completely atrophied—shriveled up and not functioning at all. Terry was referred to a kidney specialist (nephrologist) who eventually started him on hemodialysis and intravenous Epogen® (erythropoietin) treatments three times a week; each dialysis treatment took about four hours to complete.

At first Terry was so fatigued he could hardly make it in for treatment. He would come home feeling drained and wanting to sleep. After six weeks of treatments he began to feel better because in addition to the dialysis he was able to resume his daily walks with his wife Louise and was able to work in the yard again without becoming overly tired. Terry attributes his positive experience with dialysis to his wife of fifty-five years, and the team of physicians, nurses, and technicians at the dialysis center. He says he will have to remain on dialysis three times a week for the rest of his life but he is grateful for the medical advances in treatment for kidney disease available to patients today.

* * *

In response to the oxygen concentration in the blood, the kidneys increase or decrease production of a hormone called erythropoietin (EPO). EPO stimulates the production of red blood cells (RBCs) in the bone marrow. In this way the kidneys help to control the amount of RBCs and hemoglobin in the bloodstream. Damaged kidneys do not function normally and often do not make enough EPO. As a result, the bone marrow makes fewer red blood cells to circulate and anemia is the consequence.

The most prominent causes of kidney damage are diabetes mellitus and high blood pressure (hypertension). Kidney function can also be impaired by trauma, such as a direct blow to the kidney, infection or inflammation, polycystic disease, chemotherapy, radiation therapy, problems of hemolysis such as hemolytic uremic syndrome (HUS), and medications such as pain relievers or certain antibiotics, and excessive levels of metals such as mercury, lead, and iron.

Loss of kidney function can be sudden (acute) or slow to

develop (chronic) and is classified by stages. Complete kidney failure which is defined as less than 10 percent kidney function is called end stage renal disease (ESRD). Patients with ESRD must receive renal replacement therapy (dialysis or kidney transplantation) to survive. Unfortunately there are not enough donated kidneys to meet the demand for transplantation. Though the number of donated kidneys available remains relatively unchanged, the number of patients needing kidney transplantation has risen well beyond the supply. In fact, only about 6 percent of patients who need kidney transplantation receive a new kidney. When they do, these recipients must take antirejection drugs for the remainder of their lives.

Prior to total kidney failure, chronic kidney disease (CKD) may be present and undetected for years, causing a gradual loss of kidney function. People in the early stages of kidney disease may not feel sick at all. The first signs of kidney disease come late and are nonspecific, such as frequent headaches or feeling tired or itchy all over the body. The amount of urine output does not correlate to kidney function. Loss of appetite, nausea, vomiting, swollen or numb hands or feet, drowsiness, muscle cramps, darkening of the skin, and difficulty concentrating are symptoms that can occur with advanced stages of kidney disease. Chronic and debilitating fatigue, confusion, inability to concentrate, frequent infections, heart failure, elevated cholesterol, high blood pressure, and stroke can accompany kidney disease as well. In the last stage of kidney disease, there is total loss of kidney function.

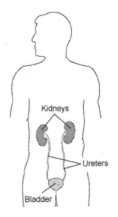

Source: NIDDK

Kidney function

The kidneys are kidney bean–shaped organs about the size of a small fist (150 grams each), located near the middle of the back on both sides just below the rib cage. The kidneys help to regulate blood pressure, control the concentration and volume of body fluids, and the level of electrolytes such as sodium, potassium, phosphorus, and calcium. The kidneys filter out waste products from the blood such as urea, uric acid, and creatinine and produce urine so that these waste products can be eliminated from the body. The kidneys also return key nutrients from the urine, placing them back into the bloodstream.

On a weight basis, the kidneys receive the highest amount of blood flow of all of the tissues in the body (about 1 quart of blood per minute), or approximately one-fifth of the total cardiac output at rest. Each day the kidneys process about 1,440 quarts of blood to sift out about 2 quarts of waste and waste products. The waste and extra water is called urine, which flows to the bladder through tubes called ureters. The bladder stores urine until it is excreted. Waste products in blood come from the normal activities of metabolism. The body uses food for energy and self-repair. After cells take what they need from food, the unused portion, waste, is deposited in the bloodstream. If the kidneys did not remove these waste products, they would accumulate in the blood and damage vital organs, especially the heart. Poor kidney function is a major contributor to the development of congestive heart failure.

Each kidney has about a million nephrons, which are tiny functioning units. In each nephron, a glomerulus, which is a very small collection of blood vessels, or capillaries, is responsible for starting the production of urine. In the glomerulus blood, water along with nutrients, electrolytes, and waste products gets sieved into the tubule, which then along its path holds on to the nutrients and most of the electrolytes, while excreting the wastes in water (this water enriched with wastes is called urine).

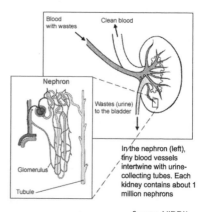

In the nephron (left), tiny blood vessels intertwine with urine-collecting tubes. Each kidney contains about 1 million nephrons

Source: NIDDK

"It was only when we were able to treat anemia that we realized many of these symptoms—if not the majority—were actually caused by the anemia and not by the kidney disease per se."

—Allen R. Nissenson, MD, FACP, Professor of Medicine; Associate Dean, Department of Medicine, Division of Nephrology, David Geffen School of Medicine at UCLA, Los Angeles, California; Director, Dialysis Program, DaVita Dialysis Center, Los Angeles, California

Anemia is common in patients with kidney disease. However, the onset, duration, and the causes of anemia in these patients can vary. Anemia may begin to develop in the early stages of renal disease, or when a patient has 20 percent to 50 percent normal kidney function. This partial loss of kidney function is often called chronic renal insufficiency. Anemia tends to worsen as renal disease progresses. End stage renal disease (ESRD), the point at which dialysis or kidney transplantation becomes necessary, does not occur until there is only about 10 percent of kidney function remaining. Nearly everyone with ESRD will experience anemia.

Iron-deficiency anemia in patients who are receiving dialysis treatment is due to blood loss from blood sampling, when needles are placed and removed, and in dialysis tubing. With blood loss there is loss of nutrients such as iron, zinc, vitamin B_{12}, and folic acid. These nutrients are key in the production of hemoglobin, the oxygen-carrying protein of the blood. According to nephrologist Paul Sakiewicz, "Iron deficiency alone affects more than 50 percent of patients on dialysis, and the estimated iron loss for these patients is 1.5 to 3 grams per year."

Anemia of chronic disease can also occur in renal disease patients as a result of inflammation due to infection from catheters or perhaps the dialysis procedure itself, which causes the level of serum ferritin (a marker for iron stored in the body's tissues) to rise. Paradoxically, this occurs while the transferrin iron saturation percentage (the iron circulating in the blood available for red blood cell production) remains low. In other words, the iron is "locked up" in the tissues and not released to the blood proteins, which carry it to the bone marrow. There is no direct treatment for anemia of chronic disease except to treat the underlying condition that is causing the inflammation.

Uncontrolled iron, or iron that is not bound or contained, can trigger free radical activity. The delicate tissues of the kidneys can be damaged severely as a result of this activity.

Diagnosing anemia

According to the National Kidney Foundation Kidney Disease Outcomes Quality Initiatives (KDOQI) Clinical Practice Guidelines, hemoglobin values are more reliable than hematocrit for determining the level of anemia in dialysis patients. Hemoglobin is the actual oxygen carrying molecule, while the hematocrit indicates the amount of red blood cells in blood. Given that the hemoglobin content per cell can vary, it is simpler and more accurate to evaluate the actual hemoglobin content rather than hematocrit alone.

The guidelines recommend a target hemoglobin of 11–12 g/ dL, which is usually a hematocrit 33 to 36 percent. An anemia workup for renal patients should include: hemoglobin/hematocrit, red blood cell indices (the size and color of the cells), reticulocyte (young red blood cells) count, and iron parameters: serum ferritin and transferrin saturation, or hemoglobin content in the reticulocytes. Additionally, a test for occult blood in the stool and serum vitamin B_{12} and folate levels may be considered.

Management of anemia

In the past, as part of the therapeutic strategy to correct anemia, physicians have administered genetically engineered erythropoietin (rHuEPO), brand names Procrit® for non-dialysis patients, Epogen® for dialysis patients, and Aranesp® for either. Recent controversy about the appropriate target hemoglobin level has affected rHuEPO use; consult with your healthcare provider about the risks and benefits of rHuEPO. Nonetheless, it is generally agreed that rHuEPO is preferable to blood transfusion. In addition to rHuEPO, iron replenishment is a standard approach for ESRD-associated anemia. For the most part, blood transfusions should be avoided in ESRD patients for a very compelling reason. Patients receiving blood transfusions can be exposed to "foreign" antigens to which they become "sensitized." By becoming sensitized to these antigens, these patients gradually lose their ability to accept a transplanted kidney, which is undesirable for someone seeking a long-term solution for their ESRD.

For hemodialysis patients, intravenous iron is usually preferred over oral iron. Iron dextran (Infed®), sodium ferric gluconate (Ferrlecit®), and ferric saccharate (Venofer®) are often used. Until several years ago, a single dose of 500 to 1,000 milligrams (mgs) was used when physicians detected iron deficiency. However, because of occasional anaphylaxis-like reactions, The National Kidney Foundation KDOQI Guidelines recommend weekly (maintenance) dosing with smaller amounts: generally 50 to 125 milligrams, depending upon the patient's needs. Maintenance dosing was developed in part because it led to a lower incidence of anaphylactoid (allergic) reactions. The new generation iron products (Ferrlecit® and Venofer®) were developed to reduce the incidence of anaphylactoid reactions to intravenous iron. This life-threatening reaction has been effectively eliminated in ESRD but other possible complications have come up in its place.

The new generation IV preparations appear to release iron more easily in the bloodstream. This requires a longer infusion time to prevent acute intoxication reactions, which can lead to hypotension (low blood pressure), arthralgia (joint pain), flushing, and nausea. Additionally, when there is oversaturation of transferrin, free iron may be associated with uncontrolled oxidation reactions. This action can damage tissues like the inside of blood vessels and may also provide an easily accessible iron source for pathogenic bacteria. Because dialysis treatments are invasive, concern about bacterial infection is constant.

Iron supplementation in peritoneal dialysis (PD) is quite different from hemodialysis. PD patients receive their dialysis treatment directly through the abdominal cavity. Most commonly this type of treatment takes place at home, so the patient does not routinely go to a clinic to receive IV iron. For this reason, most PD patients can be effectively treated with oral iron supplements and receive IV iron only when oral iron fails to sustain the serum iron concentration. Oral iron preparations may be considered for chronic kidney disease (CKD) or peritoneal dialysis (PD) patients. Proferrin® (Colorado Biolabs), a heme based oral iron supplement, may work as an alternative to iron salts if they are ineffective or poorly tolerated. Studies indicate that heme iron absorption rates are between 15 and 20 percent without erythropoietin (rHuEPO) therapy and as high as 30 percent with rHuEPO therapy even in patients with high serum ferritin values (>600 ng/ml). In one study, the change in serum iron from Proferrin® was nearly twenty-three times greater than from an identical dose of ferrous fumarate. Read more about oral, injected, or infused iron in chapter 30.

Managing iron overload

Kidney patients who are receiving frequent and regular doses of intravenous iron should be monitored for iron overload. Although serum ferritin is used to determine the levels of tissue iron, its value is affected by inflammation, making it an unreliable test for this purpose. Transferrin is the blood protein that carries iron from the intestine to iron storage sites, and from iron storage sites to the bone marrow. Transferrin is usually about 25 to 35 percent saturated with iron. When saturation of transferrin is greater than 50 percent, transferrin becomes unstable and some iron can get free. Free (unbound) iron increases the risk of infection because harmful pathogens need iron to survive and can proliferate only when there is a ready supply. The ability of some bacteria to cause infection is directly related to their ability to take iron away from transferrin. For more about iron and infection, read chapter 13.

Kidney dialysis patients are not candidates for iron chelation (binding and removal) therapy because of the potential for a serious fungal infection called mucormycosis. According to kidney disease expert Dr. Johan Boelaert, Unit for Renal and Infectious Diseases, Brugge, Belgium, "Desferal® may be problematic mainly because of the possible occurrence of a mucormycosis." In a 1991 *American Journal of Kidney Disease* article "Deferoxamine Therapy and Mucormycosis in Dialysis Patients: Report of an International Registry," Dr. Boelaert discusses his findings of a study of fifty-nine cases of mucormycosis in dialysis patients; 80 percent were receiving iron chelation therapy with Desferal®. Of the 49 dialysis patients who developed this severe infection while on Desferal®, 42 (86 percent) of these cases were fatal.

Iron overload in ESRD patients is an acquired condition caused by repeated iron infusions. This condition is managed by withholding IV iron for a period of time. When serum ferritin is 800 ng/mL or higher, with an accompanying transferrin iron saturation percentage (TS%) of 50 percent or greater, IV iron should be withheld. Iron parameters are remeasured in three months. If the serum ferritin and TS% have fallen, such that the ferritin is less than 800 ng/mL and the TS% percent less than 50 percent, the IV iron can be resumed at smaller doses. Some nephrologists will be even more conservative and not resume intravenous iron, unless the ferritin level is less than 500 ng/mL and the TS% less than 30 percent.

Taking action

Education is key. There are a number of excellent resources from which renal disease patients can learn about the various stages of kidney disease, diet, exercise, therapy, kidney transplantation, and the names of specialists (nephrologists).

Resources
National Kidney Foundation
30 East 33rd St., Suite 1100
New York, NY 10016
Guidelines: Kidney Disease Outcomes and Quality Initiatives
Tel: 800-622-9010
www.kidney.org

American Kidney Fund
6110 Executive Boulevard
Suite 1010
Rockville, MD 20852
Tel: 800-638-8299
Fax: 301-881-0898
Email: helpline@akfinc.org
www.akfinc.org

Kidney & Urology Foundation of America
1250 Broadway, Suite 2001
New York, NY 10001
212-629-9770 or 800-633-6628
Fax 212-629-5652
Email: info@kidneyurology.org

The American Association of Kidney Patients
800-749-AAKP (2257)
Ask for their free pamphlet "The Iron Story"
www.AAKP.org

National Institute of Diabetes and Digestive and Kidney Diseases (NIDDK)
2 Information Way
Bethesda, MD 20892-3570
www.niddk.nih.gov
Use the search feature with words *kidney disease*

National Kidney and Urologic Diseases Information Clearinghouse
3 Information Way
Bethesda, MD 20892-3580
Email: nkudic@info.niddk.nih.gov

Centers for Medicare and Medicaid Services
https://www.cms.hhs.gov/

20

Hemolytic Anemia

"Management of both acquired and hereditary hemolytic anemias is still very unsatisfactory. Often the only decision that can be made is whether to perform a splenectomy. In the future it is hoped that the knowledge that has been gained about these disorders in this century will make available better therapy to our patients in the next."

—E. Beutler, L. Luzzatto, "Hemolytic Anemia,"
Seminars in Hematology, 1999 36:38-47

Navy Master Chief Arthur Callahan did not know what it was like to walk through the Memphis airport metal detector without causing the annoying, and somewhat embarrassing, high-pitched squeal of the security equipment. Arthur dutifully dumped cigarette lighters, keys, pocket change, his watch, and anything else metal onto the tray provided by the attendant. His uniform prompted airport personnel to ask if he had any shrapnel or metal plates in his body. "Nope," Arthur answered as the attendant concluded a full-body examination with a hand-held wand. It would be another ten years before Arthur would get an explanation as to why metal detectors resounded as he passed through their sensors.

In 1988 Arthur was diagnosed with discoid lupus erythematosus, a type of lupus that affects the skin. The dermatologist began treating Arthur with a drug called quinacrine hydrochloride, an antimalarial drug (brand names Atabrine or Mepacrine). After about a year on the drug Arthur had become progressively weaker and very fatigued. These symptoms prompted the dermatologist to refer Arthur back to his family doctor.

His family doctor ran a number of blood tests and determined that Art was anemic and experiencing hemolysis, a condition where red blood cells are prematurely destroyed. Arthur was eventually diagnosed with Glucose-6-phosphate dehydrogenase (G6PD) deficiency, a condition that causes hemolysis as a result of some infectious illnesses or when certain drugs, such as anti-malarial drugs, antibiotics, or alcohol are ingested. The physician instructed Art to immediately stop taking the Atabrine.

Art's older brother, Paul, had been diagnosed with G6PD deficiency more than twenty years earlier, but Art did not realize that it was an inherited disorder. As far back as he could remember, Art had a yellow tint to the whites of his eyes. When he was old enough to drink alcohol, he found that he could tolerate only two drinks before falling asleep. Once, he was put into a Naval hospital because of jaundice. After a time in the hospital, his jaundice cleared up for no apparent reason. Everything would make sense after Art got his diagnosis and began to understand his condition. Alcohol, antibiotics, anti-malarial drugs, Fava beans, and several other substances can trigger hemolysis in a person with G6PD. Jaundice is one of the symptoms of hemolysis. When he drank, he triggered a hemolytic event; when he was put in the hospital he did not drink and the hemolysis stopped.

Arthur's problems were not yet completely solved. Another problem for patients with G6PD is hemosiderosis (iron overload). When his family doctor checked, Arthur's serum ferritin, a test used to determine tissue iron levels, was 2,480 (normal range for an adult male is 25–300). Also, his transferrin iron saturation percentage—another test to determine body iron—was elevated; his was 70 percent (normal is 25–35 percent). Additionally his red blood cells were larger than normal (macrocytic). Art realized that after years of setting off metal detectors in airports it was the condition of hemosiderosis—excess tissue iron—that caused the alarms to sound.

Phlebotomies are used to remove the excess iron and Arthur helps to control his condition with diet and by avoiding certain drugs. He especially watches the amount of red meat he consumes. He educated himself about his condition and has helped others in his family. As a retired U.S. Navy Master

Chief Petty Officer, Arthur Callahan thinks it is fantastic that the military is now routinely screening for G6PD deficiency because often overseas duty requires antimalaria treatment.

Editor's note: Art Callahan lost his battle with iron overload in early 2008. His story is an important one, as it has the potential to help many of the men and women of our United States Armed Forces. Read the Iron Disorders Institute memorial tribute to Art in the third-quarter 2008 newsletter *Nanograms.*

Hemolytic anemia explained

The normal life span of red blood cells (RBC), also known as erythrocytes, is about 120–125 days. New or immature red blood cells, also called reticulocytes, are released from the bone marrow. During their life cycle, red blood cells pick up oxygen-bound iron contained in hemoglobin and travel throughout the body delivering oxygen to every tissue. At the end of the 120–125 days, when the RBCs become old, they are removed from the blood by special white blood cells called macrophages.

Macrophages—present in the liver, lymph nodes, and the spleen—are unique cells that engulf bacteria and consume debris in the blood, such as old red blood cells. When red blood cells become mature they are lysed, which means "to kill." Macrophages are programmed to seek out the old red blood cells and "kill" them by internalizing and digesting. This ability is called phagocytosis. The destruction of red blood cells is called lysis. Lysis is a normal and important part of the red blood cell life cycle and is only problematic when it occurs prematurely or too rapidly.

As the red blood cells are removed, iron and heme are released from the hemoglobin to recirculate back to the liver. The heme portion of hemoglobin is of no further use and is converted to bilirubin, a bile pigment, and excreted by the liver in bile. The iron is stored as ferritin. The destruction of the red cell membrane is called hemolysis. When red cell survival is significantly shortened, hemolytic anemia is the result.

Causes of hemolytic anemia

Hemolytic anemia can occur because of intrinsic factors, extrinsic factors, or red cell metabolism defects. When the cause is intrinsic, hemolysis is due to a defect in the red blood cell itself. This type of hemolytic anemia is often inherited. Examples include beta thalassemia, sickle cell disease, hereditary stomatocytosis, hereditary spherocytosis, and hereditary elliptocytosis.

Extrinsic causes

When hemolytic anemia is caused by extrinsic means, hemolysis is due to something outside the red blood cell. The red blood cells are produced normally and are healthy but are destroyed by

- Infection
- Toxins
- Alcohol
- Medications
- Hypersplenism
- Trauma
- Prosthetic heart valves
- Vascular malformations due to abnormal coagulation within the vascular system
- Severe burns
- High blood pressure—usually due to malignancy
- Hemolytic-uremic syndrome
- "March hemoglobinuria"
- Acquired genetic disorders such as enzyme deficiencies, leukemia, or paroxysmal nocturnal hemoglobinuria (PNH) or
- Autoimmune disease

Some of these conditions are discussed in more detail in other chapters, such as infection, alcohol, leukemia, PNH, and autoimmune disease. However, central to hemolysis is the role of the spleen.

Hypersplenism

The spleen is the largest organ of the lymphatic system—the system that helps our body to fight infections. In an unborn child, the spleen is the source of both red and white blood cells. After birth, the spleen only produces lymphocytes and monocytes, two types of cells essential to defense and keeping the system cleared of debris, such as old red blood cells and bacteria.

When the spleen is enlarged (splenomegaly), it is generally due to the presence of a serious infection or increased hemolysis, where the spleen becomes hyperproductive. This is also called hypersplenism. In some cases a splenectomy, the surgical removal of the spleen, is the only way to slow hemolysis.

Once the spleen has been removed, the patient is more susceptible to infections with germs such as pneumococci, meningococci, H. influenzae, and the parasite that causes malaria. Some physicians will advise patients whose spleens have been removed to take daily doses of penicillin as a preventive measure.

Autoimmune hemolytic anemia (AIHA)

In autoimmune diseases, the body mistakes normal cells for invading pathogens and attacks the normal cells. When this attack is against the red blood cells, the result is autoimmune hemolytic anemia (AIHA). AIHAs are defined as warm-body or cold-body based on the temperature at which the autoantibodies react with red blood cells. Warm-body autoantibodies react at normal body temperature; cold-body autoantibodies react at temperatures below normal body temperature.

Cold-body autoimmune hemolytic anemia is generally associated with infection such as mononucleosis or pneumonia. Warm-body autoimmune hemolytic anemia is generally associated with diseases such as lymphocytic leukemia, autoimmune disease, reactions to drugs or foods, or problems with blood transfusions. One example of this type of anemia is Rh hemolytic anemia, also called erythroblastosis fetalis. In Rh-hemolytic anemia, the trigger is the Rh-factor in the blood.

All blood types are either Rh-positive or Rh-negative. A newborn might inherit an Rh-positive blood type from its father while the mother has an Rh-negative blood type. The mother's immune system can cause an attack on the infant's Rh-positive blood. This reaction is potentially fatal to a newborn.

Rh-immune globulin (RhIG), marketed under various brand names (one example is RhoGAM), is used to prevent the development of these antibodies. This type of product can

be given to Rh-negative expectant mothers as a precaution-
ary measure at twenty-eight weeks into the pregnancy. If the
child is Rh-positive, RhIG is administered within seventy-two
hours after delivery. The U.S. Centers for Disease Control and
Prevention estimates the incidence of Rh-hemolytic anemia to
be one case per 1,000 live born infants.

Sometimes the cause of the AIHA is unknown or idiopathic.
A person may test positive for antibodies on the red blood cells.
This confirms an autoimmune condition is present, but the cause
may not be identifiable. Idiopathic autoimmune hemolytic anemia accounts for one-half of all immune hemolytic anemias.

Microangiopathic hemolytic anemia (MAHA)

Misshapen red blood cells result from traumatic impact or
turbulence in the circulation system. This is commonly seen in
patients with prosthetic heart valves or aneurysms. The RBCs
are fragmented and look like "helmets" or "arrowheads" in
a peripheral blood smear. Blood cell indices in patients with
MAHA might include low hemoglobin, low hematocrit, and low
red cell count, but elevated red cell width (RDW), with a normal
to low mean corpuscu-
lar volume (MCV). B_{12}
deficiencies can mimic
MAHA; therefore B_{12} levels should be checked
in patients where MAHA
is suspect.

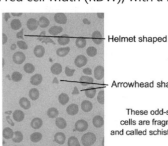

Helmet shaped cells

Arrowhead shaped

These odd-shaped
cells are fragmented
and called schistocytes.

Hemolytic–uremic syndrome (HUS)

This condition is mostly seen in infants, young children, and
pregnant women, although HUS can occur in older children
and adults of either gender.

When someone suffers from HUS, platelet aggregates are
deposited within the kidney's tiny capillaries, impairing function. Eventually, the result is renal failure. The most striking
symptom is the sudden absence of urine production.

HUS frequently occurs after a gastrointestinal (enteric) infection, such as *E. coli* bacteria (*Escherichia coli* O157:H7). HUS has

also been associated with other enteric infections, including shigella and salmonella, and some non-enteric infections.

Inherited hemolytic anemia

Two of the most common types of inherited hemolytic anemia are thalassemia and sickle cell disease. Both of these conditions are hemoglobinapathies (hemoglobin diseases/disorders), and both result in early destruction of red blood cells. Abnormal red cells cannot deliver oxygen efficiently. Abnormal cell shapes seen in peripheral blood smears of patients with hemolytic anemia include spherical (spherocytosis), oval (elliptocytosis), sickle-shaped (sickle cell anemia), fragmented (schistocytes), or mouth-like in appearance (stomatocyte).

Hereditary stomatocytosis (HS) is quite rare, with fewer than a dozen known cases worldwide. In this condition the red blood cell membrane is deficient in a protein called stomatin. This defect allows the outer portion of the red blood cell to leak and to allow excessive sodium and water into the cell, causing the cells to swell. These leaky cells have a distinct appearance under the microscope. "Stomato"

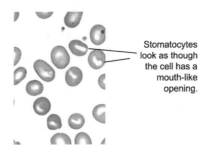

Stomatocytes look as though the cell has a mouth-like opening.

means mouth. A stomatocyte has a "mouthlike" slit, which gets its appearance because of the swelling of the cell. Though the hereditary form of stomatocytosis is rare, the acquired form is often seen in alcoholics.

Intrinsic causes

Hereditary spherocytosis is a condition of abnormal red blood cell membrane. In this condition the red blood cells are spherical rather than concave. Hereditary spherocytosis is a common form of hemolytic anemia

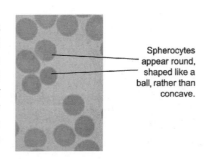

Spherocytes appear round, shaped like a ball, rather than concave.

among whites of northern European descent. In the United States the incidence is about 1 in 5,000 and has been diagnosed at all ages. Hereditary spherocytosis is generally a mild disease but symptoms to watch for, especially in children, include: increased paleness or yellow color of the skin or eyes, complaint of stomach aches or enlarged stomach, fever, vomiting, listlessness or less energy than usual with adequate sleep, decreased appetite, or brown-colored urine.

Hereditary elliptocytosis (HE), also known as ovalocytosis, is a condition in which the red blood cells are oval or elliptical in shape. The condition is found in 1 in 2,000 to 4,000 people. Elliptocytosis is generally benign; however, 10 percent of affected people may experience hemolytic crises where the red blood cells rupture, releasing their hemoglobin. Symptoms such as those listed in hereditary spherocytosis are ones that can alert a person of a hemolytic crisis.

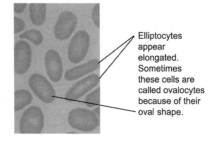

Elliptocytes appear elongated. Sometimes these cells are called ovalocytes because of their oval shape.

Red cell metabolism defects

In the development of the red cell certain proteins or enzymes are necessary to normal formation and function. When these enzymes are deficient normal red blood cell metabolism cannot take place and hemolysis of the cells occurs. Glucose-6-phosphate dehydrogenase (G6PD), pyruvate kinase (PK), or triosephosphate isomerase (TPI) are examples of enzymes that, when deficient, result in hemolytic anemia.

Glucose-6-phosphate dehydrogenase (G6PD) deficiency is an inheritable X-linked recessive disorder, which means that the gene defect occurs on the X chromosome and is usually passed to an affected male by a carrier mother. This condition is estimated to affect about 400 million people worldwide. The highest prevalence rates are found in tropical Africa, the Middle East, tropical and subtropical Asia, Papua New Guinea, and some parts of the Mediterranean.

In the United States, the incidence of G6PD deficiency is

AVOID If *G6PD* Deficient

Analgesics / Antipyretics
acetanilid, acetophenetidin (phenacetin), amidopyrine (aminopyrine), antipyrine, aspirin, phenacetin, probenicid, pyramidone

Antimalarials
chloroquine, hydroxychloroquine, mepacrine (quinacrine), pamaquine, pentaquine, primaquine, quinine, quinocide

Cytotoxic / Antibacterial
chloramphenicol, co-trimoxazole, furazolidone, furmethonol, nalidixic acid, neoarsphenamine, nitrofurantoin, nitrofurazone, para-aminosalicylic acid

Cardiovascular Drugs
procainamide, quinidine

Sulfonamides / Sulfones
dapsone, sulfacetamide, sulfamethoxypyrimidine, sulfanilamide, sulfapyridine, sulfasalazine, sulfisoxazole, sulfapyridine

Miscellaneous drugs:
alpha-methyldopa, ascorbic acid, dimercaprol (BAL), doxorubicin, hydralazine, mestranol, methylene blue, nalidixic acid, naphthalene, niridazole, phenylhydrazine, toluidine blue, trinitrotoluene, urate oxidase, vitamin K (water soluble), pyridium, quinine, thiazolesulfone, toluidine, blue trinitrotoluene (TNT)

Miscellaneous foods:
Fava beans, some people also avoid red wine, all legumes, blueberries [and yogurts containing these], soya products, tonic water, and camphor

Source: G6PD Deficiency Reference Guide
Written by Ramez Ethnasios
(G6PD email: ps98157@itsa.ucsf.edu)
Edited and Set by Chanan Zass
(Favism Site: http://www.rialto.com/favism/)

much higher among African Americans with a heterozygote frequency (carrier state with one normal gene and one abnormal gene) of 24 percent. Approximately 10 to 14 percent of the black male population is affected. The disorder may occasionally affect a few black females to a mild degree (depending on their genetic inheritance). People with the disorder are not normally anemic and display no evidence of the disease until the red cells are exposed to an oxidant or stress. Blood cells of patients with G6PD deficiency can appear blistered when observed under a microscope.

Patients with G6PD deficiency should not take any of the medications that can promote hemolysis (examples provided in the list on the previous page) without consulting a physician. They are encouraged to share this list with their physician or emergent care provider.

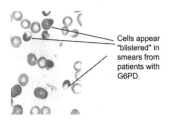

Cells appear "blistered" in smears from patients with G6PD.

Pyruvate kinase is one of the enzymes essential to the relegation of carbohydrate metabolism. Pyruvate kinase deficiency (PKD) is an inherited condition and is the second most common cause of enzymatic-related hemolytic anemia. (G6PD is number one.)

Pyruvate kinase deficiency may produce mild or severe hemolysis and anemia. Problems may first appear in a newborn as prolonged neonatal jaundice and anemia. Older children may be pale (from their anemia) and have intermittent episodes of jaundice. Occasionally PKD is not discovered until adulthood in mild cases. Prevalence of PKD is estimated at fifty-one cases per million and primarily occurs in the Caucasian population.

Triosephosphate isomerase (TPI) deficiency is an extremely rare inherited condition. Fewer than a dozen cases worldwide have been identified. Symptoms of TPI deficiency include severe progressive neuromuscular degeneration, most often first seen in infants around the seventh month of life. These infants have an increased incidence of infection with hemolysis and loss of muscle tone. The condition is mostly seen in persons of African or East Asian heritage.

Congenital dyserythropoietic anemias (CDA) comprise a group of hereditary disorders of red blood cell production. They are considered to be rare diseases, with fewer than 300 cases identified worldwide. The classical types are CDA I, II, and III. Each of these three types has in common a distinct abnormality of structure and form (morphology) of the majority of erythroblasts in the bone marrow. The types differ in inheritance patterns; consequences, such as iron overload, hemolysis, vacuoles (a clear space in the center of a red blood cell that is filled with fluid or air); and the type of morphology observed, such as binuclearity or multinuclearity (more than one nucleus) or fragmentation of the chromatin, which is the colored genetic material within the nucleus than normally remains intact.

CDA II or HEMPAS is the most common of the CDAs. The acronym HEMPAS comes from hereditary erythroblastic multinuclearity with a positive acidified-serum test. This test, which is also referred to as Ham's, is used to diagnose CDA II and another type of anemia called PNH (paroxysmal nocturnal hemoglobinuria) a rare acquired condition that also results in hemolysis.

Patients with CDA II can experience any of the symptoms associated with anemia, such as shortness of breath, weakness, and chronic fatigue. Jaundice can also be seen in these patients due to the increase in bilirubin because of ongoing hemolysis. Piebaldism, which is a lack of color or streak of white hair most commonly in the hair just above the forehead, has been observed in CDA II patients. Cirrhosis, iron overload, gallstones, and enlarged spleen may develop in CDA-II patients.

Findings include a mild microcytic (smaller than normal) anemia, and numerous bizarre and binucleated (two nuclei—normal cells have only one) normoblasts (immature red blood cells found in the red bone marrow), fragmented chromatin (the genetic coloring of a nucleus within the red cell), and the presence of an antigen to the "i red blood cell."

Iron overload occurs in CDA II patients because of ongoing hemolysis. The red cells that are produced are defective and therefore continue to be destroyed prematurely. Despite the existence of ineffective erythropoiesis with mild anemia, treatment with regular phlebotomies, in order to prevent complications of iron overload, is generally well tolerated. Splenectomy may be recommended in some cases, since the spleen plays a major role in this condition.

Blood smear of patient with CDA-II

Image courtesy of Department of Laboratory Medicine and Pathology, University of Minnesota.

fragmented chromatin

vacuoles

multi-nucleated

Congenital erythropoietic porphyria, also known as Gunther's disease, is a rare autosomal recessive disorder of heme synthesis caused by a deficiency of the enzyme uroporphyrinogen III synthetase. The condition is characterized by an accumulation of porphyrins in the bloodstream, causing hemolysis, splenomegaly, and photosensitivity, which can result in blisters or scarring of skin that is exposed to sunlight. Urine, bones, and teeth may appear pink-colored. A few patients with congenital erythropoietic porphyria have been treated successfully by transplantation of bone marrow from a normal donor.

Signs and symptoms of hemolysis

The most striking sign of intravascular hemolysis is hemoglobinuria, which is hemoglobin—free of the red blood cell—in the urine. The presence of the hemoglobin causes the urine to be dark brown or black in color. The patient is often jaundiced—a yellowing of the skin or whites of the eyes. In mild cases of hemolysis, shortness of breath, rapid pulse, weakness, and fatigue appear during or after physical exertion. If hemolysis is severe, shortness of breath, rapid pulse, increased heart rate (tachycardia or palpitations), and fatigue can be present at rest. Some patients complain of abdominal or back pain. Other signs or symptoms can include dizziness, confusion, fever, enlargement of the spleen and liver (splenomegaly and hepatomegaly), heart murmur, and hemoglobinemia (pink to brown colored plasma).

Detecting hemolytic anemia with tests

Specific tests can help to differentiate between the causes of hemolysis. For example, enzymes such as G6PD or pyruvate kinase can be measured directly in blood for deficiencies. For autoimmune related hemolytic anemia, the direct Coombs' test is used. Blood cell indices, which include white blood cells, red cell distribution width (RDW), red cell count, hemoglobin, hematocrit, mean corpuscular volume (MCV), and other tests such as blood and plasma hemoglobin levels, plasma hapto-globin level, reticulocyte count, and lactose dehydrogenase level (LDH) can be part of the analysis. The following chart includes some of the tests that a physician might use to confirm hemolysis is taking place.

Treatment for hemolytic anemia

The treatment and approach to iron replacement is defined by the cause of hemolysis. For example, in PNH and autoimmune hemolytic anemia, iron replacement or blood transfusion can trigger hemolysis; corticosteroids or immunosuppressive drugs are used.

Some hemolytic conditions become so severe that the spleen must be removed in an effort to control hemolysis. Other treatment might involve eliminating the offending agent as in the example of G6PD.

Often folate supplements are advised for patients with hemolytic anemia. Supplemental B_{12} may also be indicated, especially when autoimmune related. Folate can mask a B_{12} deficiency, therefore when checking red cell folate levels, serum B_{12} needs to be checked at the same time. When a physician

cause of anemia	TESTS THAT CONFIRM HEMOLYSIS				
	indirect bilirubin	hemoglobin & red cell count	LDH*	absolute reticulocyte count	haptoglobin
hemolytic anemia	⬆	⬇	⬆	⬇	⬇

*Serum lactose dehydrogenase
Source: http://www.nlm.nih.gov/medlineplus/ency/article/000571.htm

encounters hemolysis, malabsorption, and a folate deficiency, a B_{12} deficiency might be considered. These vitamin deficiencies are not so much the cause as the consequence of chronic hemolytic events.

Some types of hemolytic anemia, such as thalassemia and sickle cell anemia, require repeated blood transfusions. A consequence that patients with hemolytic anemia can experience is iron overload, which can occur as a direct result of hemolysis, as in the rare condition of congenital dyserythropoiesis type II, or from repeated transfusions. In the patient with hemolytic anemia, iron is absorbed normally, but due to ongoing hemolysis, the cells are destroyed and their iron content is dumped back into the system and contained in ferritin, along with the new iron being absorbed. This causes an accumulation of excess iron in the functional cells of organs in the body and is referred to as hemosiderosis. Also patients who receive repeated blood transfusions are acquiring 250 milligrams with each standard unit transfusion, which adds to the excess iron trapped in the body. The excess iron must be removed by phlebotomy or chelation therapy at some point before serious tissue iron overload develops. Vital organs such as the liver, heart, pancreas, and joints are vulnerable to excessively high iron levels and can fail if the iron overload condition is not addressed.

Newer agents such as ecaluzimab for PNH and Rituximab for autoimmune hemolytic anemia are coming into more widespread use.

Resources

There are good resources available about hemolytic anemia, especially through the National Institutes of Health Library of Medicine—www.nlm.nih.gov.

The images in this chapter are courtesy of American Society of Hematology, The National Institutes of Health. We deeply appreciate the rare image of a CDA II blood smear courtesy of Dr. Karen Lafsness, associate professor of hematology, and Phuong L. Nguyen, MD, Department of Laboratory Medicine and Pathology, University of Minnesota. Dr. Lafsness, Hematology Plus CD can be ordered through the department's website: www1.umn.edu/hema/index.html.

21

Sickle Cell Disease

"Sickle cell disease is the most common cause of hemolytic normocytic anemias in children. Because of longevity, this disease is also becoming an increasingly prevalent cause of these anemias in adults."

—John R. Brill, MD, Dennis J. Baumgardner, MD, "Normocytic Anemia,"
American Family Physician, 2000, 62: 2255–64

Deb Hill dropped the phone and raced out the door to her car. With key poised in hand, she was ready to unlock the door, jump into the driver's seat, start the ignition, and get to the school without delay. She was experienced in doing this. Her son Eli has sickle cell disease; so Deb was accustomed to medical emergencies.

The moment she entered the classroom and saw Eli she knew exactly what had happened. Eli was on the floor, and his teacher was supporting his head. Deb dropped to the floor beside her son and embraced him. Eli lay back in her arms drooling; he could not sit up. He was dazed and not himself. Deb looked up at the teacher, who was visibly shaken, and instructed the teacher to call Children's Hospital to let them know that she was on the way.

In the emergency room at Children's, Deb got word that Eli's physician was on his way. Upon arrival, the doctor ordered fluids and a blood transfusion. Deb's fifteen years as a certified medical assistant had taught her enough to know that Eli had experienced a TIA (transient ischemic attack) stroke, or a seizure.

Deb sat near Eli while he got his blood transfusion. She leaned her head back, remembering how Eli had come into her life. He was eight years old when she adopted him. Eli had been abused, neglected, malnourished, and shown very little love. He had suffered a stroke, a bad one, when he was around one year old. His second stroke was believed to have happened when he was about eight. That one caused him to be paralyzed on the left side of his body because he received no medical attention.

Before his adoption and while preparing to take Eli home, Deb read as much as she could about sickle cell disease. She discovered that about 10 percent of all sicklers have strokes. They are delayed in their growth, often contract pneumonia, and many have kidney damage and hypertension. They need fluids like crazy, more than a normal person would care to consume in a day. They need supplemental folic acid for red blood cell production; often their spleens have to be removed—Eli's had been. Sicklers often wet the bed and some lose total control of their bladder and bowel functions; this was true for Eli. Sicklers are stoic little beings. Often they experience excruciating pain when they have a sickling crisis. Most are so used to pain that when they do complain it's definitely serious.

She read (and later learned by experience) that a parent has to learn the child's facial expressions to determine the intensity of the pain. Ibuprofen can be given first; if it works you'll know by the expression. If ibuprofen doesn't work then you try a high-powered prescription for pain. You use this sparingly and pray that the pain will subside. Again you look at the face. If the high-powered prescription pain reliever doesn't work, you get to the hospital immediately for morphine, fluid, and blood. It's the stages of facial expressions that you eventually learn that help you know what to do.

Eli would recover from this stroke, but his medical adventure would continue for some time and include the diagnosis of MoyaMoya disease, another stroke, several surgeries, blood exchanges, and complicated blood transfusions, but all accompanied by an endless stream of wonderful and supportive friends, teachers, physicians, and organizations. Eli is the Iron Disorders Institute ambassador for sickle cell disease and the poster child of bravery and endurance for other children with this disease. While Eli's story is not typical, it does include many rare or unusual consequences that might be experienced by someone with sickle cell disease.

* * *

Sickle cell disease (SCD) is an inherited condition that affects the red blood cells. According to the U.S. Centers for Disease Control and Prevention (CDC), sickle cell disease is one of the most common genetic diseases in the United States. More than 70,000 people have sickle cell disease, and more than 2 million people carry the gene that allows them to pass it on to their children.

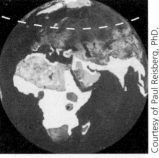
Courtesy of Paul Reisberg, PhD, Wellesley College

The disease was first noted in the United States in the November 1910 issue of *Archives of Internal Medicine*. Dr. James B. Herrick, a Chicago cardiologist, described the disease in his article "Peculiar Elongated and Sickle-Shaped Red Blood Corpuscles in a Case of Severe Anemia."

Screening for sickle cell disease in newborns is currently mandated in all fifty states and the District of Columbia. Within

Sickle   Click Art

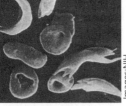
Sickle-shaped cells   Images:NIH

forty-eight hours of a child's birth, a sample of blood is obtained from a "heel stick," and the blood is analyzed for treatable diseases, including phenylketonuria, sickle cell disease, and hypothyroidism. More than 98 percent of all children born in the United States are tested for these disorders. The sample, called a "blood spot," is tested at a state public health or other participating laboratory. CDC's Environmental Health Laboratory evaluates the performance of all participating laboratories (seventy-three domestic and one or more laboratories in fifty-three other nations), ensuring that they analyze the blood spots correctly and providing technical assistance to resolve any diagnostic problems.

Each year, at least 4 million babies in the United States are tested for these diseases; severe disorders are detected in about 5,000 newborns. Accurate screening ensures that

- Affected babies are identified quickly.
- Cases of disease are not missed.
- The number of false-positive results is minimized.
- Early treatment will begin that will prevent negative and irreversible health outcomes for affected newborns.

In the case of sickle cell disease newborn screening, extremely premature infants may have false positive results because the adult hemoglobin is undetectable.

Sickle cell disease is thought to have evolved as a defense against malaria. Persons with sickle cell disease or those who are carriers of sickle cell disease rarely get malaria. Sickle cell disease is most prevalent in areas where there is a high incidence of malaria, such as Africa, India, the West Indies, and the Mediterranean. Areas in white below the dotted line on the map on the previous page indicate where there is a high prevalence of malaria.

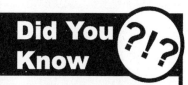

Did You Know ?!?

The reason that babies don't show symptoms of sickle cell disease at birth is because "baby" hemoglobin protects the red blood cells from sickling. At around 4 to 5 months old, the "baby" hemoglobin is replaced by "adult" hemoglobin and the cells begin to sickle.

Source: CDC NCBDDD

Normal red blood cells are disc shaped and contain hemoglobin, which contains iron. Oxygen is attached to iron that is in the hemoglobin. Sickle cells are misshapen and cannot retain oxygen. When sickle cells lose oxygen (become deoxygenated) they bend and change form. These cells become long, pointed, and crescent-shaped like a sickle, which is a tool used to cut down tall grasses or weeds.

A sickling episode and crisis explained

According to doctors of pharmacology Karen F. Marlowe and Michael F. Chicella, "Acute sickle cell pain has been described as more severe than postoperative pain and as intense as cancer pain."

A sickling episode begins when oxygen levels in the body drop due to overexertion, smoking, stress, temperature extremes (fever or hypothermia), or dehydration.

Blood vessel walls narrow. Hemoglobin S cells, which do not contain oxygen at the time (deoxygenated) become rod-like or sickle shaped. A glue-like blood vessel wall protein called thrombospondin helps the sickle-shaped cells to clump together.

These distorted cell clusters cannot get through the constricted blood vessels. This logjam of misshapen cells stabbing into the vessel walls and preventing normal red cells from getting through causes a great deal of pain.

Some normal red blood cells do get through the narrow blood vessels, but not enough to deliver the amount of oxygen needed by organs in the body. The brain, heart, lungs, liver, kidney, bone, and endocrine system all need oxygen to work properly.

Pain from a crisis is most commonly felt in the chest, abdomen, lower back, thighs, hips, and knees. Pain can also occur in the bones and is usually symmetric. Pain often begins at night. Episodes of pain can last for hours or days or even weeks, and usually follow a pattern. Most patients are pain free between episodes, but

OUCHER SCALE

Some children can point to the face that best describes how they feel.

100--- IV fluids and blood transfusion urgently needed

90---

80--- I need to go to the hospital

70---

60--- I need prescribed pain medication

50---

40--- I need pain medication

30---

20--- I hurt a little

10---

0--- I'm okay

Reprinted with permission of Mary Denyes

some patients experience fatigue and symptoms such as numbness or tingling and scleral icterus, which is a yellowing (jaundice) in the white portion of the eye.

Without adequate amounts of oxygen the brain cannot send clear messages to the body systems, so muscles get weak. Inadequate supplies of oxygen also cause the heart not to pump well. The lungs cannot expand and contract, the kidneys and liver cannot clear the body of poisons or metabolize nutrients, the sex organs won't work properly. The bony structure of the larger joints, such as the hips and the shoulders, deteriorates. The entire body system begins to break down. Pain, organ failure, and disease are the consequences.

Some of the deoxygenated sickle cells can be unsickled with oxygen, but repeated sickling and unsickling eventually damages the red cell membrane and the cells die. Premature red cell death (hemolysis) is the cause of the anemia in sickle cell disease.

The blood pH also can contribute to a crisis. The body pH is measured by the acidity or alkalinity of the body. The human body functions best with a blood pH at 7.4. If blood pH is greater than 7.4, the patient has alkalosis or alkalemia. If pH is lower than 7.4, the patient suffers from acidosis or acidemia. If the pH drops below 6.8 or rises above 7.8, death may occur. An acidic pH can initiate a sickling episode and lead to a crisis.

Many things can contribute to changes in body or blood pH. What we eat and drink can have considerable influence on pH. Inadequate fluids, too many sugary foods or soft drinks, too many foods and beverages high in caffeine, not enough fruits and vegetables in the diet, stress, certain medications, tobacco or marijuana smoking, and alcohol consumption are among the culprits that may change the body pH.

Disease can also cause acidosis. Damage to the kidney can reduce the ability of the kidneys to excrete acid, leading to acidosis. Other causes include dehydration due to inadequate intake of fluids or diarrhea, insulin deficiency due to diabetes, or inflammation of the pancreas (pancreatitis).

Once a sickling episode is triggered, events are set into motion within the patient. This cascading chain reaction results in a crisis of extreme pain, sometimes so severe that hospitalization is necessary.

Some small children may not be able to tell a caregiver that they need medical attention. The Oucher scale, developed by Mary J. Denyes, PhD, RN, and Antonia M. Villarruel, and inspired by Judith E. Beyer, PhD, RN, was designed to help young children communicate their degree of pain. Caregivers, teachers, and family members can use a series of photographs to help determine the child's severity of pain. Pointing to the photo of a serene face at the bottom of the scale, the image is described to the child as "not hurt." Continuing up the scale, each photo represents increased pain intensity, such as "a little hurt, a little more hurt, even more hurt, a lot of hurt, or the biggest hurt." The child is asked to answer the question, "How much hurt are you having right now?" by pointing to the picture that best represents their level of pain.

Most at risk for sickle cell disease are people whose ancestors come from Africa, Central America (especially Panama), Caribbean nations, India, Mediterranean countries, Near Eastern countries, or South America. Also at risk is anyone with a family history of sickle cell disease.

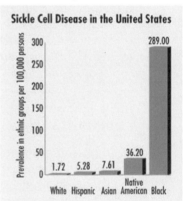

Sickle Cell Disease in the United States

Source: CDC

In the United States, an estimated 10 percent of the black population are carriers of sickle cell disease, and nearly .3 percent have the disease. According to the U.S. Centers for Disease Control and Prevention, three of every 1,000 African Americans have the genes for sickle cell disease.

Genes explained

HBB, or the hemoglobin beta gene, is the gene responsible for sickle cell disease; HBB is on chromosome 11. When the HBB gene is mutated or flawed, it can cause disease.

One HBB gene each is inherited from each parent. If a person inherits two variant (mutated or flawed) copies of this gene, he has sickle cell disease. If he inherits only one variant copy of the gene, he is a carrier of the disease. In other words, he has the sickle cell trait, but not the disease.

Inheritance of Sickle Cell Disease from Parents with Sickle Trait

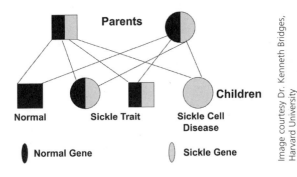

Image courtesy Dr. Kenneth Bridges, Harvard University

Two carriers can pass one variant copy each to their baby who will then develop the disease. For this reason, sickle cell disease is one of the diseases most states in the United States screen for at birth. Currently forty-one states screen all newborns for sickle cell disease and eleven screen infants of parents who are at high risk for the disease.

The common variants of sickle cell disease are homozygous sickle cell disease (hemoglobin SS disease), compound heterozygous sickle hemoglobin C disease (hemoglobin SC disease), and the sickle ß-thalassemias or Hemoglobin Barts, which indicates an alpha thalassemia trait. (Read more about thalassemia in chapter 22.)

People with sickle cell disease may have one or several of the following symptoms, findings, and complications:

Hand-foot syndrome is usually the first symptom of sickle cell disease. Swelling in the hands and feet, often along with a fever, is caused by the sickle cells getting stuck in the blood vessels and blocking the flow of blood in and out of the hands and feet. Other signs, symptoms, or findings include

- Low red cell counts
- Nausea or possible vomiting
- Weakness
- Fatigue
- Jaundice

- Shortness of breath
- Chest pain
- Stomach pain
- Short torso with long arms, legs, fingers, and toes
- Bone pain and damage to the bones
- Enlarged spleen
- Priapism (constant erection)
- Blood in the urine
- Fever
- Stroke
- Leg ulcers
- Eye damage
- Yellow eyes or jaundice
- Early gallstones
- Lung blockage
- Kidney damage and loss of body water into urine
- Blood blockage in the spleen or liver
- Delayed growth
- Frequent infections

In some patients the spleen must be removed in order to stop the chronic (ongoing) hemolysis (breakdown of red blood cells). The spleen traps red blood cells that have survived a normal life cycle, which is about 100–125 days. In anemias caused by chronic hemolysis, the life of the red cell is shortened. The spleen must work harder to recycle the red blood cells. This overwork due to an excess of red blood cells causes swelling and increased function of the spleen. In some, the swelling can be controlled with fluids, but children as young as age four might need to have their spleen removed.

"About 10 percent of children with sickle cell disease have strokes... The peak incidence is between four and six years of age... Although strokes usually occur without warning, they are occasionally preceded by severe headaches or deterioration of school performance. The sudden appearance of a limp in a child with sickle cell disease warrants careful evaluation for a neurologic cause.

—*Doris L. Wethers, MD, St. Luke's-Roosevelt Hospital Center, NY, NY*

Signs that a sickler is in need of prompt medical attention:
- Fever
- Chest pain
- Shortness of breath
- Increasing tiredness
- Abdominal swelling
- Unusual headaches
- Any sudden weakness or loss of feeling
- Pain that will not go away with home treatment
- Priapism (erection that will not go away—very painful)
- Sudden vision change

Diagnosing sickle cell disease
Besides DNA analysis, several tests are used by physicians to detect sickle cell disease.

Sickledex Hgb S is one type of blood test that can detect sickle-shaped cells. This test initially screens for sickle cell disease. If some cells are present, the doctor will perform hemoglobin electrophoresis to confirm the disease.

Hemoglobin electrophoresis identifies abnormal forms of hemoglobin. Each form of hemoglobin is electrically charged and when removed from red blood cells these cells are placed on a special paper and put into an electrical field. Different forms of hemoglobin migrate at different rates and to special locations on the paper. The bands correspond with types of hemoglobin. The quantity of hemoglobin on a specific location helps the physician know the severity of the disease. Sickle cell disease and trait, Hemoglobin C or H disease, and thalassemia major or minor can be detected using hemoglobin electrophoresis.

Persons with SS type have the most serious form of the disease; these patients will have more severe symptoms and are likely to have shorter lifespans. Persons with Barts or one sickle variant and one thalassemia variant may have serious health consequences similar to patients homozygous for SS. Those who have Hemoglobin C disease usually only experience a mild form of the disease, as do the persons with sickle cell trait.

Treatment and management of sickle cell anemia

Management of anemia for patients with sickle cell disease can differ, depending on the age of the person. Whether an adult, adolescent, or child, all sickle cell disease patients should be under the care of a medical team that understands the disease. Spouses, parents, teachers, caregivers, and friends of sicklers should read as much as they can about the disease so that they understand when a sickle cell patient is in need of medical attention and know what to do in these times.

Special attention must be given to any patient with sickle cell disease because complications can occur suddenly and be severe. Strokes and infection are two complications with potential life-threatening consequences. Therefore, preventive strategies such as prophylactic use of antibiotics are vital.

Steps to lower the risk or prevent a sickling episode:

- Avoid temperature extremes, either hot or cold
- Get plenty of fluids. For adults and adolescents: a minimum of three liters of fluids per day. Fluids help blood flow and helps prevent dehydration.
- Eat a balanced diet with lots of fresh fruits and vegetables. These foods are rich in nutrients that improve hemoglobin levels and the absorption of iron from the diet. Plus, most fresh fruits have a high water content and antioxidants, which help control oxidative stress and cell death.
- Take supplements. Some nutrients are difficult to get from the diet and people with sickle cell anemia need daily supplementation of some nutrients and therapeutic doses of others, such as B-complex, folic acid, zinc, and selenium. Always check with your physician about the proper doses for any supplements because doses will be different for patients of different ages, genders, weights, and overall health.
- Get adequate rest. Being too tired can trigger a sickling episode.
- Exercise in moderation; do not over exert.
- Avoid stressful situations or over-excitement.
- Do not smoke tobacco or marijuana or be exposed

to second-hand smoke of either of these products because use or exposure causes constriction of blood vessels (arteries and capillaries).

- If permitted to consume alcohol at all, limit intake to moderate amounts (one drink per day for females; two per day for males). Alcohol robs the body of vitamin B, dehydrates, and can cause liver damage. Some over-the-counter products such as cough syrup contain significant levels of alcohol. Check with your doctor before taking these products.

- Avoid caffeine. Caffeine is a diuretic, or a substance that makes you lose body fluids; if you lose fluids you may become dehydrated. For every cup of caffeine-containing beverage (coffee, tea, cola) consumed, a person needs about two cups of water or two servings of fruit to replace lost fluids.

Exercise for people with sickle cell disease

Some patients with sickle cell disease can do mild to moderate exercise without triggering an episode of sickling.

Not recommended: High-impact sports such as running, jogging, gymnastics, or tennis because they can result in bleeding in the joints. Contact sports such as football, wrestling, boxing, soccer, hockey, and basketball are also not recommended. Other strenuous sports such as softball, some forms of dancing, rowing, hiking, rappeling, skating, skateboarding, weight lifting, or judo should be discussed with your physician, as participation in these activities must be evaluated individually.

Recommended, depending on the condition of the bones such as the ankles, knees, and hips: Swimming, walking, aerobic walking, cycling, cross-country skiing, some forms of dancing, golf, gardening, and some resistance exercise.

Therapies and iron balance

Addressing the anemia that occurs in sickle cell disease patients is not as simple as taking extra iron pills or eating an iron rich diet. Most sickle cell patients with anemia are given routine blood transfusions with accompanying iron chelation to remove the excess iron that builds up as a result of these transfusions.

BLOOD EXCHANGE

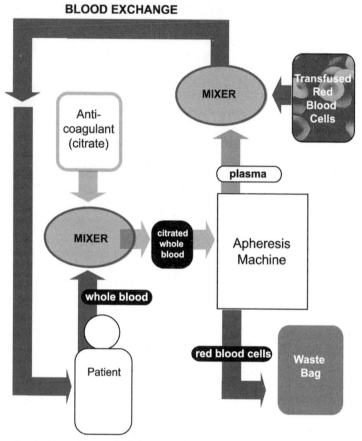

Blood exchange image adapted with permission:
Nifong TP, Gerhard GS, Bongiovanni MB. Mathematical modeling and computer
simulation of erythrocytapheresis for sickle cell disease. Transfusion. 2001;41(2):256-63.

Blood transfusion

Humans must have sufficient red blood cells to survive. Because
one consequence of sickle cell disease is a severe reduction
of red blood cells, blood transfusion is needed as a source of
healthy red blood cells. However, blood transfusion is a bit
more complicated for the sickle cell disease patient. Not only
is a blood type match needed but the donor blood must also
contain an anti-antibody. Anti-antibodies are specific to race.

Therefore, the hospital or treatment center has to find African American donors with blood types that match and that are without sickle-cell disease. Screening for this type of blood is very expensive. A sickle cell patient needing a blood transfusion usually must give twenty-four hours advance notice.

Reminder: September is National Sickle Cell Awareness Month; this is a great time to encourage eligible friends and family members to donate blood. Source: National Health Observances, www.healthfinder.gov/library/nho/nho.asp.

Iron chelation

Consequential to blood transfusion is a build-up of excess iron. Each standard unit of blood contains about 250 milligrams of iron. Iron is not easily excreted by the body and must be removed pharmacologically with chemicals formulated to bind specifically to iron. This therapy is needed to avoid organ damage, disease, or premature death caused by excessive iron build-up in the heart, liver, endocrine glands, and synovium. Read more about iron chelation therapy in chapter 33.

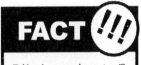

FACT !!!

Taking iron supplements will not help people with sickle cell disease. This type of anemia is not caused by too little iron in the blood; it's caused by not having enough red blood cells. In fact, taking iron supplements could harm a person with sickle cell disease because the extra iron builds up in the body and can cause damage to the organs.

Source: CDC NCBDDD

Besides blood transfusion and iron chelation therapy physicians may also prescribe:

- Painkillers (over-the-counter or prescribed) as needed
- Prophylactic penicillin to prevent serious infection such as pneumonia starting at two months of age and continuing until age six
- Medication such as nitric oxide, which can dilate blood vessels (hydroxyurea), sometimes in combination with EPO (erythropoietin)
- PCV—A special pneumococcal vaccine (called 23-valent pneumococcal vaccine) at two and five years of age (pneumococcal conjugate vaccine)

- Flu vaccine (influenza vaccine) every year after six months of age
- Meningococcal vaccine, if recommended by a doctor

Women with sickle cell disease are more likely to have problems during pregnancy that can affect their health and the health of their unborn baby. During pregnancy, the disease can become more severe and pain episodes can occur more frequently. A pregnant woman with sickle cell disease is at a higher risk of preterm labor and of having a low birthweight baby. However, with early prenatal care and careful monitoring throughout pregnancy, women with sickle cell disease can have a healthy pregnancy.

During pregnancy, there is a test to find out if the baby will have sickle cell disease, sickle cell trait, or neither one. The test is usually done after the second month of pregnancy. The risk of miscarriage is increased in procedures where genetic information is obtained from the amniotic fluid, which is the watery fluid that surrounds the developing fetus. If considering this type of testing discuss the risks with a qualified medical professional. Women with sickle cell disease might want to see a genetic counselor to find information about the disease and the chances that sickle cell disease will be passed to the baby.

Did You Know ?!?

February is the month Iron Disorders Institute asks that African Americans donate blood. Please help a child with sickle cell anemia who needs repeated blood transfusions by giving the gift of life.

Blood exchange described

Many of the serious manifestations of sickle cell disease, including acute chest pain syndrome and stroke, are due to poor blood flow and the aggregation of rigid sickled red blood cells due to the presence of hemoglobin S (HbS). Patients with sickle cell disease usually have baseline HbS levels of about 80 percent. The prevention and immediate treatment of these clinical complications often include simple transfusion or red blood cell exchange therapy (RBCX) to lower the concentration of HbS-containing red blood cells. When performing a transfusion or RBCX for the initial treatment of sickle cell disease, the primary goal is to decrease the HbS to a prescribed level, usually less than 30 percent, to improve the clinical complications.

With simple transfusion the total amount of red blood cells in the patient is increased with each transfusion, diluting the fraction of HbS-containing red blood cells. The total increase in the amount of red blood cells in the patient limits the amount of transfusion that can be given. Since the total amount of red blood cells in the patient can be kept at a constant level with RBCX, the HbS level can be reduced much more than with simple transfusion. RBCX is performed using an "apheresis machine" to separate and remove red blood cells from the patient while simultaneously replacing them with red blood cell transfusions (see illustration on page 248). The blood is removed through either a peripheral intravenous catheter (IV) or a centrally placed catheter, mixed with citrate to prevent the blood from clotting, and pumped into the apheresis machine. Within the apheresis machine the red blood cells are separated from the plasma by centrifugal force. The separated red blood cells are pumped into a waste bag, while the remainder of the patient's blood is mixed with banked red blood cells, warmed, and returned to the patient through another peripheral IV catheter or a separate port in the centrally placed catheter.

For patients on chronic transfusion programs, a primary goal is to not allow the patient's HbS level to rise above a prescribed threshold, while minimizing the risks of over-transfusion. The goal of keeping the HbS below a certain level can be accomplished by either RBCX or simple transfusion. Although both simple transfusion and RBCX are effective for preventing severe complications of sickle cell disease, these regimens are associated with iron overload, potential exposure to transfusion-transmitted infectious diseases, immunization to "foreign" blood proteins (alloimmunization), and allergic reactions. Iron overload is directly related to the amount of excess red blood cells administered as described above. The risks of transfusion-associated infectious disease, alloimmunization, and allergic reactions are directly related to the number of donor exposures.

Iron overload, one of the major complications associated with chronic transfusion regimens, can be reduced by the use of RBCX versus simple transfusion, since blood is removed and replaced rather than simply added. However, RBCX tends to require more banked red blood cell units, increasing the risks of transfusion-associated infectious disease, alloimmunization, and allergic reactions. Also, the blood exchange procedure is more costly than the blood transfusion.

Cures

Bone Marrow Transplantation (BMT) and Gene Therapy.
The only known cure for sickle cell disease is bone marrow/stem cell transplant. The cure rate is 70 to 90 percent; unfortunately only about 10 to 20 percent of patients find a compatible marrow donor. When there is a match, most times the donor is a sibling, but in some cases the donor may not be related. Often donors are located through marrow donor registries such as the National Bone Marrow Registry.

Gene therapy is the newest frontier where cures to diseases such as sickle cell disease may be found. GT is highly experimental and carefully regulated because of the many unknown consequences. Investigators have used gene therapy successfully to cure mice with sickle cell disease, but the approach would be toxic to humans.

Read more about transfusion, bone marrow transplantation, and gene therapy in chapter 31.

Resources
Contact Iron Disorders Institute for the full reprint of Eli's story or contact the Hill family directly:
Deb Hill
2305 Sam Houston St.
Knoxville, TN 37920
Email: Hillgangintn@aol.com

To obtain copies of the Oucher Scale go to:
www.oucherscale.org
www.oucher.org/the_scales.html

Read more about MoyaMoya:
www.ninds.nih.gov/disorders/moyamoya/moyamoya.htm

For more information about sickle cell disease:
www.cdc.gov/ncbddd/sicklecell/default.htm
sickle.bwh.harvard.edu/malaria_sickle.html
www.sicklecellsociety.org/information/prenatal.htm
www.sicklecelldisease.org
www.ascaa.org/support_groups.asp
www.noah-health.org
www.cdc.gov/genomics
www.wellesley.edu
www.stjude.org/

For more information about bone marrow donation:
National Marrow Donor Program www.marrow.org/

For information about screening:
www.ahrq.gov/clinic/USpstf/uspshemo.htm
www.cdc.gov/nceh/dls/newborn.htm

Test your knowledge about SCD
National Center on Birth Defects and Developmental Disabilities (NCBDDD)
www.cdc.gov/ncbddd/sicklecell/quiz/default.htm

22

Thalassemia

"The story of thalassemia is still being told. We have come so far from the heartbreaking days when children born with thalassemia major rarely lived past infancy. The medical advances of the past decades have enabled people with thalassemia to live longer, healthier and fuller lives. But there is more—much more—to be done. The Cooley's Anemia Foundation is committed to improving the care of thalassemia patients until a universal cure is found. Then, and only then, can the book on thalassemia be closed."

— *Gina Cioffi, Esq., Executive Director, Cooley's Anemia Foundation*

Even though Karen was nearly twenty years older than eight-year-old Gargi, Gargi referred to Karen as her "special friend." Gargi, now twenty-eight, remembers things about Karen that at the time didn't make sense. Karen used to drink Diet Pepsi; she still lived at home; and her dad always came with her to the treatment center where she and Gargi got blood transfusions. Besides their friendship, they shared the experience of an inherited blood disorder called thalassemia major. The disorder is one of abnormal hemoglobin production, and people with thalassemia require frequent blood transfusions to survive.

Karen and Gargi spent many hours together on the pediatric floor of a private hospital in New Jersey. Every two weeks

Did You Know ?!?

Fifty percent of patients with thalassemia major die of a heart attack before the age of thirty-five, primarily due to iron-related heart failure.

they received their transfusions in a converted waiting room. They were companions for the day since a transfusion of two units takes four to five hours to complete. On one trip to the hospital Karen was not there. Gargi learned that Karen had died of heart failure, a common cause of death in people with thalassemia major.

Gargi realizes how similar her life could be to Karen's. She understands now that Karen drank diet products because she had developed diabetes as an adolescent because of iron damage to the pancreas—a problem not uncommon in thalassemia. Gargi also developed diabetes when she was sixteen.

Prior to the approval of a drug called Desferal® (deferoxamine) in the late 1970s, iron overload was the reason that most children with thalassemia died in their late teens to early twenties. When Gargi was first diagnosed in 1975, her parents feared the worst when they got the grim news. Her diagnosis of thalassemia had eluded doctors for a while because the disorder was easily confused with other conditions such as iron-deficiency anemia.

Her mother says that as a toddler Gargi stopped laughing and walking and reverted to crawling. Originally doctors thought that she had iron-deficiency anemia and she was given iron pills. These failed to work and the doctors pursued other tests, including tests to rule out leukemia. Eventually the doctors performed hemoglobin electrophoresis and a bone marrow biopsy that provided the diagnosis of thalassemia major when Gargi was seventeen months old. (Note: Bone marrow biopsy isn't necessary to diagnose thalassemia, though it could be needed to rule out some alternatives for some cases.)

The diagnosis came as a complete shock to Gargi's parents as they had never heard of this disorder before. What was even more confusing for them was the idea that this disease came from both of them, and that other family members likely had the condition. Thalassemia is a genetic disorder that is recessive; therefore both parents must be "carriers" in order to pass the disease on to their child. A single copy of an abnormal globin gene, which can be caused by any of hundreds of varieties of mutations, by itself does no harm. However, when two abnormal genes are present, the red cell doesn't have enough hemoglobin to carry oxygen to cells of the body.

Gargi's first experience with chelation therapy began when she was seven. At the time (the early 1980s) she had to stay in the hospital for an entire week so that doctors could monitor her iron excretion and tolerance to the drug Desferal®. Gargi thought the doctor was joking about having to sleep with a needle in her stomach all night. Frightened and skeptical, she absolutely refused to participate in this "experimental" therapy. Gargi's father, in an effort to convince her that the procedure was not painful, pulled his shirt up and stuck the needle in himself. A wide-eyed Gargi, seeing him tolerate the pain and hearing him say that he would stick himself every day if necessary, reasoned that if he could do it then so could she.

Her only problems with therapy occurred when she was a teenager. Desferal® ideally is infused over an eight- to twelve-hour period of time as often as seven days a week, if the iron overload is severe. Desferal® is given at night when the patient tends to move around less and because the infusion takes about eight hours. Initially, Gargi received Desferal® five nights a week for eight-hour infusions. As she got older she slept less and less and often didn't allow the Desferal® treatment to run the full eight hours. Additionally, she started to have social engagements on Friday and Saturday nights, and she would come home late and not want to do Desferal® at all. Issues of how treatment would interfere with vacation or when staying overnight at a friend's house began to grow in importance.

Gargi was confused, frustrated, and scared. Iron overload is fatal, and people with thalassemia know it. Still, compliance to her therapy was a problem for her. Besides the social limitations, administration of Desferal® can be very painful. After the infusion is over people are often left with a swollen infusion site surrounded by an inflamed rash. Also, Desferal® can remain under the skin and not be absorbed. This is because it is a very large molecule that does not form a solution easily. This causes painful swelling and scar tissue. Further, there is no immediate positive result from the Desferal® treatment. It takes months for many patients to feel better. Together all of these problems can deter the most compliant and determined patient from having their treatment.

Gargi remembers her experience as a roller coaster of compliance and non-compliance. There were many periods of time when she ignored Desferal® altogether, pretending that thalassemia didn't even exist in her life. She recalls a scene when her parents were in her bedroom and opened her dresser drawer where she kept her chelation products. The horrified but scared look on their faces is something she will never forget. They realized that there were weeks and months where Gargi had ignored her treatment.

Today, Gargi is an advocate for people with thalassemia. She has served as a volunteer for the Cooley's Anemia Foundation, and is presently pursuing a career in law. She was recently awarded a fellowship program from the prestigious New York/New Jersey–area law firm Gibbons, Del Deo, Dolan, Griffinger, and Vecchione. Gargi continues to receive blood transfusions twice a month and Desferal® five times a week, twelve hours per treatment. She says if there is one thing she hopes to impress upon people it is to remain compliant. She realizes that it is difficult to expect a person to trust in a medication, especially when they see their friends, older and younger, die around them. Until other therapies are available, however, chelation is the only way to prolong life for people with thalassemia.

Thalassemia explained

Thalassemia is an inherited disorder. It is sometimes called Mediterranean anemia, or Cooley's anemia, named after the physician who first diagnosed it. Thalassemia is a hemoglobinopathy, which is any disorder of the hemoglobin. In some types of thalassemia, red blood cells are destroyed prematurely, which results in simultaneous anemia and iron overload. Excess iron that is released from the prematurely destroyed red blood cell collects in the tissues of major organs such as the liver, joints, pancreas, pituitary, and the heart. Iron overload is further increased because of the repeated blood transfusions needed to treat the anemia.

Thalassemia is commonly found in people of Mediterranean, Southeast Asian, South Asian, Middle Eastern, Chinese, and Caribbean origins. It is a disease that arose in areas of the world where malaria is endemic. In Southern Africa as a result of malaria, people developed sickle cell anemia, and in Asia and the Mediterranean people developed thalassemia. Because of increased immigration to the United States and because of inter-marriage, thalassemia is increasing in newly immigrant popula-tions as well as becoming common in other ethnicities such as Hispanics and Latinos.

The genes involved are those that control the produc-tion of proteins known as globins, contained in hemoglobin. Hemoglobin productions involve two sets of genes on dif-ferent chromosomes, which produce two different pairs of proteins. One set is alpha, the other is beta. Each hemoglobin molecule contains these sets of proteins: two alpha and two beta. Hemoglobin properly binds and releases oxygen when two alpha proteins are connected with two beta proteins. The gene for alpha globin is located on chromosome 16, and the gene for beta globin is located on chromosome 11. Depending on the makeup of genes inherited from the par-ents, thalassemia occurs when one or more of the genes fails to produce protein.

When the beta globin gene is defective, beta thalassemia results; when the alpha globin gene is defective, alpha thalas-semia results. If one of the beta globin genes is defective, the amount of beta globin in the cell is nearly normal; this condition is called thalassemia minor. If both genes are defective, no beta globin protein is produced; this condition is thalassemia major. (Sometimes the clinical symptoms of a person with both defec-tive genes are not quite so dire, resulting in a condition known as thalassemia "intermedia"—between major and minor.)

E-beta thalassemia is a hemoglobinopathy (disorders charac-terized by structural alteration of globin chains). E-beta thalas-semia is caused by one beta globin mutation and Hemoglobin E (a structural variant of beta globin). This combination of genes causes an intermediate form of hemolytic anemia.

People most at risk for thalassemia major or minor or interme-dia are those of Mediterranean (Greek, Italian), Middle Eastern, African, Indian, and Southeast Asian descent. Hemoglobin E is more common in southeast Asians, especially in Cambodia, Laos, and Thailand.

Patients with thalassemia major might become symptomatic

as infants. In the first year or two of life and in the absence of transfusion, a child can demonstrate severe anemia and expansion of the facial and other bones. These children may be pale or jaundiced, have a poor appetite, fail to grow normally, or have an enlarged spleen, liver, or heart.

Diagnosing thalassemia

To differentiate between iron deficiency and beta thalassemia trait, the red blood cell indices can be helpful. The hemoglobin concentration and the red cell count will generally be lower in iron deficiency. The distinguishing finding in beta thalassemia is a hemoglobin electrophoresis with the finding of elevated Hgb A2 and F. Both will be increased in beta thalassemia trait without iron deficiency and will be normal or decreased in alpha thalassemia and isolated iron-deficiency anemia. There are several formulas to help in office screening, but they are also based on the assumption that the child is not iron deficient. Usually iron deficiency can be ruled out using free erythrocyte protoporphyrin (FEP), transferrin saturation, or ferritin as a screening test in children who have a hypochromic microcytic anemia.

The Mentzer index was developed to help distinguish thalassemia from iron deficiency. It is calculated by dividing the red blood cell (RBC) count into the mean corpuscular volume (MCV).

Mentzer Index = MCV / RBC

Index <13 = Thalassemia
Index >13 = Iron-Deficiency Anemia

MCV Cutoffs for Microcytic Anemia	
Age in years	Cutoff
1-2	<77 fl
3-5	<79 fl
6-11	<80 fl
12-15	<82 fl
>15	<85 fl

Source: US Centers for Disease Control & Prevention
American Academy of Family Physicians

If the quotient is less than 13, thalassemia is more likely, and if the quotient is greater than 13, iron deficiency is more likely.

Often, a physician will look only at the MCV in order to rule out the presence of thalassemia trait. In general, if the MCV is greater than 80, the individual does not carry trait; if it is less than 80 and the individual is not iron deficient, s/he may be a thalassemia trait carrier. Further tests—

hemoglobin electrophoresis and quantification of hemoglobin A2 and hemoglobin F—can then help to determine if the individual is indeed a trait carrier.

Hemoglobin electrophoresis identifies abnormal forms of hemoglobin. Thalassemia major or minor, sickle cell disease and trait, and Hemoglobin C or H disease can be detected using electrophoresis.

Thalassemia minor occurs in heterozygotes, or those who carry the thalassemia trait. These individuals are mostly asymptomatic, although some may experience an occasional mild anemia. People with thalassemia intermedia fluctuate between being asymptomatic and having symptoms as severe as those associated with thalassemia major. Diagnosis of thalassemia intermedia is usually made after a period of observation; the decision to transfuse is often a complex one.

Anyone of Mediterranean, Middle Eastern, Southeast Asian, South Asian, Chinese, or Caribbean descent of childbearing age should be tested to see if they are a carrier, so that they can make informed decisions about family planning.

Treatment and iron management

Patients with the more serious forms of thalassemia require repeated blood transfusions. Each unit of blood contains about 250 milligrams of iron. Iron cannot be excreted by the body; therefore, excesses that are gotten from the repeated transfusions are stored in vital organs along with the iron present because of hemolysis. The excess iron can cause an entire host of secondary complications for people with thalassemia, including heart failure, liver disease, diabetes mellitus, hypothyroidism, and hypoparathyroidism.

Aggressive monitoring of body iron burden is key to the survival and well-being of a chronically transfused patient. There are several methods of iron assessment. The easiest, most affordable, and most common method is a serum ferritin test. This involves drawing a small sample of blood and testing for its ferritin content, which is an important iron-storage protein. Ferritin tests are useful for measuring gross iron overload or dramatic reduction in iron levels, but are limited when attempting to finely measure actual organ storage of iron. Several factors can affect test results: inflammation or infection of the liver, liver disease (such as fibrosis or hepatitis), hemolysis or breakdown of red blood cells during the blood draw or due to rough handling of the sample, vitamin C deficiency, or even too much alcohol the night before a test. Ferritin tests remain an approximation rather than an accurate indicator of iron stores.

A second method of measuring body iron burden is the liver biopsy, a direct sampling of iron loaded tissue. The method is an invasive procedure, sometimes involving a short hospital stay. As a result, many patients are reluctant to get a liver biopsy and are worried about its safety. However, a recent study from Italy, where thalassemia is extremely prevalent, showed that of 1,000 patients biopsied over five years, no complications occurred. This is due in part to improved ultrasound technology, which allows physicians to see the liver before the procedure.

A third, very accurate method of measuring iron is through MRI-based technologies, utilizing measurement techniques known as "R2" and "T2." R2 measurements provide a picture of the amount of iron in the liver, while T2* helps to assess cardiac damage related to iron overload.

In the United States, there are currently two approved iron chelators for use in removing transfusional iron overload. Desferal® (deferoxamine) is prescribed for administration via subcutaneous infusion, typically over an eight- to twelve-hour period, five to seven nights per week. In 2005, an oral chelator, Exjade® (deferasirox), was approved. Exjade is a pill that the patient dissolves in water or juice and drinks, and is designed to be administered once a day.

Outside of the United States, a second oral chelator, Ferriprox® (deferiprone), is available in many countries. Ferriprox® has been used both as a monotherapy and in combination with Desferal®. As of this writing, Ferriprox® has not been approved by the U.S. Food and Drug Administration for use in the United States.

Experimental therapies

Bone marrow transplantation has resulted in a cure for some patients with thalassemia major. Italian investigators studied the reversibility of cirrhosis in six patients who were cured of thalassemia with bone marrow transplantation. When they compared liver biopsies of these patients done prior to and following transplantation, the reversal of cirrhosis in these patients was confirmed. Bone marrow transplantation procedure is complicated as exact marrow matches are needed for the procedure. Also there are risks and post-transplantation consequences such as infection due to the immunosuppressive medications used and possible rejection.

Gene therapy is also being investigated as a possible curative approach, following successful experiments in curing thalassemia in animal models. One Phase I trial was recently launched in Europe, and it is thought that several laboratories in the United States will soon be in the position to begin Phase I trials.

One of the most critical issues that families with thalassemia face is compliance with therapy. For those on Desferal®, the routine nightly process of using the pumps can become tiresome, especially for young patients, and they may opt to disregard instructions and skip doses. This practice seriously increases the risk of early heart failure, as well as the development of other serious complications. Similarly, some patients experience similar compliance issues with Exjade®, which can also lead to serious complications.

Patients who follow therapy as prescribed and who observe diets that can reduce the amount of iron absorbed increase the potential for longer life expectancy and better quality of life.

Contact the Cooley's Anemia Foundation to learn more about thalassemia, emerging therapies, patient support, and how to locate a major thalassemia treatment center.

Resources

For more information about thalassemia contact:

Cooley's Anemia Foundation
330 Seventh Ave., #900
New York, NY 10001
800-522-7222
Tel: 212-279-8090
Fax: 212-279-5999
www.cooleysanemia.org
info@cooleysanemia.org

Thalassemia Action Group (TAG)
330 Seventh Ave., #900
New York, NY 10001
800-522-7222
Email: TAG@cooleysanemia.org

Thalassemia Treatment Centers in the United States:

Children's Healthcare of Atlanta
404-785-3614
www.choa.org

Children's Hospital and Research Center at Oakland
510-428-3347
www.thalassemia.com

Children's Hospital, Boston
617-355-8246
www.childrenshospital.org

Children's Hospital, Los Angeles
323-361-4132
www.childrenshospitalla.org

Children's Hospital, Philadelphia
215-590-2197
www.chop.edu

Children's Memorial Hospital, Chicago
773-880-4618
www.childrensmemorial.org

Children's Medical Center, Dallas
214-456-6102
www.childrens.com

Texas Children's Hospital, Houston
832-822-4242
www.texaschildrens.org

Weill Medical College of Cornell University
212-746-3404
www.med.cornell.edu

Portions of this chapter were generously provided by the Cooley's Anemia Foundation and the Children's Hospital Oakland website: www.thalassemia.com.

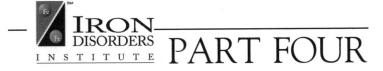

PART FOUR

Uncommon and Rare Causes
of Anemia

23

Aplastic Anemia

"Aplastic anemia can strike anyone of any age, sex, race, or gender, anywhere in the world."

—*Aplastic Anemia & MDS International Foundation, Inc.*

At the age of twenty-five, Adrian Menapace first noticed symptoms that would eventually lead to a diagnosis of aplastic anemia. While playing tennis, Adrian felt as though she could not catch her breath. She began to see black spots in front of her eyes. Thinking that she might be iron deficient, she made an appointment for a medical checkup. Upon seeing the results of her complete blood count, Adrian's physician immediately admitted her to the hospital—all of the counts were dangerously low.

Over the next week, Adrian experienced a confusing and worrisome array of procedures and medical terminology, with little explanation of what was happening. She received many units of platelets and packed red blood cells and was told that she might be "pre-leukemic." A CAT scan showed a mass in the abdomen, which might be a malignant tumor that would require resection of various organs.

A laparoscopy revealed that this "mass" was actually a harmless blood clot. Finally, a bone marrow biopsy was suggestive of aplastic anemia.

Parts of this chapter reprinted with permission of Aplastic Anemia & MDS International Foundation, Inc., from Aplastic Anemia: Basic Explanations, *contributors: Dr. Neal Young of the National Institutes of Health, Dr. Bruce Camitta of the Medical College of Wisconsin, and Dr. Yvette Ju. © 2002 by Aplastic Anemia & MDS International Foundation, Inc.*

Adrian was told that, at her age, a bone marrow transplant offered the best hope for survival. However, neither of her siblings were matches. In 1987, antithymocyte globulin (ATG) had recently ceased to be an experimental drug for treatment of aplastic anemia, and cyclosporine was not yet in common use. Adrian was treated in the hospital with a twelve-day course of ATG and high-dose prednisone. Throughout this period, seeking a better understanding of her condition, Adrian read what medical literature she could find on aplastic anemia. She grilled every medical professional she came in contact with but found the statistics and much of the feedback from doctors to be very discouraging.

The response to ATG was gradual. Transfusions continued along with Decadron, but after three months the blood counts had not improved. However, four to six months after ATG therapy, the blood counts began to rise very slowly. Nine months after therapy the red cells, platelets, and white cells were approaching the lower limits of normal range. At this time Adrian returned to work.

Adrian was fortunate in that she did not require further treatment or transfusions and has been able to lead a normal life for the past fourteen years. She recalls how many things have changed since her diagnosis and treatment. Facing the challenge of this illness brought her family closer together. It also changed some of her personal ideas about what is important in life.

Eventually, Adrian went back to school and earned a nursing degree. In this role her personal experiences with the health-care system continue to serve others who are newly diagnosed. She points out that patients today face more encouraging prospects than she did fifteen years ago. Hematologists have refined BMT (bone marrow transplantation) and medications such as ATG and cyclosporine. New and adjuvant therapies, such as Epogen® and Neupogen®, still in developmental stages when she was diagnosed, are now readily available.

Also, newly diagnosed patients have access to sources of support and information that were not nearly as available fifteen years ago. AA&MDSIF provides literature, information on treatment decisions, and patient support services so that no one with this diagnosis need feel confused and isolated.

Adrian is encouraged by the progress being made in the medical and scientific community, which promises more refinements and developments in the near future. As a volunteer patient contact, Adrian Menapace often speaks with newly diagnosed patients over the phone. She says she is happy and grateful to be able to provide encouragement by sharing her story.

Aplastic anemia explained

Aplastic anemia (AA) was identified in 1888 when distinguished German pathologist Dr. Paul Ehrlich studied the case of a pregnant woman who died of bone marrow failure. The term "aplastic anemia" was first used in 1904. Aplastic anemia is relatively unusual and most hematologists have only seen a few cases.

In aplastic anemia the body stops making enough of all three types of blood cells: red cells, which contain hemoglobin and deliver oxygen throughout the body; white cells, which help fight infections; and platelets, which help clot our blood when we are bleeding.

Within the bone marrow, a red spongy substance in the center of the bones, are stem cells that manufacture these three types of blood cells. Stem cells are also able to replace themselves as needed by creating exact duplicates of themselves. Normally our bone marrow is like a factory churning out as many blood cells as we need. For example, if we get infections, the bone marrow steps up production of white cells. If we start bleeding, then it makes more platelets.

In patients with aplastic anemia there are not enough stem cells in the bone marrow. In most cases, the immune system has turned against the marrow and destroyed the stem cells. Aplastic anemia is thus an autoimmune disease with similarities of pathophysiology to diseases in childhood like diabetes, ulcerative colitis, and multiple sclerosis. New stem cells are no longer being produced, and the remaining stem cells are working less effectively, so the levels of red cells, white cells, and platelets begin to drop. If the levels drop too low this can result in fatigue and anemia (low red cells); bleeding in the skin, mouth, and from the nose; or heavy periods (low platelets); and/or an increase in the number and severity of infections (low white cells).

Symptoms

Listed below are some symptoms of aplastic anemia; however, experiencing one or more of these does not necessarily indicate that you have the disease since all of these symptoms can occur with other conditions. It is essential to consult a physician for a professional diagnosis.

- Increased bleeding
- Bruising
- Petechiae (pinpoint red spots on the skin)
- Increased susceptibility to infections
- Shortness of breath
- Fatigue
- Decreased alertness
- Shortened attention span
- Unusually pale skin color
- Dizziness
- Lingering illness

One problem that affects over one-half of all aplastic anemia patients is paroxysmal nocturnal hemoglobinuria (PNH). There is lab evidence that PNH exists in most aplastic anemia cases without showing symptoms. In PNH red blood cells are broken down by the body, with the products of this breakdown appearing in the urine.

Aplastic anemia and myelodysplastic syndromes (MDS)—similarities and differences

There are many similarities between aplastic anemia and myelodysplastic syndromes (MDS), and patients share many of the same symptoms. Both groups suffer from anemia and reductions in the number of platelets and white blood cells. However, aplastic anemia is more prevalent among young people, while the incidence of MDS increases with age. Some aplastic anemia patients progress into myelodysplastic syndromes.

Physicians sometimes have difficulty initially telling the two apart. One type of MDS, the hypoplastic form (hypoplastic referring to a decrease in cell growth), looks very similar to severe aplastic anemia. A hematologist—a doctor who specializes in blood disorders and is experienced in treating these diseases—can usually determine which one is present by careful examination of the marrow cells.

The biggest difference between the two diseases is that in aplastic anemia the bone marrow is producing normal blood cells but isn't making *enough* of them (hypoplastic bone marrow); in MDS the bone marrow may be stuffed with cells (hyperplastic bone marrow), but most of these cells are derived from an abnormal stem cell. This means they do not function properly as mature "differentiated" cells. The end result is similar to aplastic anemia—not enough of the right sorts of cells for each job.

Diagnosis

Diagnosis begins with your doctor reviewing your symptoms and history, including possible exposure to toxins and other risk factors. As a first step your physician will order a complete blood count (CBC), a simple blood test, usually taken from an arm vein, which gives a profile of the blood's components. Blood cell levels normally stay within a certain range. If your blood cell levels fall below normal ranges this may indicate aplastic anemia. To confirm the diagnosis your doctor will need to examine a sample of your bone marrow under a microscope. A bone marrow aspiration is done by removing a small amount of marrow through a needle. If blood cell counts in the sample are significantly below standard levels and the remaining cells look normal, you may have aplastic anemia. A hematologist or pathologist should examine the sample to confirm the diagnosis. A bone marrow biopsy, in which an intact piece of marrow is removed, is done to get a more precise picture of the marrow's blood cell production. Other tests (chromosomal analysis, liver function tests, PNH tests) may also be needed to rule out alternative causes of bone marrow failure.

Types of aplastic anemia

Doctors classify aplastic anemia into three categories: moderate, severe, and very severe. Although basic symptoms, treatment, and medication are similar for all patient groups, the time frame for administering certain treatments will vary according to severity. The prognosis for recovery also depends on severity of the disease. Most doctors use the following criteria, defined in 1975 by a leading hematologist, Dr. Bruce Camitta, and his team.

Moderate aplastic anemia (MAA) is the classification for those who have significantly reduced blood counts but not as reduced as occurs in severe aplastic anemia. In many cases doctors will not prescribe treatment for moderate aplastic anemia patients but will simply monitor blood counts. Moderate aplastic anemia may remain unchanged for many years. Sometimes it is detected during a routine physical exam, or it may be discovered if it escalates to severe aplastic anemia, as it begins causing more symptoms.

Severe aplastic anemia (SAA) is defined by a marrow cellularity (blood cell production) of less than 25 percent and at least two of the following: a neutrophil count less than half a billion per liter (<500/mm3); a platelet count less than 20 billion per liter (<20,000/mm3); a reticulocyte count less than 20 billion per liter (<20,000/mm3).

Very severe aplastic anemia (VSAA) is defined by a neutrophil count of less than 0.2 billion per liter (<200/mm3).

Causes and risk factors
Aplastic anemia can strike anyone of any age, sex, race, or gender, anywhere in the world. In Western countries the incidence of aplastic anemia is about two cases per million people per year (or approximately 500 new cases in the United States per year). These estimates are not precise, however, because aplastic anemia is not a reportable disease. Aplastic anemia is two to three times more common in Asian countries.

In most cases the exact cause of aplastic anemia is unknown; conditions without an identified cause are termed "idiopathic." High doses of radiation and cytotoxic chemotherapy can produce aplastic anemia. Aplastic anemia can follow exposure to environmental toxins (such as benzene), some medications, and certain viruses. Acquired aplastic anemia is not contagious nor is it hereditary.

Prognosis

Aplastic anemia is a serious illness that requires immediate medical attention. Progress is being made every day to increase the effectiveness of both standard and experimental treatment options, and the prognosis for affected patients has improved dramatically in the past ten years. Aplastic anemia treated with only blood transfusions was frequently a fatal illness. Now however, the standard treatments described below—bone marrow transplant and immunosuppressive drug therapy—have response rates of 70 to 90 percent. Treatments are being refined all the time, as research continues and our understanding of the disease keeps growing. It is important to remember, though, that statistics are only indicators—all patients react to their illness and treatment differently. The likely course of the disease will vary greatly depending on specific circumstances.

Treatments

Bone marrow transplant: For children and young adults with severe aplastic anemia, a bone marrow transplant may be the best treatment option and will successfully cure the disease in 70 to 90 percent of cases. Bone marrow transplants are most effective in young, healthy patients with a matched family donor. If you don't have a perfect match within your family, a search can be made of bone marrow registries to find a matched unrelated donor (MUD). MUD transplants are about half as successful as sibling related transplants. Alternative donor transplantation may be an option to consider early, since it takes time to locate a donor and make arrangements. The success rate of unrelated donor transplants is no more than 50 percent because of increased risk of rejection of the graft, and increased risk of graft-versus-host disease (GVHD), a complication in which the new marrow reacts against the patient. The severity of GVHD can range from mild to life-threatening, and its incidence is higher among older patients and in mismatched transplants. GVHD can be prevented or treated with medication, or by removing T-lymphocytes, a type of white blood cell, from the donor's bone marrow.

Before transplantation is performed, unhealthy cells in the bone marrow are destroyed to make room for the healthy transplanted stem cells. The pre-treatment also suppresses the patient's immune system to allow the new marrow to grow. The transplant process itself is fairly straightforward. About one tablespoon of donor marrow is given by intravenous transfusion for every kilogram of the patient's body weight. The body should then start making its own new, healthy blood cells in about two to four weeks. In 5 to 10 percent of patients the new bone marrow does not grow.

The outcome of transplantation can be affected by a number of factors. If there is a prolonged interval between diagnosis and transplantation, or if the patient has received multiple blood transfusions or experienced serious infections, this can lower the chances of success.

Immunosuppressive drugs: Considered standard initial treatment for older patients and for all patients without a matched family donor, the response rate of immunosuppressive drugs is 70 to 80 percent. The treatment is generally tolerated well and usually requires only brief hospitalization. However, responses are less complete and the need to repeat treatment more common than in patients treated with bone marrow transplantation. Also, the risks of developing leukemia or MDS later in life are higher, with the combined risk of such complications between 15 to 20 percent according to various studies. The generally accepted thinking about aplastic anemia is that the patient's immune system is reacting against the bone marrow, interfering with its ability to make blood cells. Immunosuppressive drugs are believed to counter this problem by reducing the immune response, allowing the bone marrow to once again make blood cells. The two immunosuppressive drugs most frequently used to treat aplastic anemia are antithymocyte globulin (ATG) and cyclosporine. The most effective immunosuppressive treatment for aplastic anemia today uses ATG combined with cyclosporine and corticosteroids.

Antithymocyte globulin (ATG—a horse or rabbit serum) targets T-lymphocytes—the cells that are responsible for destroying or suppressing the stem cells of patients with aplastic anemia. Horse ATG is typically given intravenously over four days for approximately four hours a day and rabbit ATG for five days. This schedule may vary depending on your needs or the particular methods of your doctor or hospital. ATG therapy used alone is helpful about half the time. When it is used in conjunction with cyclosporine, the chances of the treatment working increase to about 70 percent and higher. If it is successful, ATG will usually eliminate the need for transfusions within two to three months, and you will feel well. Blood counts rise within several months, some rising dramatically, some more slowly. Response times can vary greatly, however, and some patients experience delayed response times up to nine months or even longer. Blood counts, however, may still be below normal. Some patients who respond to ATG may need to have treatment again because of falling blood counts. Some patients who do not respond to ATG the first time will respond if the treatment is repeated.

ATG has a number of side effects. You should discuss these with your doctor. Less serious side effects include fever, chills, and hives. A rare but severe side effect is anaphylaxis, a life-threatening allergic reaction. Patients may be skin tested to determine if they are likely to develop allergies. If you are, you can still receive ATG therapy, but you will need to undergo a procedure called desensitization, in which small, gradually increasing doses of ATG are given, reducing the body's allergic reaction to the drug. Serum sickness is another type of reaction against a foreign protein. If it occurs it usually begins about one to two weeks after the first dose of ATG or ALG, causing rash and joint and muscle aches. Corticosteroids are usually given to patients to reduce the chances of getting serum sickness or its severity.

Cyclosporine is given with ATG and is another immunosuppressive drug that targets T-lymphocytes. Cyclosporine used alone is less successful than ATG alone, and less successful than ATG used in combination with cyclosporine. Cyclosporine comes in liquid and pill forms. The first doses will be based on your body weight. Subsequent doses will be adjusted based on the amount of the medicine in your blood. Too much of the drug will cause side effects and too little won't be effective.

Cyclosporine has side effects that you should discuss with your doctor. Two of the most serious side effects are kidney damage and high blood pressure. Both of these problems, however, are usually easy to manage and reversible. You may need to take a blood pressure lowering medication while on cyclosporine as well as a supplement of magnesium. You will generally need to continue taking cyclosporine for months or even years. If you have a stable, positive response to the drug, your doctor will gradually decrease the dosage.

The usefulness of other immunosuppressive drugs, including cyclophosphamide, is being studied. Although encouraging responses have been seen, cyclophosphamide's use should be considered experimental.

Growth factors are normal body products that encourage production of blood cells. Although most people with aplastic anemia already have unusually high levels of growth factors in their blood, very high medicinal doses may occasionally help the bone marrow to work better.

Growth factors have been most successful in increasing production of white blood cells. Granulocyte-colony stimulating factor (G-CSF) and granulocyte macrophage-colony stimulating factor (GM-CSF) have been the most effective growth factors for increasing white cell production. To date, use of growth factors like erythropoietin to increase red blood cells and platelets has not been particularly successful in patients with aplastic anemia.

It is important to remember that growth factors do not cure aplastic anemia. Rather, they may help damaged bone marrow to work better until other treatments have a chance to reverse the processes causing the marrow damage.

Other treatments

Most people can be effectively treated by one of the above treatments. If none of these treatments are effective, however, there are several other options available. These include other immunosuppressive drugs and marrow stimulants (cytokines) such as stem cell factor and hormones (androgens). Many of these approaches are considered experimental and are available only at university-affiliated medical centers conducting clinical trials of these treatments. Certain types of bone marrow transplants are also under investigation.

Peripheral blood stem cell transplantation. Peripheral blood stem cell transplantation is increasingly used in hematologic disorders, including aplastic anemia. However, research is still being done to determine its effectiveness with aplastic anemia. In this procedure the stem cells are harvested from the bloodstream of the donor rather than from the bone marrow. Peripheral blood stem cells appear to be as effective as bone marrow stem cells in patients with leukemias; however, in patients with aplastic anemia, peripheral blood stem cell transplants appear to be slightly less effective. Recently, stem cells harvested from fetal cord blood have been used for transplantation.

Autologous transplants. Recently a small number of autologous transplants have been performed on patients who did not have matching donors but did have some healthy stem cells of their own. In this type of transplant the bone marrow stem cells are removed from the patient and then reimplanted in them after "contaminating" unhealthy cells have been destroyed with chemotherapy. This approach should be considered experimental.

Blood transfusions

If red blood cell or platelet levels are low, patients may need to receive transfusions. Important advice about transfusions: do not ask close family members to donate red blood cells or platelets until after a bone marrow transplant has been done or ruled out. This is because if a family member turns out to be the best bone marrow donor, a prior donation from a family member could reduce the chances for a successful transplant.

Blood products used for transfusion are usually treated in some way (such as being irradiated or filtered) to remove leukocytes. These measures reduce the risk of certain complications from transfusion—irradiation minimizes the risk of graft-versus-host disease, while leukocyte filters decrease the risk of sensitization to proteins present in the transfused blood product, and also reduce the risk of transmitting cytomegalovirus. Irradiation and filtering are important in cases where the patients are severely immunosuppressed.

Blood transfusions are an important aspect of treatment for immediate problems associated with bone marrow failure. They may be given after aplastic anemia is initially diagnosed and before the treatment of choice is determined, or may be used as a supportive measure when there has not been full response to treatment. They are not effective as a long-term treatment strategy for the following reasons:

1) Red blood cells can be given indefinitely but are not a substitute for definitive treatment. They are easy to match and remain in the body for months, but if you receive regular red cell transfusions damaging amounts of iron will begin to collect in key organs such as the heart and liver. This is called iron overload. Untreated, this can lead to severe organ damage that can be fatal. Iron can be removed by treatment with metal chelators such as Desferal®.

2) Platelets last only a few days, which means you would require several transfusions a week. In addition, your body's immune system can eventually learn to recognize and destroy transfused platelets.

3) White blood cells have a very short life span of only a few hours and cannot be administered routinely or to prevent infections. White cell transfusions may be used in severe infections that have not responded to antibiotics.

Wellness

Apart from specific treatments and medications, there are actions you can take or avoid so that you can have the optimum level of wellness possible for you. Here are some of the main dos and don'ts:

1) Avoid contact with toxic substances that can be ingested, inhaled, or absorbed through the skin. Do not take any type of medication, supplements, vitamins, or herbs without first consulting with your doctor.

2) If you have low red cell counts you should avoid excessive exercise, going to high altitudes, or any activity that causes chest pain, severe shortness of breath, or a fast heart rate. However, some form of regular exercise is important to your physical health.

3) If you have low white cell counts you may be more likely to catch bacterial infections. You should try to avoid cuts on your skin and on the lining of your mouth or throat, which can lead to these types of infection. Dental work and burns from

hot food are two common causes of damage to the lining of the mouth and throat. Practice good dental hygiene to reduce the risk of infection and take steps to avoid contagious illnesses by staying away from sick people and crowds. Keeping minor infections from becoming more serious is very important. Be alert to early symptoms of infection—fever or increased fatigue can be warning signs, and you should report these promptly to your doctor.

4) If you have low platelets you should avoid activities that could result in injuries. If you develop severe headache or severe or persistent pain anywhere, which could indicate a bleeding problem, you should notify your doctor.

5) It is important to report any symptoms of low blood counts to your doctor so that treatment can be adjusted as necessary.

Emotional issues

When you are diagnosed with aplastic anemia, you may feel shock, anger, and fear, and even relief at learning what is wrong. You will need to make time for medical treatment and administration. And everyday life must go on for you and your family. Although all this may seem overwhelming, many other patients in the same situation have come through to lead full lives, often becoming stronger as individuals and as families. Two booklets that may help: *Families Coping with AA & MDS* and *Managing Treatment Decisions*. Also contact the AA&MDSIF to be put in touch with other patients who are glad to share their successful treatment experiences with others.

Resources

For a complete packet of information on aplastic anemia and related bone marrow failure disorders, or to speak with a patient educator, please contact:

Aplastic Anemia & MDS International Foundation, Inc.
P.O. Box 310
Churchton, MD 20733
Toll Free: 800-747-2820
Tel: 410-867-0242
Fax: 410-867-0240
Email: help@aamds.org
www.aamds.org

Patient Literature:

Aplastic Anemia Basic Explanations. Annapolis, MD: Aplastic Anemia & MDS International Foundation, 2003.

Families Coping with AA & MDS. Annapolis, MD: Aplastic Anemia & MDS International Foundation, 2002.

Iron Chelation Therapy in Aplastic Anemia, MDS & PNH. Annapolis, MD: Aplastic Anemia & MDS International Foundation, 2002.

Managing Treatment Decisions. Annapolis, MD: Aplastic Anemia & MDS International Foundation, 2003.

24

Myelodysplastic Syndromes (MDS)

In 1990 Robert Carroll was diagnosed with MDS/RA after having gone to his doctor for a routine checkup, which included a complete blood count (CBC). Test results showed all three of his blood lineages were severely depressed. Because Robert looked and felt great, he decided that there was no need to worry his wife by telling her about the lab findings. Besides, he reasoned that perhaps the culprit was faulty lab equipment! Robert was referred to a hematologist/oncologist who did a bone marrow biopsy. When the results came back, he was given the diagnosis of MDS. Robert had always told his wife that he wouldn't want to know if he had a life-threatening disease, but when faced with the real possibility of a life-threatening condition, his attitude changed.

Robert and his wife began to read about MDS. They found

Portions of this chapter reprinted with permission of Aplastic Anemia & MDS International Foundation, Inc., from *Myelodysplastic Syndromes: Basic Explanations*, contributors: Dr. David Araten of Memorial Sloan Kettering Cancer Center and Dr. Yvette Ju. © 2002 by Aplastic Anemia & MDS International Foundation, Inc.

what they read about the disease discouraging, but they continued to search for information and groups that offered support. Additionally, Robert sought a second and third opinion.

After the reconfirmation that MDS was the proper diagnosis, Robert returned to the first doctor for treatment. This physician explained to Robert that observations and periodic blood transfusions were all he could offer in the way of managing the condition as it progressed. Robert decided to look for an expert, a hematologist who primarily works in MDS research and takes a limited number of patients.

Robert was successful in finding a hematologist. He remembers May 11, 1991, very well. On this day he carried a two-inch-thick folder of medical documents and research articles he had accumulated into the MDS expert's office. His wife was right by his side. The hematologist needed only a few moments to look through what Robert had brought with him. She was able to answer every folder-related question he asked, admittedly just to test her knowledge of MDS in general, and matters relating specifically to his diagnosis.

From the beginning, his way of coping with this disease was to be well informed, to investigate new treatments, and to continually confer with his doctor as to the next course of action. Robert says that he refuses to let his life change because of MDS. He did not retire; he continued his career as a educator and pursued numerous hobbies.

Robert has been transfusion dependent for almost twelve years. His advice to others with this condition:

> Every patient with MDS is different. Because it is still a very rare disease, many doctors know very little about it, and most have never had an MDS patient. They are learning that some patients progress rapidly while others live many years with the disease and die from other causes. Not too long ago it was referred to as "pre-leukemic," a term no longer used because only about 35 percent of MDS patients actually transform to acute leukemia. Knowing that we are all different and we don't follow the same progression rate gives me cause to be optimistic—something I

wish I had known when first diagnosed. At first the classification system painted a bleak picture of how long I could survive. It turned out to be wrong, not only for me, but for thousands of MDS patients. Sound advice to newly diagnosed MDS patients is to immediately learn as much as possible about this disease. Partner with your doctor on a plan of treatment. It might be supportive therapy with a wait-and-see attitude, or perhaps an aggressive approach to try and cure the disease.

Robert's complete story, "MDS: A Gift," by Robert F. Carroll, EdD, can be read on the Aplastic Anemia & MDS International Foundation website under the section "Victory Letters."

What is MDS?

Myelodysplastic syndromes (MDS) are rare and potentially fatal blood diseases that occur when the body starts incorrectly manufacturing the three types of blood cells—white, red, and platelets—resulting in malformed, immature cells. MDS was described as a "pre-leukemic" condition in the early 1930s. It is now understood, however, that most patients will not develop leukemia. The first group of patients was codified in 1955 and myelodysplastic syndromes were not treated as a separate group of disorders until 1976. Many terms were used to describe this disease: refractory anemia, preleukemia, oligo-blasticleukemia, myelodysplastic anemia, and hematopoietic dysplasia. There are five recognized types of MDS as well as several variants.

MDS explained

Your body has three types of blood cells: red cells, which deliver oxygen throughout the body; white cells, which help fight infections; and platelets, which help clot your blood when you are bleeding. Within your bone marrow, which is a red spongy substance in the center of your bones, are precursor cells, the earliest forms of which are stem cells. Stem cells are also able to replace themselves as needed by creating exact duplicates of themselves. Normally your bone marrow is like a factory churning out as many blood cells as you need. For example, if you get an infection the bone marrow steps up production of white cells. If you start bleeding, the bone marrow makes more platelets and red cells.

But in patients with MDS, something causes a defect to occur in one of the stem cells within the bone marrow. From that point forward all of the cells produced by that stem cell carry that same defect. This defect somehow allows that particular stem cell to have an advantage over all the other stem cells in the bone marrow. It is able to produce more cells and ones that stay around longer. These cells eventually crowd out and overwhelm the normal, healthy cells. However, despite their apparent success in the marrow they are actually less able to produce blood cells, which result in low blood counts.

A helpful analogy

Think of the bone marrow as a busy car factory with many different assembly lines, turning out lots of different models from a single basic chassis. In our example, the basic chassis is the stem cell. MDS develops when for some reason one of the assembly lines puts out a single defective chassis. This causes all the other lines to shut down. Soon only this one assembly line is working. It's doing overtime, but every chassis it produces is faulty. In other words, this defective stem cell ends up making most or all of the cells in the bone marrow. The cells it produces are all defective and in many cases they don't mature. Like a pile-up on the assembly line, immature cells also pile up in the bone marrow. Then just around the time they should be released into the bloodstream, most of them self-destruct. For this reason, MDS patients usually do not have enough cells in the bloodstream, a condition known as cytopenia. The cells that do mature and reach the bloodstream often don't work as well as normal cells. These deficiencies or defects may cause a number of symptoms.

Symptoms

The following are some symptoms of MDS; however, experiencing one or more of these does not indicate that you have the disease, since all of these symptoms can occur with other conditions: weakness, anemia, fatigue, palpitations, dizziness, headaches, irritability, bruising, increased bleeding, frequent infections, lingering illnesses, and unusually pale skin color. It is vital to consult a physician for a professional medical diagnosis. Anemia (the condition that results from having low red blood cell levels) is responsible for the most common symptoms of MDS—symptoms such as fatigue and lightheadedness. Bleeding complaints are also frequent, because of the blood's poor clotting ability. Paroxysmal nocturnal hemoglobinuria (PNH) is a separate disorder, which MDS can mimic. Since PNH is often treated differently from MDS, patients should be tested for PNH in appropriate cases (by the Ham's test or flow cytometry) at the time of diagnosis of MDS. Low blood counts and certain abnormalities in the marrow can be seen in both disorders. Distinctive features of PNH include darkened urine (a result of red blood cell breakdown) and a tendency to form inappropriate blood clots. These blood clots can result in leg swelling, shortness of breath, headache, abdominal pain or swelling; breakdown of red cells can cause yellow discoloration of the eyes or skin. It is particularly important that patients with such symptoms be tested for PNH.

MDS and aplastic anemia—similarities and differences

There are many similarities between myelodysplastic syndromes and aplastic anemia, and patients share many of the same symptoms. Both groups suffer from anemia and reductions in the number of platelets and white blood cells. The incidence of both diseases increases with age. It is estimated that about 25 percent of aplastic anemia patients develop MDS. Physicians sometimes have difficulty initially telling the two apart. The hypoplastic form of MDS looks very similar to severe aplastic anemia. A hematologist (a specialist in the treatment of diseases of the blood) can usually determine which one is present by careful examination of the appearance of the marrow cells. The biggest difference between the two diseases is that in aplastic anemia the bone marrow is producing normal blood cells, but it isn't making enough of them (hypoplastic bone marrow); in MDS the bone marrow may be stuffed with cells (hyperplastic bone marrow), but these cells are cloned from an abnormal stem cell. This means they do not function properly as mature differentiated cells. The end result is similar to aplastic anemia—not enough of the right sort of cells for each job.

Diagnosis

The symptoms of MDS are similar to those of many other diseases. Also, in the early stages of MDS people often don't show any symptoms at all. This means that the disease can be very difficult to diagnose. It is not uncommon for it to be discovered accidentally during a routine physical exam or a blood test. A doctor's diagnosis begins with a review of the patient's symptoms and history, including possible exposure to toxins and other risk factors. As a first step, your physician will order a complete blood count (CBC), a simple blood test, usually taken from an arm vein, that gives a profile of the blood's components. Blood cell levels normally stay within a certain range. If your blood cell levels fall below normal ranges this may indicate MDS. If a doctor suspects MDS he or she will examine a sample of the person's bone marrow under a microscope to confirm the diagnosis. This sample is taken by removing a small amount of marrow through a needle, usually from the pelvic bone. This is known as a bone marrow aspiration. A biopsy may also be done at this time, which involves the removal of an intact piece of bone marrow for examination. These samples sometimes undergo cytogenetic testing to determine if there is a change in chromosomal profile.

In MDS the bone marrow will show visible abnormalities in the appearance of one or more of the three types of blood cells. In most cases, the bone marrow will be full of cells, or hypercellular, which would not occur in a healthy person. Also, the chromosomes—the genetic "blueprints" in each of our cells that determine the cell's characteristics—of the bone marrow cells may be abnormal. Only a knowledgeable hematologist can confirm the diagnosis of MDS, determine the exact subtype, and rule out alternative causes of bone marrow failure.

Types of MDS

The most common means of classifying the different types of myelodysplastic syndromes is the FAB system, which was developed by a team of French, American, and British research-ers in the 1970s. To determine which of the five basic forms of MDS a patient has, the type and volume of the immature blood cells ("blasts") that are found in the bloodstream and bone marrow are examined.

Refractory anemia (RA): Less than 5 percent blasts in bone marrow, less than 1 percent blasts in bloodstream, cytopenia in at least one cell line (usually red cells), and normal or hypercel-lular bone marrow.

Refractory anemia with ringed sideroblasts (RARS): Less than 5 percent blasts in bone marrow, less than 1 percent blasts in bloodstream, cytopenia (usually red cells), and more than 15 percent of marrow red cell precursors are "ringed sideroblasts." In RARS, the developing red cells found in the bone marrow cannot use the iron necessary to produce hemoglobin. Iron forms a visible dark ring in the developing red cell, providing the name ringed sideroblast. RA and RARS are the most com-mon types of MDS, and patients experience the fewest side effects and usually have a longer prognosis. RARS is sometimes associated with excess body iron, even in patients who have not received transfusions.

Refractory anemia with excess blasts (RAEB): 5 to 20 per-cent blasts in bone marrow, less than 5 percent blasts in blood-stream, and cytopenia of at least two types of blood cells. Note that normal bone marrow carries less than 5 percent blasts. However, when MDS mainly affects white cells, this count can exceed 35 percent.

Refractory anemia with excess blasts in transformation (RAEB-t): 21 to 30 percent blasts in bone marrow, more than 5 percent blasts in bloodstream, and cytopenia of at least two types of blood cells. If the blast count continues to increase, this form of MDS usually develops into acute myelogenous leukemia (AML).

Chronic myelomonocytic leukemia (CMML): 5 to 20 percent blasts in bone marrow and less than 5 percent blasts in bloodstream. Monocytes, a type of white cell, multiply in abnormal quantities, which can progress to acute leukemia. The course of patients with CMML varies greatly. CMML may not be a single disease but a mixture of disorders that need to be separated from one another.

In addition to these five classifications of MDS, there are several variants. One of these is hypoplastic MDS, in which the bone marrow reveals a decrease in the numbers of cells, in contrast to the more common appearance of MDS, which is hyperplastic 5q minus Syndrome. This syndrome is probably more similar to aplastic anemia and is likely to respond to immunosuppression. This is another variant that is distinguished by a characteristic abnormal chromosome, higher platelet counts, and a better prognosis, as is MDS with fibrosis, in which the marrow has a fibrous appearance due to an increase of reticulin, a type of collagen found in the marrow. Therapy-related myelodysplastic syndrome (t-MDS) is another, in which the development of MDS is related to chemotherapy or radiation therapy. This latter syndrome has the worst prognosis and should lead to a consideration of bone marrow transplantation soon after diagnosis. The classification of MDS is complex, and is an area where your physician can be helpful, both for clarifying the type or variant involved, and in explaining the treatment implications.

The current WHO classification of myelodysplastic syndromes is shown below:

- Refractory Anemia (RA)
- Refractory Anemia with Ring Sideroblasts (RARS)
- Refractory Cytopenias with Multilineage Dysplasia (RCMD)
- Refractory Cytopenias with Multilineage Dysplasia and Ring Sideroblasts (RCMD-RS)
- 5q minus Syndrome
- Refractory Anemia with Excess Blasts (RAEB)

If the bone marrow contains more than 20 percent blast cells, this now satisfies the diagnosis of acute myelogenous leukemia.

Chromosome defects
Researchers have discovered that about half of all MDS patients have clearly recognizable defects in their chromosomes. These defects are believed to be caused by the disease, not inherited. The number and type of chromosomal defects that a patient

has can reveal information about the progression of the disease. Patients who do not have chromosome defects generally do better than those who have them. Certain types of defects, isolated loss of Y, 5q, or 20q chromosomes, indicate that a person will have a mild or less severe form of the disease. Abnormalities of chromosome 7 or complex chromosomal changes with three or more defects point to a more severe form of MDS.

Causes and risk factors

MDS can affect people of any age, gender, or race, anywhere in the world. In most cases the cause of myelodysplastic syndromes is unknown (or idiopathic), but there are some instances in which the disease can be traced to a specific cause. For example, some patients will develop MDS after receiving intensive chemotherapy or radiation treatment for another disease. In addition, long-term or heavy exposure to the chemical benzene has been linked to an increased risk of developing myelodysplastic syndromes. Pesticides and other chemicals may also increase a person's risk. MDS is not contagious and with very rare exceptions is not inherited.

The incidence of myelodysplastic syndromes in the United States is estimated from 10,000 to 20,000 annually, based on European studies. This is equivalent to 40 to 80 cases per million population per year, or one person out of approximately 12,000 to 25,000. These estimates are not precise, however, because MDS is not a reportable disease—that is, the Centers

Evaluating Myelodysplastic Syndromes
INTERNATIONAL PROGNOSTIC SCORING SYSTEM

Prognostic Variable	Risk Group Score Value					
	0 Low	0.5 Intermediate I	1.0	1.5 Intermediate II	2.0	>2.5 High
Bone Marrow Blasts	<5	5-10%	—	11-20%	21-30%	
Karotype	Good		Intermediate		Poor	
Cytopenias	0-1 lineages		2-3 lineages			

Source: Greenberg P, Cox C, LeBeau MM, et al: International scoring system for evaluating prognosis in myelodysplastic syndromes. *Blood* 1997, 89:2079

for Disease Control and Prevention (CDC) do not require that the cases be reported to them. AA&MDSIF maintains a volunteer registry, the only one in the world. MDS can strike anyone at any age, even children. However, it is most frequently diagnosed in people sixty to eighty years old. In recent years, though, there has been an increase in the number of cases for younger people. The development of the diagnostic criteria for MDS is relatively recent, so that MDS, as a diagnosis, is increasing. MDS is considered to be somewhat more common in men than in women.

Risk levels and prognosis

Recently researchers have developed several scoring systems to identify the risk level of patients. These systems use the percentage of blasts in bone marrow, presence of chromosome abnormalities, and blood counts to predict disease progression. Determining which risk group a person falls into can help in deciding on the best course of treatment. The scoring system most frequently used is the International Prognostic Scoring System (IPSS). It considers the three factors that together have been found by research to be the best predictors of disease outcome: the percentage of bone marrow blasts (immature blood cells); the karyotype (profile of chromosomal abnormalities); and the extent of cytopenias (deficiencies of cells in the blood). For this cytopenia component, the IPSS considers, specifically, how many types (lineages) of cytopenia the patient has among the possible three (red cells, white cells, and platelets). The scoring ranges from 0 to 2.0, with 0 as the best score.

Myelodysplastic syndromes are not a single disease but a group of disorders, which means that symptoms and disease progression vary. People with milder forms may live for many years with few or no problems. Unfortunately, the life expectancy for many people in the highest-risk group is only around six months. It is important to remember, though, that these statistics are only indicators—all patients react to their illness and treatment differently. The likely course of the disease will vary greatly depending on your specific circumstances. You should discuss your situation with your doctor and together determine your prognosis. Keep in mind that new and aggressive treatment options are being developed that are improving the quality and quantity of life for patients with all types of MDS.

Risk of developing leukemia

In some cases MDS will progress over time to become acute leukemia. This can take months or years. However, the majority of cases will not turn into acute leukemia. The type of MDS a person has is a very good indicator of whether acute leukemia will develop. Acute leukemia will occur eventually in about 11 percent of RA patients; 5 percent of RARS patients; 23 percent of RAEB patients; more than 48 percent of RAEBt patients; and 20 percent of CMML patients.

Treatment options

Supportive care: Though there are several treatment options for patients with MDS, an important common denominator is excellent supportive care. This entails management of fevers that may occur while the white blood count is low—a situation that requires immediate medical attention in an emergency room and prompt administration of a broad spectrum antibiotics. Along side antibiotics, fever with a low white count may be treated (or prevented) with growth factors to stimulate the production and prolong the circulation time of the critical white cells—called neutrophils or granulocytes. Many patients require transfusions of red cells or platelets. Sometimes erythropoietin can reduce red cell transfusion requirements. Blood counts would need to be monitored closely in such patients.

It is important to be sure that the patient has adequate body stores of vitamin B_{12} and folic acid and to monitor iron levels for excess or deficiency. Because MDS tends to affect older individuals, close attention to other medical problems is important. Thus one should choose a physician who is available and has coverage for "off-hours" and who is able to work closely with other specialists.

Your treatment should be tailored to the type of MDS that you have, the severity of the disease, and your age and overall health. For some people a bone marrow transplant can cure the disease. Unfortunately, MDS most often strikes older people who are not ideal candidates for a transplant. For those who don't qualify for a transplant there are several other treatment options. If the MDS is not severe, and blood counts are relatively close to normal, the doctor may recommend simply keeping an eye on the disease and not undertaking specific treatment. Some MDS patients go many years without treatment and have few ill effects. It is very important, though, to continually monitor the disease.

Other treatment options include chemotherapy and experimental medications, which are particularly helpful for people in an advanced stage of MDS. In some cases these treatments are capable of producing short-term remission during which time there will be no symptoms of MDS and no evidence of leukemia cells.

Bone marrow transplant: If you are considering a transplant you should carefully discuss the benefits and risks with your doctor. As noted earlier, bone marrow transplantation is an option in younger, healthier patients and in many cases will cure myelodysplastic syndromes. The optimum age for transplant patients is fifty-five and younger. In recent years, however, doctors have begun successfully performing transplants on older patients who are in good health. This is most often done in cases where the patient has a high likelihood of developing leukemia.

Identical twins or a brother or sister who has a perfect bone marrow match with the patient are the best candidates to be donors. If there isn't a perfect match within the family a search can be made of bone marrow registries to find a matched unrelated donor (MUD). Recent data suggests that the patient's own bone marrow may be used to perform autologous transplants in selected cases.

A transplant involves destroying the patient's marrow and replacing it with that of the donor. This requires high doses of chemotherapy and/or radiation, to kill cells in the marrow that might cause MDS to return after the transplant or that might cause rejection of the donor's marrow (as can happen with kidney transplants). The chemotherapy and/or radiation can damage vital organs—which older patients are less able to withstand. This is part of the reason for the age limitation on transplantation. The transplant process itself is fairly straight-forward. About one tablespoon of donor marrow is given by intravenous transfusion for every kilogram of the patient's body weight. The body should then start making its own new, healthy blood cells in about two to four weeks. In 5 to 10 percent of patients the new bone marrow does not grow. In such cases a repeat transplant is necessary after additional immune suppression.

In some cases, the new marrow will react against the patient. This is called graft-versus-host disease (GVHD). The incidence of GVHD is higher among older people and in mismatched transplants. Severity may range from mild to life-threatening. Graft-versus-host disease can be treated with medication, or by removing T-lymphocytes from the donor bone marrow. This procedure—called T-cell depletion—may increase the upper age limit for transplantation somewhat. If GVHD does occur, treatments to suppress the immune system may be helpful.

People who are at high risk of developing leukemia tend to have a higher relapse rate after transplantation. About one-third of such patients are typically cured. People who are at low risk for developing leukemia tend to have a low relapse rate after a transplant and the survival rate is greater than 50 percent.

Peripheral blood stem cell transplantation: Peripheral blood stem cell transplantation (PBSCT) is increasingly used in hematological disorders. In this procedure the stem cells are harvested from the bloodstream of the donor rather than from the bone marrow.

Autologous: Peripheral stem cell transplantation in which the patient's own peripheral stem cells are used, rather than a donor's), is a relatively new treatment approach for MDS. It is considered an alternative therapy for elderly patients or patients who do not have a suitable donor.

Mini-transplants: Also called non-myeloablative trans-plants, and transplant-lite, this procedure uses a less toxic pre-treatment regimen than is used for the standard bone marrow transplant. Some of the patient's stem cells coexist with the donor stem cells for some time after transplantation, thereby decreasing the chances of developing severe graft-versus-host disease. It is used more frequently in older patients, although its usefulness in younger patients who have not responded to standard treatments is being researched. Mini-transplants are still considered experimental for treatment of aplastic anemia.

Growth factors: Growth factors are normal body products that stimulate the production of blood cells. Growth factors don't eliminate MDS, but by increasing blood counts they can often limit the need for transfusions in some patients.

There are a number of different types of growth factors that are used both individually and in combination. Erythropoietin (trade names Epogen® and Procrit®) has been successfully used to stimulate red cell growth in some MDS patients. Recently researchers have been able to improve the effectiveness of erythropoietin by combining it with another growth factor called granulocyte-colony stimulating factor (G-CSF, Filgastrim, Neupogen®) or granulocyte-macrophage-colony stimulating factor (GM-CSF, Sargramostim, Leukine®). The combined treatment has been successful in generating red cell production in as many as 40 percent of patients. Given by itself G-CSF has been successful in stimulating white cell production in some patients. Erythropoetin treatment is more likely to work in patients whose endogenous erythropoetin level is relatively low. Response rates are high in those with levels <200 and response is unlikely if level is >500.

Many other growth factors are in the process of being developed and tested. Not all patients respond to growth factors. Those who do respond usually need to receive them on an ongoing basis.

Immunosuppressive drugs: This family of drugs, including antithymocyte globulin (ATG, a horse serum)—or the comparable European antilymphocyte globulin (ALG, a rabbit serum)—and cyclosporine, has been very successful in treating aplastic anemia, but not nearly as effective against MDS. The effects of ATG or ALG in MDS patients are short-lived, lasting on average about ten months. This therapy is used most often on patients with hypoplastic MDS, which is the form of the disease that most closely resembles aplastic anemia, for which immunosuppressive drugs are one of the standard treatments. Immunosuppressive drug therapy also has been successful in treating people with earlier stages of MDS (RA).

In MDS, the immune system may play a role in the disruption of blood cell production, with certain white blood cells reacting against the bone marrow, interfering with its ability to make normal blood cells. This appears to be why immunosuppressive drugs, which target those white cells, are helpful in some cases.

Immunosuppressive drugs have a number of side effects. You should discuss these with your doctor. Less serious side effects include fever, chills, and hives. A rare but severe side effect is anaphylaxis, a life-threatening allergic reaction. All patients who receive ATG or ALG should be pretested to determine if they are likely to develop anaphylaxis. If you are, you can still receive ATG or ALG therapy, but you will need to undergo a procedure called desensitization, in which small, gradually increasing doses of ATG or ALG are given, reducing the body's allergic reaction to the drug. Serum sickness is another type of reaction against a foreign protein. If it occurs it usually begins about one to two weeks after the first dose of ATG or ALG, causing rash and joint and muscle aches. Steroids are usually given to patients to reduce the chances of their getting serum sickness or the severity of it if it does occur. Two serious side effects that can occur with the use of cyclosporine are kidney damage and high blood pressure, although these can be managed with medication.

Differentiating agents: One of the problems in people with MDS is that their blood cells don't mature and specialize. As a result most cells die without leaving the bone marrow. However, even abnormal cells can be helpful to the body if they mature and are released into the blood. The process that causes a blood cell to go from being immature to mature is called differentiation.

Differentiating agents are a type of medication that can, in some cases, force the defective stem cell to work more efficiently, producing more mature blood cells and fewer immature ones. So far the success of these agents has been limited, but there are some patients who have benefited from them: Interferons, HMBA, HHT, 5-Aza-cytidine, Cytosine arabinoside (Ara-C), Amifostine, Butyrates, Haem arginate, Retinoids, vitamin A, retinoic acid, all-trans-retinoic acid, 13-cisretinoic acid), and vitamin D3. Some of these agents may decrease the blood counts—particularly the white count—before they have a beneficial effect. Therefore, the patient may need to be monitored closely for the development of fever. Recently, a drug called Decitabine has been used with some promising preliminary results. These agents should be given as part of a clinical trial.

A new use may have been found for an old drug, thalidomide. Use of this drug was discontinued decades ago because of extensive birth defects in children born to women taking this drug during pregnancy, and this drug must never be given to pregnant women or women who might become pregnant. It is not known how it works for certain cancers, and we still have to learn for which types it may be effective. Because MDS resembles cancer in some ways, thalidomide has been tried and shown to reduce transfusion requirements in some patients with MDS. However, there are many side effects of this drug besides birth defects (including sedation, blood clots, nerve damage, gastrointestinal upset, and rash) and patients taking this agent need close medical monitoring. This agent should be given as part of a clinical trial. A thalidomide derivative, lenalidomide (Revlimid®), is better tolerated and extremely effective, especially in individuals with MDS who have the 5q minus chromosome abnormality.

Five-azacytidine, also called azacytidine or Az-C, is a hypomethylating agent, influencing the expression of genes in the MDS cells, and may generate a more normal pattern of gene expression. Patients may experience lower blood counts but also better control of MDS cells. A Phase III study of azacytidine showed 60 of 99 patients met criteria for response or improvement. Several treatments are now FDA approved for MDS; lenalidomide for 5q minus and azacytidine and decitabine for all forms of MDS.

Chemotherapy: Another treatment that is being used in some cases is low- and high-dose chemotherapy given by injection or in pill form. Various chemotherapy agents, used alone or in combination, are given to kill fast-growing abnormal blood cells that are potentially leukemic. Data suggest that in some MDS patients low-dose chemotherapy can slow down the production of blood cells by the defective stem cell. This allows the few remaining normal stem cells to repopulate the bone marrow, which leads to a rise in normal blood cells. Unfortunately, the effects are usually short-term and don't occur in the majority of patients.

Approximately 40 to 60 percent of MDS patients go into remission after receiving high-dose chemotherapy. The remission, however, doesn't last long, and the chemotherapy can produce some serious side effects. High-dose chemotherapy is most often used in patients who are high-risk or those who are candidates for a bone marrow transplant. As with any treatment approach, discuss the risks and benefits with your doctor so that you can make informed decisions about your health care.

Blood Transfusions

Supportive care, including transfusions, is an important aspect of treating MDS. Many patients need periodic transfusions to maintain red blood cell and platelet levels. While blood transfusions do not cure disease, they can help alleviate symptoms and contribute to overall health. Important advice about transfusions: do not ask close family members to donate red blood cells or platelets until after a bone marrow transplant has been done or ruled out. This is because if a family member turns out to be the best bone marrow donor, a prior donation from a family member could reduce the chances for a successful transplant.

Blood products used for transfusion should be irradiated and filtered to remove leukocytes. These measures reduce the risk of certain complications from transfusion—irradiation minimizes the risk of graft-versus-host disease, while leukocyte filters decrease the risk of sensitization to proteins present in the transfused blood product, and also reduce the risk of transmitting cytomegalovirus. Ideally, patients who have not been exposed to cytomegalovirus who are candidates for BMT should receive transfusion products that have been checked and found to be negative for cytomegalovirus. Irradiation and filtering are important, unless your doctor has good reasons why these precautions are not necessary.

Chelation therapy: Since excess iron can accumulate in patients receiving transfusions and in patients with RARS, infusions of a non-chelation drug, deferoxamine, is sometimes suggested.

Blood transfusions are a short-term solution to deal with immediate problems associated with bone marrow failure. They are not effective as a long-term treatment strategy for the following reasons:

Red blood cells are easy to match and remain in the body for about four months, but if you receive regular red cell transfusions, damaging amounts of iron will begin to collect in key organs such as the heart and liver. This is called iron overload. Untreated, this can lead to severe organ damage that can be fatal.

Platelets last only eight to ten days, which means you would require several transfusions a week. In addition, your body's immune system can eventually learn to recognize and destroy transplanted platelets.

No effective method has been developed for routine transfusion of white blood cells because of their short life span of only a few hours. White cell transfusions may be used in severe infections that have not responded to antibiotics.

Wellness

Apart from specific treatments and medications, there are actions you can take or avoid so that you can have the optimum level of wellness possible for you. Here are some of the main do's and don'ts: Avoid contact with any chemicals or toxins that can be ingested, inhaled, or absorbed through the skin, including gasoline, kerosene, paint, solvents, pesticides, and cleaning agents. Do not take any over-the-counter medications, including aspirin, or any prescription medicine, vitamins, herbs, or other products without the approval of your hematologist.

If you have low red cell counts you should avoid excessive exercise, going to high altitudes, or any activity that causes chest pain, severe shortness of breath, or a fast heart rate. However, some form of regular exercise is important to your physical health.

If you have low white cell counts you may be more likely to catch bacterial infections. This is a particular risk in patients with a neutrophil count (granulocyte count) of less than 1,000. Since bacterial infections can be rapidly fatal if not treated, patients should have a thermometer on hand and know how to use it. Oral or tympanic temperatures are easily taken and rectal temperatures are to be avoided. If the temperature is greater than 38°C (100.4°F) the patient should go immediately—even in the middle of the night—to the nearest emergency room. The standard procedure is for prompt medical evaluation, blood cultures to be taken, and intravenous broad spectrum antibiotics if the neutrophil count is less than 1,000.

It should be noted that some patients with MDS have dysfunctional neutrophils despite normal counts. Patients in whom this is suspected should be treated if they had low neutrophil counts.

You should try to avoid cuts on your skin and on the lining of your mouth or throat, which can lead to these types of infection. Dental work and burns from hot food are two common causes of damage to the lining of the mouth and throat. Practice good dental hygiene to reduce the risk of infection, and take steps to avoid contagious illnesses, by staying away from sick people and crowds. Avoid suppositories, enemas, rectal exams, or rectal temperatures. Keeping minor infections from becoming more serious is very important. Be alert to early symptoms of infection—fever or increased fatigue can be warning signs, and you should report these promptly to your doctor.

Depending upon the platelet count, light exercise may still be permitted. Activities with a potential for head injury are a particular concern. Patients with low platelet counts should not take drugs that affect the function of platelets. This includes aspirin, Motrin®, Advisl, ibuprofen, Naprosyn, Indocin, or similar anti-inflammatory drugs. If you develop severe headache or severe or persistent pain anywhere, which could indicate a bleeding problem, you should notify your doctor.

It is important to report any symptoms of low blood counts to your doctor so that treatment can be adjusted as necessary.

Emotional issues

When you are diagnosed with MDS, you may feel shock, anger, and fear, and even relief at learning what is wrong. You will need to make time for medical treatment and administration.

And everyday life must go on for you and your family. Although all this may seem overwhelming, many other patients in the same situation have come through to lead full lives, often becoming stronger as individuals and families. AA&MDSIF publishes two booklets that can help: *Families Coping with AA & MDS* and *Managing Treatment Decisions*. Also contact the AA&MDSIF to be put in touch with other patients who share their successful treatment experiences with others.

Resources
For a complete packet of information on myelodysplastic syndromes contact:

Aplastic Anemia & MDS International Foundation, Inc.
P.O. Box 310
Churchton, MD 20733
Toll Free: 800-747-2820
Tel: 410-867-0242
Fax: 410-867-0240
Email: help@aamds.org
www.aamds.org

Patient Literature:

Families Coping with AA&MDS. Annapolis, MD: Aplastic Anemia & MDS International Foundation, 2002.

Iron Chelation Therapy in Aplastic Anemia, MDS & PNH. Annapolis, MD: Aplastic Anemia & MDS International Foundation, 2002.

Managing Treatment Decisions. Annapolis, MD: Aplastic Anemia & MDS International Foundation, 2003.

Myelodysplastic Syndromes Basic Explanations. Annapolis, MD: Aplastic Anemia & MDS International Foundation, 2003.

MDS Foundation

US Patient Liaison: Audrey Hassan
Patientliaison@mds-foundation.org
P.O. Box 353, Crosswicks, NJ 08515
Phone: 800-MDS-0839
Outside the US only: 609-298-6746
Fax: 1-609-298-0590
www.mds-foundation.org/

25

Sideroblastic Anemia

"Named for the Greek words for iron and germ, sideroblastic anemia is one of the principal types of iron-utilization anemia. Abnormal, iron-saturated red cells are present in the blood of people who have this disease. Although the iron circulates normally from the plasma to the bone marrow, where new red blood cells are created, it is not properly incorporated into new red blood cells."

—*Dr. Joseph F. Smith,* Medical Health Encyclopedia

Leah Robin knows what it means to have a health issue that involves the entire family. She remembers back to the 1970s, when her mother, grandmother, and both of her brothers were diagnosed with thalassemia intermedia on the basis of red blood cell smears. Although the family didn't know it at the time, that diagnosis was incorrect. In 1992 Leah's mother, Ellen, had her hemoglobin count checked and it had declined steeply. A bone marrow aspiration was performed and on the basis of the findings, her mother was diagnosed with MDS (myelodysplastic syndrome). The physicians who treated her thought that she had MDS in addition to thalassemia intermedia. She was given pyridoxine (vitamin B_6) and her hemoglobin level improved and remained stable.

But her diagnosis of MDS was also incorrect. In 1998, Leah's brother Paul became ill and was hospitalized with low hemoglobin counts and an enlarged spleen. His physicians concluded that he had inherited sideroblastic anemia (SA). Then her brother David was tested, and his doctors came to the same conclusion. The physicians now believe that the first diagnosis of thalassemia intermedia was incorrect for all family members and that the problem has been inherited SA only.

Ellen's SA has been controlled exclusively through pyridoxine. However, both brothers received additional supportive care, including red blood cell transfusions, pyridoxine, folic acid, and erythropoietin. They were both diagnosed with iron overload and were treated with chelation therapy using deferoxamine and deferasirox. Both brothers received splenectomies that reduced the number of red blood cell transfusions they needed but caused other problems, such as high platelet counts and blood clots. Neither brother was able to work fulltime. In 2008, Paul died of peripheral vascular and cardiac disease related to SA.

Leah helps other people with SA every day. She volunteers for organizations that address anemias and bone marrow failure and provide advice and support for people diagnosed with these illnesses and their caregivers.

Definition of sideroblastic anemias

Sideroblastic anemias (SA) are characterized by two common symptoms: (1) the body is impaired in its ability to use iron to synthesize heme to form hemoglobin; (2) this results in iron that collects around the nuclei of immature red blood cells (called ringed sideroblasts). People who have SA are likely to experience anemia ranging from mild to severe, and are also likely to have iron overload. SA is diagnosed on the basis of symptoms that may be caused by several underlying disorders. Those disorders have varied courses, severities, and treatments; therefore it is very important for people affected by SA to work with their medical care providers to determine the type of SA that they have.

Medical researchers have proposed several ways to classify the sideroblastic anemias. Some forms of SA are inherited or acquired; some are nonreversible or reversible. Inherited SA is present from birth and acquired SA occurs sometime later in life. Nonreversible SA can be treated and sometimes cured, but the cause of the condition cannot be eliminated. In contrast, reversible SA can be treated in a way that reverses the cause of the symptoms.

Inherited SA may result from mutations of the X chromosome, autosomes, or mitochondrial chromosomes. To date, the most common form of inherited SA is X-linked (the X chromosome is one of two chromosomes that determines gender). A rare second form of X-linked SA is associated with ataxia (a condition in which the brain does not keep track of the position of the limbs relative to the body, resulting in lack of coordination and unsteadiness of gait). Autosomal SA is the result of a mutation in one or more of the non-sex-linked chromosomes. Mitochondrial SA occurs when there is a mutation of the mitochondrial chromosomes. The mitochondria have their own set of DNA that is inherited only from the mother and replicates independent of the cellular DNA. Some disorders that include SA are caused by mitochondrial mutations, such as Pearson's Syndrome. Congenital sideroblastic anemias are also present from birth, but medical care providers cannot detect a familial history of SA. As the classification chart of the types of sideroblastic anemia on the next page indicates, there are no forms of inherited SA that can be reversed, although the symptoms may be treated. When mutations that lead to SA exist along with mutations that lead to hereditary hemochromatosis, the symptoms of SA are more severe and the disease progresses more quickly.

The chart lists types of SA that are acquired and nonreversible, also called acquired idiopathic sideroblastic anemias. Acquired idiopathic sideroblastic anemia is one of the myelodysplastic syndromes (MDS). It often occurs among older adults, in contrast to the inherited forms that are often present since childhood. Their symptoms may include SA, but may affect all three types of blood cells. These are bone marrow malignancies in which some faulty stem cells improperly produce mature blood cells. These faulty stem cells have a reproductive advantage over healthy stem cells and produce a disproportionate number of inferior mature blood cells that lead to SA, among other problems (these are called clonal disorders). The genetic mutations that occur among people with MDS can be similar to those occurring in inherited forms, particularly SA with ataxia. Acquired nonreversible SA is more aggressive than the inherited disorders, and may progress to leukemia. However, the aggressiveness of these disorders is variable. One group of people with

Classification sideroblastic anemias

	Nonreversible	Reversible
Inherited	X-linked Autosomal Mitochondrial Congenital	None
Acquired	Myelodysplastic Syndromes (MDS)	**Environmental Exposures** Copper deficiency Pyridoxine (vitamin B6) deficiency Lead overload Zinc overload Alcoholism **Drugs** Copper chelating drugs Ethanol Isoniazid Cycloserine Penacillamine COL-3 Busulfan

MDS may have a form of the disorder called pure sideroblastic anemia (PSA) in which only their red blood cells are affected. The course of PSA is slower than that of other kinds of MDS and less likely to transform into leukemia. (To find out more about these disorders, see chapter 24, Myelodysplastic Syndromes.)

One type of acquired reversible SA comes from environmental exposures, such as nutritional deficiencies in copper, pyridoxine, or ingestion of toxic levels of lead and zinc, or from alcoholism or hypothermia. Other forms of acquired reversible SA come from certain drugs, including some copper chelators (drugs that bind to copper to remove it from the body), ethanol, some drugs to treat tuberculosis, some antibiotics, and some drugs used in cancer treatment.

Symptoms

People with SA experience general symptoms related to anemia including fatigue, low ability to tolerate exercise, dizziness, chest pain, headache, and irritability. Some people with SA may also have enlarged spleens (called splenomegaly), which result in tenderness in the abdominal area. They may also experience symptoms related to iron overload. People with acquired nonreversible SA may experience iron overload because they are receiving blood transfusions in the course of being treated. In contrast, people with inherited SA may have iron overload without ever having a blood transfusion. Iron overload may include disorders that result from damage to internal organs, such as cirrhosis of the liver and diabetes. These symptoms are very general and may indicate a number of possible disorders other than SA, and therefore careful diagnosis by medical care providers is necessary.

Diagnosis and treatment

The most commonly accepted method to diagnose SA is to take a sample of bone marrow, obtained through a bone marrow biopsy, and examine it for ringed sideroblasts. If the number of ringed sideroblasts is greater than 15 percent of the immature red blood cells, then a diagnosis of SA may be called for. Medical care providers look for other changes in nucleated red blood cells as well; they are typically abnormally small (microcytic), although some people with SA have abnormally large red blood cells. Red blood cells are also pale (hypochromic), and they may be abnormally shaped (poikilocytosis). A subset of people with SA have elevated platelet counts (thrombocytosis).

Typically, people with SA have decreased levels of hemoglobin, and the red cell distribution width (that is, variation in size of red blood cells) is increased. Iron panels typically reveal increased serum iron and ferritin levels, and decreased transferrin levels. The chart on the next page provides similarities and differences of sideroblastic anemia and other iron-loading conditions.

Medical care providers may also need to determine whether organ damage has occurred from iron overload. Among people with acquired nonreversible SA, genetic abnormalities may be

iron panel	IRON PANEL TESTS					
	Serum Iron	Serum Ferritin	Transferrin Iron Saturation Percentage	Total Iron Binding Capacity (TIBC)	Transferrin	Serum Transferrin Receptor
Hemochromatosis	⬆	⬆	⬆	⬇	⬇	NORMAL TO LOW
Iron Deficiency Anemia	⬇	⬇	⬇	⬆	⬆	HIGH
Sideroblastic Anemia	⬆	⬆	⬆	⬇	⬇	NORMAL TO HIGH
Thalassemia	⬆	⬆	⬆	⬇	⬇	HIGH
Porphyria Cutanea Tarda	⬆	⬆	⬆	⬇	⬇	NORMAL
Anemia of Chronic Disease (ACD)	⬇	⬆ OR NORMAL	⬇	⬇	⬇	NORMAL
African Siderosis	⬆	⬆	⬆	⬇	⬇	NORMAL TO LOW

present and may change during the course of that disorder. Each form of acquired nonreversible SA has its own specific set of signs and symptoms.

There are two kinds of treatment for SA: supportive treatments that reduce the occurrence of symptoms, and curative treatments to put symptoms into remission or cure the disorder. Most people with SA get supportive treatments; the range of curative treatments is limited. More information about treatment for acquired nonreversible SA is available in chapter 24, Myelodysplastic Syndromes.

Supportive treatments for all forms of SA include pyridoxine (vitamin B₆), which may raise hemoglobin levels of people with SA and is effective in about one-third of people with inherited SA. Hemoglobin levels may also be raised through the use of a hormone that increases red blood cell production, called erythropoietin. Among some people with acquired nonreversible SA, the effectiveness of erythropoietin may be increased by also using another hormone called G-CSF that stimulates growth of white blood cells. Transfusion of red blood cells may also be necessary to maintain hemoglobin levels. Among people with acquired nonreversible SA a range of other supportive treatments may be necessary.

An equally important form of supportive treatment is the management of high levels of iron. Two types of iron chelation drugs are used: deferasirox and deferoxamine. Deferasirox is an oral medication that is a suspension, meaning that a tablet is dissolved in a liquid that is drunk. Deferoxamine is slowly infused through a pump or bolus injection, often for ten to twelve hours a day for five or six days a week. Iron chelation drugs may also be administered following blood transfusions. There is some evidence that removal of excess iron may increase the effectiveness of pyridoxine treatment. Management of organ damage because of iron overload may also be necessary.

Few effective curative treatments are available. For inherited SA there are few curative options; a few cases have been reported in which a bone marrow transplant has successfully cured inherited SA. For acquired nonreversible SA there are more curative options including chemotherapies that sometimes result in remission of the SA. Many of the chemotherapies are experimental treatments. Bone marrow transplant has also been successful in curing acquired nonreversible SA, but sometimes this procedure cannot be used because people with this disorder are older adults for whom the procedure poses too great a risk. A promising procedure is nonmyeloablative bone marrow transplant (also called "mini-transplant"), that can be used with somewhat older adults. Correcting the environmental factor that led to the disorder can usually cure people with acquired reversible SA, such as changes in diet and environment or discontinuing drug use.

Diet and exercise

There are relatively few guidelines for diet and exercise for people with SA. People with SA may wish to avoid foods rich in iron and that are iron fortified to help minimize or avoid iron overload. Dietary supplements such as vitamins, minerals, and herbal remedies may be useful (such as pyridoxine) but should be used only in consultation with medical care providers. Some dietary supplements may interact badly with other medications that people with SA must take and others may be harmful if they are taken in high doses. Because other disorders such as diabetes may be secondary to iron overload, people with SA may have special dietary considerations. People with SA are encouraged to exercise, but keeping in mind that their tolerance for exercise may be reduced if their hemoglobin levels are low. Like diet, some people with SA may need to exercise to manage other related disorders.

Who is at risk

SA is a set of rare disorders and therefore it is difficult to determine who may be at risk for them. A few of the X-linked and mitochondrial mutations responsible for inherited SA have been discovered, but less is known about the mutations for autosomal SA. Some families in which there is a history of SA may benefit from genetic testing and counseling to determine their risk for these disorders and help in making reproductive decisions.

Other risk factors for SA are environmental factors that, like the inherited causes, are incompletely understood. These disorders may be caused by exposure to environmental toxins, such as benzene or cancer therapies, but their causes are not fully known. The best known risk factors are those for acquired reversible SA. Medical care providers who diagnose SA should first check for the environmental factors and drug exposures that can produce these types of SA.

Resources

There are several helpful resources to provide information and support for people affected by SA, which includes both patients and their caregivers:

Aplastic Anemia and MDS International Foundation
P.O. Box 310
Churchton, MD 20733
Tel: 800-747-2820
Fax: 410-867-0240
www.aamds.org

Genetic Alliance
4301 Connecticut Ave. NW, Suite 404
Washington, DC 20008-2369
Tel: 800-336-GENE (4363)
Tel: 202-966-5557
Fax: 202-966-8553
www.geneticalliance.org

Leukemia and Lymphoma Society
1311 Mamaroneck Ave., Suite 310
White Plains, NY 10605
Tel: 800-955-4572
www.leukemia-lymphoma.org

National Family Caregivers Association
10400 Connecticut Avenue, Suite 500
Kensington, MD 20895-3944
Tel: 800-896-3650
Tel: 301-942-6430
Fax: 301-942-2302
www.nfcacares.org

National Organization for Rare Disorders
55 Kenosia Avenue
P.O. Box 1968
Danbury, CT 06813-1968
Tel: 800-999-6673
Tel: 203-744-0100
Fax: 203-798-2291
www.rarediseases.org

Patient Advocate Foundation
700 Thimble Shoals Blvd., Suite 200
Newport News, VA 23606
Tel: 800-532-5274
Fax: 757-873-8999
www.patientadvocate.org

Leah Robin can be reached at:
leduck@bellsouth.net

26

Hypoplastic Anemias:
Diamond Blackfan, Pearson's, Transient Erythroblastopenia of Childhood (TEC), and Fanconi Anemia

---

"The Diamond Blackfan Anemia (DBA) Registry of North America is a detailed database of patients with DBA from the United States and Canada. To date, 354 patients have been registered. From this database an analysis of the outcome of hematopoietic stem cell transplantation for DBA was undertaken. The survival for HLA-matched sibling versus alternative donor transplant was approximately 87.5 percent versus 14.1 percent."

—A. Vlachos, N. Federman, C. Reyes-Haley, J. Abramson, J. M. Lipton. "Hematopoietic Stem Cell Transplantation for Diamond Blackfan Anemia: A Report from the Diamond Blackfan Anemia Registry." Bone Marrow Transplant 27 (2001): 381–86

Jayson and Michelle Whittaker are frequently in the news, especially in the United Kingdom. Their son Charlie has Diamond Blackfan anemia and his only hope of survival depends upon getting a bone marrow transplantation. The problem lies with how the Whittakers wish to secure the stem cells needed for transplantation.

Normally cord blood taken from a sibling is HLA typed to determine a match with the patient. Dr. Adrianna Vlachos, who maintains a Diamond Blackfan anemia database in the United States, reports preliminary findings from more than 350 patients with DBA who participated in stem cell transplantation. In her analysis she found that when children receive stem cells from a HLA compatible sibling they have about an 87 percent chance of successful transplantation. Those children who were HLA typed with stem cells from non-family members had about a 14 percent chance of survival.

This sobering statistic has motivated the Whittakers to seek permission from the Human Fertilisation and Embryology Authority (UK) to screen embryos fertilized in vitro (outside the womb). In the process, a number of eggs are taken from the mother and fertilized outside the womb with the father's sperm. Some of the embryos will begin to grow. After a few days, a sufficient number of cells are available to "screen" for specific genetic material. An embryo that genetically matches the patient awaiting transplantation is implanted into the mother's womb and a normal pregnancy takes place. At birth, the stem cells are harvested from the cord blood and transplanted into the patient.

This process is called embryonic selection, and in the UK it requires a license obtained through the Human Fertilisation and Embryology Authority (HFEA). However, the HFEA still considers this procedure illegal for very basic reasons. Embryonic selection is allowed in the UK when a condition can be confirmed with genetic testing, as is the case for beta thalassemia. In fact, the HFEA approved embryonic selection for a family whose child has beta thalassemia and was a candidate for bone marrow transplant. In the case of Charlie Whittaker, however, the HFEA denied a license for the procedure because the gene or genes that cause Diamond Blackfan have not been completely determined.

The Whittaker story exemplifies the importance of registries such as the one maintained by Dr. Vlachos and the need for more research into a better understanding of genetics.

* * *

Diamond Blackfan anemia (DBA) is a rare, inherited hypoplastic condition. In hypoplastic anemias one or more types of blood cells are affected as compared with aplastic anemia, where all types of cells are affected. The number of DBA cases worldwide is estimated at 600 to 700 with birth prevalence of about 7 in 1,000,000. Its cause is unknown, although exposure to certain toxins and genetics is considered the primary cause. Both males and females are affected in equal numbers. Variations on chromosome 19 are seen in about 25 percent of cases and in 10 to 20 percent of cases other members of the family are affected. A second gene variation on chromosome 8 has also been identified; however, in a study of seven families with DBA, the presence of variations on either chromosome 8 or 19 were not found, suggesting that there are other genetic variations contributing to the disorder.

Nuchal translucency, swelling at the back of the fetal neck, was noted in two cases at twelve weeks into the pregnancy. This type of swelling is highly suggestive that the baby will have Down Syndrome or a major heart problem or both, two possible consequences for children with DBA. Nuchal translucency is an abnormality observed with an ultrasound. According to Joseph A. Worrall, MD, RDMS, "Nuchal translucency must be done between eleven weeks and thirteen weeks six days menstrual gestational age. The swelling is transient and may be gone if you look after fourteen weeks."

In DBA, the bone marrow lacks the ability to convert from fetal hemoglobin to normal adult hemoglobins and therefore there are too few or a complete absence of red blood cells. The failure to switch from fetal to adult hemoglobin causes a relatively benign disorder called Hereditary Persistence of Fetal Hemoglobin. High fetal hemoglobin levels are the consequence of many states in which there is disordered erythropoiesis.

Diamond Blackfan anemia may be mistaken for transient erythroblastopenia of childhood (TEC), Fanconi anemia, or Pearson Marrow-Pancreas syndrome. The differences are often determined by onset of disease and specific blood tests. In Diamond Blackfan anemia the condition is acquired during childhood with the onset within the first month of life; the others are congenital.

Symptoms and physical signs
Waxy pallor of the skin and mucous membranes is characteristic;

in some cases the skin may be bronzed due to the iron buildup. When there are problems of hemoglobin development and reduced access to oxygen, the body increases its absorption of iron in an effort to get more oxygen. Some of the excess iron that cannot be used for hemoglobin is placed in ferritin, a storage protein contained throughout the body including the brain. Patients with DBA will eventually develop a buildup of iron in various tissues.

Other symptoms observed in the DBA patient can include: hemorrhages into the eyes and skin, physical defects such as abnormalities of the thumbs or heart, or short stature. A child with this condition can also present with some of the typical symptoms related to anemia such as chronic fatigue, irritability, pallor (paleness), heart arrhythmia or murmur, and fainting. If iron overload is present, problems such as endocrine abnormalities, including hypothyroidism, hypoparathyroidism, and primary and secondary hypogonadism and growth hormone (IGF-I) insufficiency may occur.

Diagnosing Diamond Blackfan

A complete blood count and iron panel accompanied by other tests for fetal hemoglobin and specific enzymes are used in the diagnosis. The red blood cells of DBA patients are usually macrocytic (abnormally large), with elevated levels of folic acid and vitamin B_{12} due to an increased need for these nutrients. Elevated fetal hemoglobin (Hb F) and increased levels of enzymes adenosine deaminase (ADA) and orotidine decarboxylase (ODC). RBC precursors are severely reduced in the bone marrow while other marrow elements are usually normal. Serum iron levels are elevated.

Treatment

Steroid medication, usually prednisone, is the first line of treatment. About 70 percent of pediatric patients with Diamond Blackfan anemia will respond to this treatment. However, most of these children will have to take steroid medication for life. When a patient does not respond to treatment with steroids, blood transfusion is used. Regular blood transfusions will supply the needed red blood cells but with each transfusion there are

250 milligrams of iron. Normally, the body uses the iron when making new red blood cells, but since the person with DBS anemia is not making many cells the iron builds up. Some type of iron chelation therapy, such as Desferal® (deferioxamine) will eventually be needed to remove the excess iron.

Bone marrow transplantation is presently the only cure for DBS and there is encouragement for increased awareness for Diamond Blackfan. On October 3, 2001, Representative Carolyn McCarthy (D-NY) introduced H.R. 3014, the Diamond Blackfan Anemia (DBA) Act. This legislation would require the director of National Institutes of Health (NHLBI), in coordination with the Office of Rare Diseases, to expand and intensify research and related activities on DBA.

Pearson's syndrome

This form of congenital hypoplastic anemia may be initially confused with Diamond Blackfan syndrome, Fanconi, or transient erythroblastopenia of childhood (TEC). There are similarities between the conditions. In patients with Pearson's, the red cells are macrocytic (abnormally large), and both fetal hemoglobin and the enzyme adenosine deaminase are elevated. However, patients with Pearson's have catastrophic multiorgan failure with metabolic acidosis at birth or shortly afterwards, which affects the bone marrow, gastrointestinal system, kidneys, liver, and pancreas. Sideroblastic anemia occurs because of the buildup of iron in the mitrochondria. Pearson's syndrome is generally diagnosed in early infancy where the patient's symptoms and findings include failure to thrive, a reduction of all types of blood cells (pancytopenia), diarrhea, weakness, and neurologic problems such as seizures, unstable gait (ataxia), or stroke-like episodes.

Pearson's is due to deletion of a part of the mitochondrial DNA. The mitochondria is the energy-producing or functioning portion of the cell. There is no cure for Pearson's, and the disorder is very complicated and difficult to treat. Bone marrow transplantation might be beneficial. Patients do not usually survive beyond the age of three, often due to complications from diabetes, infection, or liver failure.

Transient erythroblastopenia of childhood (TEC)

Transient erythroblastopenia of childhood (TEC) is an acquired hypoplastic anemia involving a decrease in red blood cell (RBC) production. The cause is not known but TEC frequently follows a viral infection. The condition can occur at any age and generally disappears within one to two months. TEC can be differentiated from Diamond Blackfan and other hypoplastic anemias, because of time of onset and differences in blood tests. In TEC the mean corpuscular volume (MCV), fetal hemoglobin (HbF), and enzyme adenosine deaminase (ADA) levels are normal for the patient's age. Blood transfusions are used to treat severe cases of anemia.

Fanconi anemia

Fanconi anemia is an inherited hypoplastic anemia characterized by reduced production of all types of blood cells in the body. Fanconi is sometimes called a "chromosome breakage" condition. This means that people with Fanconi anemia have an unusually high number of breaks along their chromosomes. Onset of the disease is seen at as early as three and as late as twelve; age eight is the average age of diagnosis. In rare cases symptoms do not appear until adulthood. Patients with Fanconi anemia rarely live beyond their teens or early twenties. Some of the symptoms that are present are extreme fatigue and frequent infections, and the first signs may be nosebleeds and bruising. Patients with Fanconi have an increased incidence of cancers of the blood (leukemia).

There are cases, however, when the disease is evident at birth through a variety of birth defects which include:

- Thumb and arm anomalies: misshapen or missing thumbs or an incompletely developed or missing radius (one of the forearm bones)
- Skeletal anomalies of the hips, spine, or ribs
- Kidney problems
- Skin discoloration (café-au-lait spots); portions of the body may have a suntanned look
- Small head or eyes
- Mental retardation or learning disabilities

- Low birth weight
- Gastrointestinal difficulties
- Small reproductive organs in males
- Defects in tissues separating chambers of the heart

Approximately 1 in every 87 Ashkenazi Jews is a carrier of Fanconi anemia. Both parents have to pass the gene change for the child to have Fanconi anemia. If two carriers for Fanconi anemia have a child that child has:

- One in four chance of having Fanconi anemia
- Two in four chance of being a carrier
- One in four chance of neither having Fanconi anemia nor being a carrier

Unaffected siblings of individuals with Fanconi anemia have a greater chance of being carriers. Carriers can be detected through blood tests. In Ashkenazi Jews the changed gene is located on chromosome number 9. By looking for the specific gene change that is seen in Ashkenazi Jews with Fanconi anemia, it is possible to achieve a detection rate of approximately 83 percent in that population.

Once pregnant, a diagnosis of Fanconi anemia is available using samples collected from amniocentesis, a procedure where a needle is inserted through the abdomen to obtain amniotic fluid. Frequent screening can ensure early detection and diagnosis of cancers that are often associated with Fanconi anemia.

Treatment

Treatment for Fanconi anemia is primarily preventive. In order to detect cancers early, individuals with Fanconi anemia should arrange for frequent screenings. In addition, avoidance of exposure to the sun and to other agents that may damage the chromosomes is crucial.

Individuals with Fanconi anemia may pursue bone marrow transplantation on an experimental basis; however, to date, there is no consistently effective treatment.

Androgen replacement can stimulate blood cells or platelets

and is effective in about half of the cases. Growth factors can sometimes stimulate the production of white blood cells. Gene therapy is on the horizon, with clinical trials specific to inherited bone marrow failure syndromes underway at the National Cancer Institute.

Content in this publication is not intended to be a substitute for professional medical advice, nor is it intended to replace the services of a medical professional or impair the patient–healthcare provider or caregiver relationship. Content in this publication should be used as information only and be discussed with a medical professional who is qualified to diagnose and treat your condition. Iron Disorders Institute, all contributors, and the publisher of this book are not responsible for the content on websites listed in the resources, nor do we endorse products promoted on such sites. We advise you to always seek the advice of a qualified health provider before making any changes to diet, supplementation, or starting any new treatment. Any application of the information or recommendations in this book is made at the reader's discretion.

Resources
For additional information about Fanconi:
Center for the Study and Treatment of Jewish Genetic Diseases
UPMC Health Systems
Contact: Erin O'Rourke, MS
University of Pittsburgh Dept of Human Genetics
E-1658 Biomedical Science Tower
Pittsburgh, PA 15261
Toll Free: 800-334-7980
Email: eorourke@helix.hgen.pitt.edu
We appreciate permission to reprint by Erin O'Rourke
Fanconi information provided on her website:
www.mazornet.com/genetics/fanconi_anemia.htm

National Foundation for Jewish Genetic Diseases, Inc.
250 Park Avenue, Suite 1000
New York, NY 10017
Tel: 212-371-1030

Fanconi Anemia Research Fund, Inc.
1801 Wilamette Street, Suite 200
Eugene, OR 97401
Toll Free: 800-828-4891
Tel: 541-687-4658
Fax: 541-687-0548
www.fanconi.org

National Organization for Rare Disorders
55 Kenosia Avenue
P.O. Box 1968
Danbury, CT 06813-1968
Tel: 203-744-0100
Fax: 203-798-2291
www.rarediseases.org

Organizations related to Diamond Blackfan anemia:
Diamond Blackfan Anemia Registry
Attn: Adrianna Vlachos, MD
Schneider Children's Hospital
Division of Pediatric Hematology/Oncology and Stem Cell
Transplantation
269-01 76th Avenue
New Hyde Park, NY 11040
Toll Free: 888-884-3227
Tel: 718-470-3460
Fax: 718-343-4642
www.dbar.org

**National Center on Birth Defects and
Developmental Disabilities (NCBDDD)**
www.cdc.gov/ncbddd

NIH/National Heart, Lung and Blood Institute
31 Center Drive MSC 2480
Bethesda MD 20892-2480
Tel: 301-592-8573
www.nhlbi.nih.gov

Websites that may be of interest:
   www.familyvillage.wisc.edu/lib_dba.htm
   www.bloodjournal.org
   www.nhlbi.nih.gov/studies/hematol.htm
   www.diamondblackfan.org.uk
   www.obgynsono.com/nt.html
   www.dbar.org
   www.fanconi-anemia.co.uk
   www.fanconi.org
   www.letthemhear.org
   www.marchofdimes.org

27
Paroxysmal Nocturnal Hemoglobinuria (PNH)

"The distinct and rather peculiar characteristics of paroxysmal nocturnal hemoglobinuria (PNH) have puzzled hematologists for more than a century."

—*Genes and Diseases 2002, National Center for Biotechnology Information*

Thirty-one-year-old Rebecca finishes the last of the letters she is preparing to mail to others with her condition, paroxysmal nocturnal hemoglobinuria (PNH). She looks across the room at her husband, Brian, and two children, ten-year-old Joshua and seven-year-old Marilyn, and realizes how fortunate she is. Women with PNH are advised not to have children because of the serious risks. Some are even given the option of "selective termination," something Rebecca thinks about as she arranges the mass mailing she is about to send out to PNH patients around the world.

Rebecca got her diagnosis of PNH in August of 1998, slightly more than a year after her son Ryan was stillborn at twenty-eight weeks of gestation.

The first sign that anything was wrong during this pregnancy was when Rebecca found blood in her urine. Her physician

Parts of this chapter reprinted with permission of Aplastic Anemia & MDS International Foundation, Inc., from *PNH Basic Explanations*, by Dr. Jaroslaw Maciejewski, MD, PhD, Cleveland Clinic Taussig Cancer Institute. © 2002 by Aplastic Anemia & MDS International Foundation, Inc.

suspected the problem was kidney stones, but tests did not support this suspicion. Urinary tract and kidney infections were ruled out. She was, however, anemic; her hemoglobin was 10.6 g/dL. Also, her platelet count was low. This sounded vaguely familiar to Rebecca—she remembered being anemic and having low platelets when she was pregnant with Marilyn, her second child.

She was given iron pills (325 milligrams) and was told to take them three times a day. As with her other two pregnancies the iron pills made her sick to her stomach, so she took them at night before bedtime, thinking that she could sleep through the nausea.

At twenty-eight weeks gestation, she realized that she hadn't felt movement for several days. Rebecca knew something was wrong. At the hospital an ultrasound confirmed the death, and Rebecca and Brian faced the grim choice of inducing labor or allowing labor to commence spontaneously. They chose to induce labor and the procedure was scheduled for the next morning, July fourth. The doctor sent Rebecca home with some sleeping pills for her and her husband, which they took gratefully.

In the early hours of the following morning, the day the inducement was to be performed, Rebecca went into labor. It was questionable whether or not she and her husband would make it to the hospital before the delivery occurred. Between contractions, a somewhat panicked and barefooted Brian maneuvered Rebecca into his car—a classic 1966 Chevelle—which he pushed to the limit, racing toward the hospital, running red lights along the way.

Today, Rebecca is reminded of that ride every time she gets into Brian's car. She still has difficulty with the memory of those events, but can now put together many pieces of the puzzle that provide clues to her PNH disorder in hopes that she can help others with this condition.

She looks back over the previous ten years to the birth of her first child. This birth had been routine. She was given iron even though her labs were normal. The iron made her sick—queasy and nauseated—so she stopped taking them. After Joshua was born but before getting pregnant with Marilyn, her second child, Rebecca began to have migraines and she noticed odd bruising on her legs. She wondered how she had gotten so many bruises without remembering injuring herself. She took pain pills for the headaches and disregarded the bruises.

After becoming pregnant with Marilyn, things were more complicated; her labs were consistently abnormal. Hemoglobin ranged between 9.4 g/dL and 10.6 g/dL, and platelets 41,000 to 71,000 were very low (normal range is 150,000–440,000). Clues to her PNH disorder were emerging, but not yet fully understood. As with her first pregnancy Rebecca was given iron pills—325 milligrams twice a day. Again, the pills made her sick.

After losing Ryan but before she was diagnosed with PNH, Rebecca endured many painful migraines and blood clots—deep vein thrombosis (DVT)—in her legs.

At first she thought the pain in her legs was due to a pulled muscle, but when her leg began to swell and the pain increased, Brian took her to the emergency room, where the clots were detected. One clot had blocked the main artery in her left leg and she realized that she could have died as a result of this experience. She was given Heparin shots in the belly and then Coumadin. Both drugs are anticoagulants (blood thinners).

Living with the new fear of what blood clots can do, Rebecca had daily, then weekly, blood draws to check her clotting time. If too thick, she would have another clot; if too thin, she could bleed to death. The constant worry if her blood was too thick or too thin brought on panic attacks. Besides the panic, episodes of dark urine, jaundice, abdominal pain, and excruciating migraines, compounded by the grief of losing her son, brought on a series of mood swings—crying spells, emotional outbursts, anger, and frustration filled Rebecca's days.

Eventually some labwork revealed that she might have some form of hemolytic anemia. She was referred to a hematologist who diagnosed her with autoimmune hemolytic anemia (AIHA). Initially the test for this condition had been inconclusive, but sometimes with AIHA this can happen.

Rebecca was started on prednisone, a corticosteroid, but her chronic anemia prevailed. Prednisone can give a person energy, but in Rebecca's case, she felt mentally "revved up" but lacked the physical energy to do anything about it. Daily exercise, long walks, and snow skiing gave way to chronic fatigue and frustration. Rebecca, a once happy, energetic young woman became a bloated, anxious, and depressed person who felt life was not worth living. Her faith and the love of her husband and two children were the only things that kept her going.

After a few months, the decision to remove her spleen was made, because often patients with AIHA are cured once the spleen is removed. Following the splenectomy, Rebecca was taken off prednisone. She was no longer taking an anticoagulant and within months developed pain in her other calf. This time Rebecca knew exactly the cause of her leg pain. Caught in the early stages, she was able to get prompt treatment for the clot. With this episode, her hematologist was beginning to suspect PNH. He ordered a CD59 test. CD59 is a molecule found on the surface of blood cells; it plays a role in controlling hemolysis and is decreased in patients with PNH. This test provided the diagnosis.

Rebecca sought the help of PNH specialist Dr. Lucio Luzzatto of Memorial Sloan Kettering Cancer Center in New York City. Consulting with Dr. Luzzatto, Rebecca began to receive blood transfusions, which improved her condition. She still suffers from periodic migraines and upper right quadrant pain, which is attributed to microembolisms (tiny blood clots). She watches for the first signs of infection, taking care to get treatment early. She continues to have blood transfusions and is now mindful of transfusion-dependent iron overload, which is now being monitored.

In all, Rebecca feels she is in now in charge of her condition, rather than her condition being in charge of her life. To help others, she began an email support group which has grown to nearly 130 subscribers—all people with PNH or family members with the condition.

What is PNH?

PNH is a rare but potentially serious blood disease that affects people of all ages. Although some of the features of this disease, such as hemolysis inside of the blood vessels or appearance of red urine, have been known for over 100 years, many aspects of PNH remain a mystery. As with other "orphan" diseases, the progress in their understanding is slow. For physicians and scientists who study this disease, it is often frustrating that they are only able to give limited answers and explanations to many of the questions that PNH patients have.

Only recently have we learned the complicated mechanisms and pathologic relationships leading to the development of this disease. Despite recent advances, much more research is needed to fully clarify all the aspects of this disease. Many specialists believe that research on the development of PNH in the bone marrow will also be helpful in understanding other diseases of the blood system such as aplastic anemia and leukemias. Because PNH is such a rare disease, rigorous clinical trials at institutions seeing numerous PNH patients produce the best chance of developing effective treatments and cure. This is why it is important that patients participate in the clinical trials whenever possible.

PNH explained

First one must understand the mechanisms of PNH in order to understand the symptoms. PNH is not inheritable. It develops from an acquired mutation in the genetic material of the most immature bone marrow cells, called stem cells. These bone marrow stem cells are responsible for the steady supply of blood cells because they produce three types of blood cells: red cells, which deliver oxygen to the tissues; white cells, which fight infections; and platelets, which clot the blood.

In PNH, the mutation in the genetic material of a stem cell affects a specific gene called PIG-A. Due to this mutation, the enzyme required for attaching many important proteins on the surface of the blood cells is missing, and the affected stem cell is producing defective mature blood cells that "spread" the disease. Red cells, white cells, and platelets produced by the diseased stem cell all carry the defect that causes symptoms associated with this disease. We do not know what causes the mutation of the stem cell in PNH. We also do not know why the defective PNH stem cell outgrows "normal stem cells that allow the diseased blood cells to progressively replace normal cells."

Symptoms

General. The presence of defective marrow and blood cells are responsible for the symptoms in PNH. PNH produces a variety of clinical symptoms but not all patients will experience every possible complication and the disease may show different degrees of severity in each patient. It is very important that patients understand the course of their disease and individual prognoses can be difficult to predict. Generally, low red cell count with low hemoglobin levels (in conjunction with low platelet and white cell count) can either be a result of increased destruction of blood cells, or a decreased production in the marrow (a hallmark of marrow failure states). While in PNH, the destruction of red blood cells is the most important factor leading to anemia; in some patients, production of red cells in the marrow is impaired and destroyed red cells are not sufficiently replaced.

Hemolysis. Lack of certain proteins on the surface of red cells (produced by the mutated bone marrow stem cell) makes the cells susceptible to being more easily destroyed (hemolysis). This process is mediated by a complicated system of serum proteins called "complement." Under normal circumstances, complement serves as an antimicrobial defense factor and kills microorganisms. Healthy red cells are equipped with surface proteins that make them resistant to the action of complement. However, in PNH, red cells lack these proteins and are susceptible to destruction by complement. When PNH red cells are destroyed, they release hemoglobin, which is the red pigment of blood. Hemoglobin is excreted in the urine, causing its red or coca-like discoloration, which is a characteristic sign of PNH. More importantly, this destruction of red cells can result in anemia. Depending on the severity of hemolysis, patients may experience headaches, ear ringing, palpitations, heart racing, fatigue, and sleepiness. Severe anemia may result in fainting spells and could possibly lead to a heart attack. Usually, destruction of PNH red cells continues at a certain individual rate and the bone marrow can compensate for it with an increased production. Unfortunately, the bone marrow of some PNH patients may not be able to produce enough red cells so patients experience more severe anemia and may even require transfusions. In addition to ongoing hemolysis, several unknown factors may cause a dramatic increase in destruction of PNH cells, often referred to as a hemolytic crisis. Some known factors to cause hemolytic crisis are other diseases and stress.

Blood clots. Because PNH stem cells can also produce defective platelets, PNH platelets can be a source of serious and often fatal complications. It is believed that in PNH, the lack of certain (currently still unknown) proteins from PNH platelets increases their propensity to form undesired blood clots—a condition termed thrombosis. Clots can be carried by the blood flow to the lungs, resulting in a very serious condition called lung embolism. Blood clots may also lead to serious complications and possible death when they block the blood flow in vital organs such as the liver, spleen, intestine, or brain. The symptoms of blood clots in legs or arms include pain, swelling and redness or bluish discoloration. Symptoms of clots in internal organs depend upon the organ affected. Clots in the liver may cause abdominal pain, feeling of fullness, chest pain, or yellow discoloration of skin and eyes. A blood clot that has traveled to the lungs can cause shortness of breath, cough with bloody sputum, chest pain, palpitations, and pain when a patient takes deep breaths. Formation of blood clots in PNH is very unpredictable; some patients may experience these clots quite frequently while other patients never have any. As the exact mechanism leading to thrombosis is not known, there are no ways to predict who is at greatest risk. Clearly, patients who had an episode of thrombosis in the past have a greater risk to experience repeated episodes.

Marrow failure/defective blood production. In many PNH patients, the marrow will sufficiently compensate for the destruction of red cells in the bloodstream. These patients will also show an adequate production of platelets or white cells. However, many studies have demonstrated that PNH marrow is not working properly even if the decrease in blood counts is not evident. PNH patients may develop more or less severe marrow failure similar to those of aplastic anemia. The reasons for the marrow failure in PNH are not clear. However, we know that PNH occurs frequently as a complication of aplastic anemia (in earlier estimates up 10 percent of AA patients) and many patients (30 to 40 percent) with aplastic anemia may harbor PNH stem cells and produce PNH blood cells. Evidence for PNH cells can be also detected in some patients with MDS.

Impaired production of platelets will result in a decreased platelet count, also referred to as thrombocytopenia, which depending on its severity may lead to bleeding and bruising. External bleeding may cause blood loss and anemia while internal bleeding may result in serious complications such as a stroke.

Decreased white cell production impairs the body's ability to fight infections. The risk for serious bacterial and fungal infections dramatically increases when the number of granulocytes in blood decreases to below 500 per μL. Patients with low numbers of white cells have to be aware that they need to seek medical attention when they experience fever or other symptoms of infection. For a PNH patient, a quick administration of antibiotics during an infection may be life saving.

PNH and aplastic anemia

As mentioned above, PNH is closely related to aplastic anemia. Many aplastic patients have different degrees of PNH involvement. PNH may develop from aplastic anemia, or aplastic anemia and low counts might be a complication of PNH. Specialists believe that aplastic anemia sets the conditions that are advantageous for the growth of PNH stem cells and allows for the development of PNH. It is possible that the clarification as to why PNH and aplastic anemia so frequently occur together might help us to understand the causes for these diseases and, hopefully, develop new specific treatments.

Diagnosis

Symptoms of hemolysis and anemia, together with the discoloration of urine especially evident in the morning, are characteristic signs of PNH. However, in the setting of low blood counts, the diagnosis may be more difficult. Historically, diagnosis of PNH was established by using the Ham's test. In this test, destruction of patient's red cells by complement in a test tube is measured. Because in patients with ongoing hemolysis most of the PNH red cells are destroyed in the bloodstream, the Ham's test is very insensitive. Currently, new, more sensitive tests are being used, which rely on the measurement of missing proteins on the patient's white cells using an instrument called a flow cytometer (PNH flow cytometry). These advanced testing techniques can identify even a tiny number of PNH cells. In addition to helping with diagnosis, these tests have helped doctors recognize that PNH cells may be found much more frequently than previously thought, and that many patients with aplastic anemia show evidence of asymptomatic PNH.

In addition to the specific diagnostic tests for PNH, measurements of numbers of red blood cells and hemoglobin levels are important for the determination of the severity of hemolysis, blood loss, or bone marrow dysfunction. All these factors may affect the hemoglobin levels and the severity of anemia. However, in order to know whether the anemia is due to hemolysis or impaired red cell production, reticulocyte count should be measured. Reticulocytes are young red cells, and their numbers, when high, will tell you and your doctor that your marrow is working properly and anemia in this setting is most likely due to the red cell destruction. While the number of platelets will be helpful to see whether a patient is at risk for bleeding, decreased platelet production in PNH also is a sign of the defective function of bone marrow. Similarly, if marrow is not working properly, the number of white cells will be decreased. Severe depression in white blood cell count may predispose to life-threatening infections (the detailed description of thrombocytopenia and low white cell counts can be found in the aplastic anemia brochure listed at the end of this chapter).

Other blood tests may also be useful. The severity of ongoing hemolysis may be measured using LDH—a protein that is set free when red cells are destroyed. High LDH values are consistent with hemolysis. Similarly, low levels of a protein, called haptoglobin, are also indicative of hemolysis. In addition, it is also important to determine iron levels to establish whether a patient is iron deficient or in an iron overload state.

Treatments

Because PNH is rare, there are only very few scientifically established facts about the best way of treating this disease. Generally, there are two ways of treatment—bone marrow transplantation and more conservative treatments. The decision of which treatment option to use should be discussed in great detail between the doctor and patient. The AA&MDSIF brochure *Managing Treatment Decisions* will be of value in asking questions about treatments.

Conservative treatment. Principally, there are no specific agents to treat PNH. Care management of patients with hemolysis, with and without signs of bone marrow failure, may differ. In patients with typical hemolytic form, many doctors advocate that flare-ups of hemolysis should be treated with courses of steroid hormones, such as prednisone. There are no scientific proofs that this strategy is really effective, but it is believed that steroids may decrease the destruction rate of red cells. Chronic usage of steroids is even more controversial as such therapy has many toxic side effects. In any case, if administered on a chronic basis, all attempts should be made to use the lowest possible dose and to limit the duration of treatment. Transfusions may be needed for acute decreases in hemoglobin or on a periodic basis when the patient's decrease in hemoglobin level is steady. Transfusion is a routine procedure and its toxicity may be less than that of a chronic steroid administration. However, many patients feel emotional resistance toward transfusions. The risks involved in a single transfusion are very low and administration of blood is not a "magic mark" that indicates progression to a more advanced and severe stage of the disease.

As explained above, PNH may increase the propensity for blood clots. Generally, routine blood thinners are not uniformly recommended unless patients have experienced an episode of thrombosis because many patients may never have this complication. Generally, thromboses are treated with infusion of the blood thinners (such as heparin) into the vein and, after acute symptoms have resolved, with chronic administration of oral blood thinners such as Coumadin. Most doctors will recommend long-term blood thinner therapy with Coumadin but it is not entirely clear whether such therapy is really effective in preventing further blood clots. In addition, blood thinners may be complicated in patients whose platelet count is low; the risk of bleeding may be higher than that of thrombosis.

Immunosuppressive therapy may be of benefit to patients whose blood counts are low due to decreased blood cell production (and/or whose marrow is empty). As explained in the previous paragraphs, low reticulocyte count (reticulocytes are immature red cells that indicate that marrow is working) can show that marrow is not working properly; hemolysis with normal compensatory red cell production would be otherwise accompanied by a high reticulocyte count.

Other signs of defective marrow function include low platelet and white cell count. Under such circumstances, similar to typical aplastic anemia, immunosuppressive treatments may be beneficial. These treatments include antithymocyte globulin (ATG) and cyclosporine. Cyclosporine given alone has not been very effective. Immunosuppressive treatments do not eliminate the PNH cells, but they may improve the function of the bone marrow and help to compensate for the destruction of the blood cells. More information on this therapy can be found in the AA&MDSIF brochure *Aplastic Anemia: Basic Explanations* or on the AA&MDSIF website. Good supportive care is very important and may affect the comfort of living and survival. In addition to the direct treatment of hemolysis, folic acid and iron may help bone marrow to replace destroyed red cells. Many PNH patients lose large amounts of iron in urine, which can result in iron deficiency. On the other extreme, if they receive many transfusions, they can develop iron overload. This is why it is important that iron status be continually monitored and appropriate therapy instituted when needed.

Bone marrow transplantation. Bone marrow transplantation offers the only known curative therapy for PNH. However, the decision to undergo this complicated procedure must be thoroughly researched and all potential risks discussed between the doctor and patient. Many aspects influence the success of this procedure; therefore, each case must be individually evaluated to determine if it is a viable treatment option. There are several types of transplants and each has a different prognosis. Best results are achieved in younger patients with a matched sibling donor. Unfortunately, only a minority of patients will have such a donor. Transplantation performed with marrow from unrelated donors has a much greater risk of serious and chronic complications. Patients must decide for themselves if they want to risk a transplant or continue their current conservative care based on the severity of their symptoms.

Eculizumab (Soliris®, Alexion Pharmaceuticals, Inc.) is a newly approved drug for the reduction of hemolysis in patients with PNH. Prescribing information for this agent includes a boxed warning describing the risk for serious meningococcal infection and the need for meningococcal vaccination prior to treatment. According to the Soliris website, in clinical trials, patients who were treated with eculizumab experienced a reduction of symptoms and chronic hemolysis, fewer blood clots, improvements in anemia, and a reduced need for blood transfusions.

Patient assistance is available through the SOLIRIS OneSource™ team, which is a group of registered nurses who will work with patients, healthcare providers, and health insurance providers to help with answers to questions about this therapy. OneSource can also help patients with information about alternative resources if insurance is not adequate.

Prognosis

The course of PNH varies in patients. PNH may be chronic with only mild symptoms or it can be a disabling disease with frequent hemolytic crises and a regular need for transfusions. Of course, unexpected complications, such as development of aplastic anemia or occurrence of blood clots, may affect survival. The most common deadly complication of PNH is occurrence of blood clots in vital organs. With a good supportive care, however, PNH patients can live with their disease for many years.

Wellness

Apart from specific treatments and medications, there are some actions you can take to have the optimum level of wellness possible for you. Do not take any over-the-counter medications, prescription medications, supplements, vitamins, or herbs without first consulting with your doctor. If you have low red cell counts you should avoid excessive exercise, going to high altitudes, or any activity that causes chest pain, severe shortness of breath, or heart racing. Some doctors believe that heavy anaerobic exercise may contribute to acidification of blood and induce hemolysis. If you have low platelet count or are taking blood thinners, you should avoid activities that could result in straining or injuries. If you develop headache or persistent pain anywhere, which could indicate a bleeding problem, you should notify your doctor. If you have low white cell counts you may be more likely to catch a bacterial infection. Be alert to any symptoms of infection—fever or increased fatigue can be warning signs, and you should report these promptly to your doctor.

Emotional issues

When you are diagnosed with this disease, you may feel shock, anger, and fear, and even relief at learning what is wrong. You will need to make time for medical treatment and administration. Everyday life must go on for you and your family. PNH is a chronic disease and you should not schedule your entire life around the disease. Although this may seem overwhelming and impossible, many other patients with the same condition have come through to lead full lives, often becoming stronger as individuals and as families. See Patient Literature at the end of this chapter for booklets that can help.

Resources

Patient Literature:

Families Coping with AA&MDS. Annapolis, MD: Aplastic
Anemia & MDS International Foundation, 2002.

Iron Chelation Therapy in Aplastic Anemia, MDS & PNH.
Annapolis, MD: Aplastic Anemia & MDS International
Foundation, 2002.

Managing Treatment Decisions. Annapolis, MD: Aplastic
Anemia & MDS International Foundation, 2003.

PNH Basic Explanations. Annapolis, MD: Aplastic Anemia &
MDS International Foundation, 2002.

For a complete packet of information on PNH, contact:

**Aplastic Anemia & MDS International Foundation,
Inc.**

P.O. Box 310

Churchton, MD 20733

Toll Free: 800-747-2820

Tel: 410-867-0242

Fax: 410-867-0240

Email: help@aamds.org

www.aamds.org

*Mission: AA&MDSIF serves as a resource for patient assistance,
advocacy, and support; provides educational materials and medical
information; and supports research to find effective treatments for
Aplastic Anemia (AA), Myelodysplastic Syndromes (MDS); and related
bone marrow failure diseases.*

Blood and Marrow Transplantation:

America's Blood Centers

725 15th Street NW, Suite 700

Washington, D.C. 20005

Tel: 202-393-5725

Fax: 202-393-1282

www.americasblood.org

Blood and Marrow Transplant Information Network (BMT InfoNet)
2310 Skokie Valley Road, Suite 104
Highland Park, IL 60035
Tel: 888-597-7674
Fax: 847-433-4599
www.bmtinfonet.org

National Bone Marrow Transplant Link
20411 W. 12 Mile Rd., Suite 108
Southfield, MI 48076
Toll Free: 800-546-5268
www.nbmtlink.org/

National Marrow Donor Program
3001 Broadway Street Northeast, Suite 100
Minneapolis, MN 55413-1753
Toll Free: 800-627-7692
www.marrow.org

Clinical Trials Listings:
CenterWatch
100 N. Washington Street Suite 301
Boston, MA 02114
Tel: 617-948-5100
Fax: 617-948-5101
www.centerwatch.com

National Library of Medicine/National Institutes of Health
8600 Rockville Pike
Bethesda, Maryland 20894
Toll Free: 888-346-3656
www.clinicaltrials.gov

Insurance and Legal Issues:
   Patient Advocate Foundation
   700 Thimble Shoals Blvd., Suite 200
   Newport News, VA 23606
   Toll Free: 800-532-5274
   Fax: 757-873-8999
   www.patientadvocate.org

Hemophilia and von Willebrand's

Hemophilia and von Willebrand's disease are two inherited bleeding disorders due to problems of coagulation (blood clotting). In these conditions, patients have missing or poorly functioning clotting factors. Hemophilia is carried on the X chromosome (one in the pair of chromosomes that determines gender), therefore most patients with hemophilia are males, although in rare cases hemophilia can occur in females. Von Willebrand's is seen mostly in females, although males can have the disease.

Hemophilia is an inherited bleeding disorder that affects 18,000 persons in the United States. The disorder results from deficiencies in blood clotting factors and can lead to spontaneous internal bleeding and bleeding following injuries or surgery. These bleeding episodes can cause severe joint damage, neurological damage, damage to other organ systems involved in the hemorrhage, and, in rare cases, death. Treating the bleeding episodes involves the prompt and proper use of clotting factor concentrates. The two most common types of hemophilia are Factor VIII Deficiency and Factor IX Deficiency. Factor VIII Deficiency, also called classic hemophilia or hemophilia A, occurs in about 1 in every 10,000 live male births in the United States. Factor IX Deficiency, also called hemophilia B or Christmas Disease, is more rare.

brand disease is one of the most common inherited
g disorders."

*—American College of Obstetricians and Gynecologists Committee on
Gynecologic Practice. ACOG committee opinion. Von Willebrand
Disease in Gynecologic Practice.* International Journal
of Gynaecology and Obstetrics, 2002

Linda was eleven years old when she started her menstrual
cycle. At first her periods were very irregular; often she would
skip months. When she did have a period, it would last sometimes as long as ten days. Menstrual flow was always very
heavy and extremely painful. Linda remembers taking aspirin
and Midol® to help alleviate the pain, not realizing that those
medications were contributing to the heavy bleeding. When
she was thirteen, her physician put her on birth control pills
to help regulate the cycles, which caused Linda to bleed more
heavily than before.

Linda remembers that as a teenager she dreaded her period
because she feared the embarrassing events that were certain
to take place. Her bleeding was so heavy that frequently her
clothing would become saturated, which was a horrifying
experience for a young woman. To prevent these awkward and
embarrassing situations, Linda wore dark-colored clothing and
carried extra sanitary supplies, in large quantities. She recalls
the most terrifying times were the high school days where she
had to participate in physical education class. Her teacher did
not understand. Believing that Linda was trying to get excused
from the class, the gym teacher often lectured Linda and forced
her to participate.

A few years into her marriage, Linda, twenty-four years old
at the time, was diagnosed with infertility problems and endometriosis. After years of trying to conceive, she and her husband adopted two children. Linda describes them as beautiful,
happy, and healthy. She had wanted children very much, but
often she lacked the energy to play with them. Her life seemed
always to revolve around the bleeding.

Vacations were never easy to plan, because she never knew
when she would start a period, how long it would last, and
how debilitated she would be during the experience. She would

remain at home the first few days of her period because she feared hemorrhaging and bleeding through her clothing. Linda suffered through many weak and painful days, never able to lead a normal life like other women. She rarely had the strength to clean her house or to grocery shop, and there was no hope of having a regular job. She tried to compensate. After her period was over, even though she was weak, she would push herself to try to interact with her family and to resume normal activities.

Through all of this Linda continued making trips to the gynecologist. She reported details to him, always stressing that she found it difficult to believe that it was normal for her to bleed so heavily. The gynecologist thought Linda was exaggerating her situation, telling her that women couldn't bleed that much, she must be like her mother, or he would say that she would just have to learn to live with the periods.

Disgusted and frustrated after several years of trying to cope, Linda decided to change gynecologists. This decision was the first step toward getting a diagnosis. Linda says that meeting her new gynecologist changed her life. Finally she had found a doctor who truly listened to her concerns and firmly believed that she did not need to live with so much pain. After going through a very thorough diagnostic process, her gynecologist suspected a bleeding disorder. He referred Linda to a hemophilia treatment center, one of 123 nationally recognized and funded comprehensive centers for the care of women with bleeding disorders. After meeting with the staff and reviewing her family and medical history and completing a series of blood tests, she was diagnosed with von Willebrand disease, a relatively common inherited bleeding disorder.

Prior to being diagnosed Linda had a number of surgical procedures, including oral surgery to remove her wisdom teeth, removal of a ganglion cyst from her wrist, and gall bladder surgery. She looks back on these surgeries and considers herself fortunate to have had no post-operative complications.

Once diagnosed, she agreed to have an endometrial ablation to help alleviate the menorrhagia (heavy periods) and fibroids that she had developed. Having a bleeding disorder meant that she needed to be medicated with DDAVP-IV before and after the operation.

Following this procedure, Linda recovered fairly well and life seemed to be going along smoothly. The surgery temporarily stopped her periods and relieved the pain. Linda says she never missed having a period and enjoyed being pain free. That all changed within eight months. During the summer, Linda began having lower abdominal pain. After a few months of trying different pain medications, her gynecologist discussed the possibility of her having adenomyosis, a benign but invasive growth into the lining of the uterus. A hysterectomy was recommended and scheduled that autumn. Surgery was moved up, however, because before the end of summer, Linda had a sudden hemorrhage and the hysterectomy had to be performed.

Linda shares her experience in the hopes that it will help others. Her only advice to women suffering with some of the symptoms that she had is this: "You know your body better than anyone. If you don't get answers to your questions, continue asking until you are 100 percent satisfied with the results!" Linda concludes, "To say that vWD has been life altering would be an understatement; but I also would say that I feel better knowing what I'm dealing with and have been able to lead a better life. Having a bleeding disorder is not the end of the world; I have learned so much about my disorder and feel very empowered with the knowledge!"

(Note: Although this patient reported irregular periods among her symptoms, vWD does not cause irregularity, but rather only heavy menstrual bleeding. This patient could have tried intranasal DDAVP before having surgery.)

Von Willebrand disease explained

Von Willebrand disease (vWD) is named after Dr. Erik von Willebrand, who first identified it in 1926. An estimated one in 1,000–1,500 Americans have vWD, ranking it as the most common known bleeding disorder, more prevalent than hemophilia. Many sufferers of vWD remain undiagnosed. The disorder affects all ethnic groups, men and women equally, and is found throughout the world. It is sometimes referred to as "pseudohemophilia."

Von Willebrand disease is caused by a deficiency in a blood

protein called von Willebrand factor (vWF). This factor is necessary for normal clotting; it is like the "glue" that holds the platelets together. People with insufficient amounts of vW factor do not clot properly and this results in bleeding. It differs from hemophilia, which is a condition caused by a deficiency in the activity of coagulation factor VIII. Hemophilia and von Willebrand are only two causes of clotting factor disorders. Others include deficiencies of the other coagulation factors (I, II, V, VII, IX, XI, XIII) and disorders of platelet function as well as disorders of fibrinolysis.

There are several known types of von Willebrand disease:

Type 1 is the most common and the mildest form; 80 percent of all cases are type I. These patients do not have enough von Willebrand factor.

Type 2 is further classified as type IIa or type IIb and affects about 20 percent of cases. Patients with Type II produce a von Willebrand factor that does not function properly.

Type 3 is the most severe form of the disease. One to three per million can be affected. In this type, the patient produces little to no von Willebrand factor.

Pseudo (or platelet-type) von Willebrand disease resembles Type IIb von Willebrand disease, but the defects are in the platelets, rather than the von Willebrand factor.

Von Willebrand can be inherited or can occur spontaneously with no family history of the disease. While men and women can be affected by vWD equally, women are more symptomatic given the known challenges to hemostasis in terms of monthly menses and childbirth. The reason for this is unknown.

A child has a 50 percent chance of inheriting the disease if either parent has von Willebrand. This is known as dominant inheritance; recessive inheritance means that a child would have to inherit two variant copies of a gene—one copy from the mother and one copy from the father—to have the disease. Gene variations are found on autosomal or sex-linked chromosomes. When sex-linked, a disease is passed by the mother if the variation is on the X chromosome and by the father if the variation is on the Y chromosome. The X and the Y chromosomes make up the 23rd pair in the complete set of chromosomes inherited. The other 22 pairs make up the autosomal sets. The gene variation for vWD is on chromosome 12, which means that it is an autosomal, rather than a sex-linked inherited disorder.

Symptoms

Heavy menstrual bleeding (menorrhagia) is a common symptom for women with vWD. Typically they report changing their protection 30 to 120 minutes on their heaviest day, note clots greater then the size of a quarter, and are low in iron. Many women who have gone through gynecological treatments such as endometrial ablations, Dilation and Curettage (D&Cs), and even hysterectomies were found to have undiagnosed vWD. Other symptoms include easy bruising (at least weekly and atraumatic and larger than a size of a quarter); prolonged bleeding from cuts (> 5 minutes), frequent and prolonged (> 10 min) nosebleeds; and prolonged bleeding following surgery, childbirth, or dental work.

Diagnosing vWD

A primary care physician who encounters a patient with symptoms of vWD can refer the patient to a hematologist. The type of vWD is determined based on laboratory findings. Due to the high variability of the disease, no single diagnostic test can be used to diagnose von Willebrand disease. A number of tests are used in order to confirm the diagnosis and identify subtypes of the disease. It sometimes takes several days to receive all the test results, which include the following:

- Factor VIII activity
- Ristocetin cofactor activity
- vWF:Antigen

Additional tests my include closure time, vWF multimers, and ristocetin induced platelet aggregation.

Treatment

Depending on the type of vWD a person is diagnosed with, the physician will determine what form of treatment is advisable for the patient. Treatment is sometimes not necessary for minor bleeding; for more serious bleeding there are several forms of treatment.

Desmopressin (DDAVP®)

Desmopressin acetate (brand DDAVP®) is a synthetic hormone that causes von Willebrand factor to be released from storage sites in blood vessels.

Desmopressin can be administered intravenously (injected into a vein), subcutaneously (injected under the skin), or as a nasal spray called Stimate. A patient is tested to see which form of desmopressin works for them.

Stimate nasal spray works well for most individuals and is more convenient to use than the injectable forms of DDAVP®. If the hematologist prescribes the nasal form of desmopressin, the patient will want to make sure that the pharmacist dispenses Stimate nasal spray and not DDAVP® nasal spray. DDAVP® nasal spray is used to treat other conditions such as bed wetting, though it may not be strong enough to be effective in treating bleeding disorders.

Factor VIII concentrates are commercially prepared compounds derived from human plasma. Synthetic forms are also available. The dosage is dependent on the degree of factor deficiency, the weight of the patient, and the level of factor VIII inhibitors.

Hemophilia centers

Many people with bleeding disorders can receive comprehensive care from a hemophilia treatment center (HTC). The staff of most HTCs consists of hematologists, nurses, social workers, dentists, and physical therapists. These professionals work as a team to help patients manage every aspect of their condition.

Taking action

Yearly checkups are scheduled that include a thorough physical examination and laboratory tests, particularly a Hct and ferritin in the menstruating female. These visits are extremely important to a patient's health. Not only do these routine visits keep the doctor up-to-date on any medical problems a patient might be having, but it also gives the patient an opportunity to learn more about the condition, which can improve the quality of life.

Physical activity

People with vWD are encouraged to exercise. Information about physical activity is available through various treatment centers and organizations such as the National Hemophilia Foundation by calling 800-42-HANDI.

Medications

Before taking any medications, vitamins, or herbs, a patient needs to check with the doctor to make sure that the drug or supplement will not interfere with platelet function. Bleeding disorder patients are advised to avoid taking any over-the-counter medications that could interfere with platelet function.

Emergency care

Emergencies can happen and patients need to be prepared for these occasions. Not all emergency and medical professionals are familiar with vWD. When traveling, it is wise to carry a letter from the physician or treatment center that explains this bleeding disorder and the type of treatment needed for such an emergency. It is also an added help for the emergency department staff if the patient wears some form of medical alert necklace or bracelet, in the event a patient is unconscious or cannot convey details to the emergency staff. Patients should also take care to have the telephone numbers of their treatment center and primary care physician so that emergency staff can obtain details promptly.

any new treatment. Any application of the information or recommendations in this book is made at the reader's discretion.

Resources

Suggested reading:

Von Willebrand Disease: Just the FAQs, published by the National Hemophilia Foundation.

A Guide to Living with von Willebrand Disease, by Renee Paper, RN, with Laureen A. Kelley
Published and distributed by Aventis Behring, LLC
King of Prussia, PA
For copies of the book call: 888-508-6978
www.stimate.com/Resources/supportMaterials.aspx

For a list of local chapters of the National Hemophilia Foundation and the locations of various treatment centers contact:

The National Hemophilia Foundation
116 West 32nd Street, 11th Floor
New York, New York 10001
Toll Free: 800-42-HANDI
Tel: 212-328-3700
Fax: 212-328-3777
Email: info@hemophilia.org
www.hemophilia.org

MedicAlert
2323 Colorado Avenue
Turlock, California 95382
Toll Free: 888-633-4298
Fax: 209-669-2450
www.medicalert. org

Mary M. Gooley Hemophilia Center
1415 Portland Avenue, Suite 500
Rochester, NY 14621
Tel: 585-922-5700
Fax: 585-922-5775
www.hemocenter.org

Another website to visit to learn about genetics:
www.ncbi.nlm.nih.gov

To find a center near you:
www.ahfinfo.com

VWD, hemophilia, and other clotting factor conditions:
www.med.unibs.it/~marchesi/clottingdisorders.html
www.medal.org

For information and resources on bleeding disorders visit the website for National Center on Birth Defects and Developmental Disabilities (NCBDDD), hereditary blood disorders: www.cdc.gov/ncbddd/hbd.

29

Hereditary Hemorrhagic Telangiectasia (HHT)

"HHT is often misdiagnosed because it masquerades as many disorders."
—*Robert I. White Jr., MD, HHT Medical Advisory board, Chair*

Adapted from a personal case history of a young female

My entire life I have had nosebleeds, many lasting as long as two hours, and I continue to have at least one daily, if not more. I cannot tell you how many doctors have misdiagnosed my continual bouts with anemia throughout the years. The doctors were convinced that my continual and habitual anemia was caused by too much loss of blood during menstruation, severe nosebleeds, or because I was simply not getting enough iron. I had my nose cauterized many times, went to see doctors thinking I had a "blood clotting" problem. I was told to take more iron, eat more liver, beef, etc. My dad passed away four years ago of colon cancer. He had all the symptoms I had but was never diagnosed.

Before getting the correct diagnosis, I was always extremely tired and very cold. I remember once when it was over 100 degrees outside, I was wearing a sweater and still could not get warm. I have been diagnosed with thyroid disease, iron-deficiency anemia, and was finally admitted to the hospital for blood transfusions when my hemoglobin dropped to 6.2.

The above case history is courtesy of the HHT Foundation.

Shortly after the transfusions, after I had returned home, I began to notice blood in the toilet when I went to the bathroom, and I immediately thought the worst: *I have colon cancer like my dad did.* I saw a gastroenterologist who didn't waste any time. He ordered a colonoscopy and endoscopy of the upper portion of my digestive system. Within ten days of my visit he told me that he cauterized more than 30 blood vessels in my colon, duodenum, and stomach. He then told me that he thought I had HHT but wanted me to see an ENT (ear, nose, and throat specialist) right away. My visit to the ENT produced the same results. He cauterized my nose and asked me, "Have you ever been diagnosed with Osler-Weber-Rendu syndrome?" He then showed me all the telangiectases in my mouth, which I had noticed all over my stomach, arms, and hands long before understanding what was happening to me.

HHT explained

HHT is a genetic (inherited) bleeding disorder characterized by abnormal blood vessels that frequently results in bleeding. These abnormal blood vessels, called telangiectasias, are fragile and susceptible to rupture and bleeding. The genetic basis for HHT is slowly being unraveled, but the disease is not curable. Treatment is focused on palliating bleeding vessels and correcting iron-deficiency anemia, which virtually all HHT patients have. HHT is also known as Osler-Weber-Rendu syndrome in the medical literature. About one in ten thousand people in the United States have HHT.

We in the HHT community shy away from the term "bleeding disorder" since many of the manifestations of HHT are not bleeding (e.g., hypoxemia, strokes, and brain abscess). In addition, many people equate "bleeding disorder" with coagulopathy, which of course is not the problem with HHT. We prefer to say that it is "a genetic disorder characterized by abnormal blood vessels that frequently results in bleeding."

The genetic basis for HHT

In HHT, the small blood vessels (capillaries) are malformed or absent and direct connections occur between arteries and veins. Genetic studies indicate that a deficiency of protein called endoglin exists in HHT, although how this deficiency leads to abnormal blood vessel formation is unexplained. Actually, mutations to ALK-1, SMAD4, and at least two other genes may result in HHT. The malformed blood vessels (telangiectasias) are easily traumatized and bleed easily. Telangiectasias are present on the surfaces of most tissues, and HHT patients may have multiple sites of bleeding.

HHT symptoms

The major symptom of HHT is bleeding. HHT bleeding may be clinically obvious, as in nose bleeding (epistaxis), which occurs in 90 percent of HHT patients. Usually bleeding in HHT patients increases with age; that is, younger people may have minimal bleeding, but after age forty, bleeding symptoms usually become more serious. This is likely due to the formation over time of larger numbers of telangiectasias.

Red blood cells contain iron, and when iron loss exceeds iron absorption from the diet, iron-deficiency anemia develops. HHT patients may have anemia that ranges from minor to severe. Body tissues in anemic patients do not receive adequate oxygen. This results in the typical symptoms of anemia, including fatigue, shortness of breath, and a generalized "low energy level."

HHT patients may have other symptoms. Larger lung (pulmonary) telangiectasias, called arteriovenous malformations (PAVM), occur in one-third of patients, occasionally leading to significantly low oxygen levels. These patients may also experience coughing up blood (hemoptysis), stroke, and brain abscess. Special X ray tests such as helical CAT scans, pulmonary angiography, and MRI scans are useful to diagnose these blood vessel malformations. The best screening test for pulmonary AVM is contrast echocardiography. Telangiectasias may occur in the brain, potentially resulting in a hemorrhagic stroke. The inner surface of the bowel, such as the upper intestine or colon, may contain telangiectasias which may cause gastrointestinal bleeding. Although up to 80 percent of HHT patients have GI telangiectases, gastrointestinal bleeding only occurs in 25 to 50 percent of HHT patients. Frequently, the patient may not be aware that they are losing blood in their stool, unless a stool test for blood is done. Larger amounts of bleeding from the gastrointestinal tract may lead to obvious changes in the patient's stools, from black, tarry stools (melena) to frank, rectal bleeding.

Diagnosis of HHT

The clinical diagnosis of HHT is usually obvious. Patients will have the characteristic telangiectasias on their lips, fingers, inside of the mouth, etc. The telangiectasias will blanch with pressure. HHT patients will almost always have a positive family history of bleeding, and usually often the diagnosis will have been previously made in another family member.

A diagnosis of definite HHT can be made if a patient has three or more of the following criteria: spontaneous recurrent nose bleeds; multiple mucocutaneous telangiectasias present about the face, mouth, or fingers; the presence of PAVM or gastrointestinal telangiectasias; and a positive family history of the disorder. HHT is likely or suspected if two of the above findings are present.

Physicians usually evaluate HHT patients in the setting of bleeding and/or anemia. Coagulation (clotting) tests are normal with the exception of anemia. Additional laboratory tests to evaluate the anemia will indicate iron deficiency. Certain research centers can evaluate the specific genetic (DNA) defect, but this is not necessary for diagnosis.

Treatment of HHT

The two major targets of treatment of HHT are to stop bleeding and to correct the anemia. Other treatment issues may be useful and are discussed below.

Bleeding in HHT patients may be emergent, requiring hospitalization or an emergency room visit, or less urgent, perhaps requiring a clinic visit. For example, patients may have massive blood loss from nose bleeding (epistaxis), necessitating intervention by an otolaryngologist (ear, nose, and throat specialist) who may need to pack the bleeding nostril. On the other hand, minor bleeding from the nose may be conservatively treated at home by the patient applying pressure to the bleeding nostril. In some patients, nose bleeding may be prevented or lessened with the use of humidification and nasal lubricants. (Most patients need other treatments for nosebleeds.)

Gastrointestinal bleeding may require endoscopic evaluation (either upper or lower endoscopy) to identify the site of bleeding, which can be cauterized (burned) by the endoscope. Occasionally patients may require surgical removal of severely affected areas of their bowel to prevent massive bleeding. Unfortunately, neither surgery nor cautery is curative, since new telangiectasias will usually develop with time.

Correction of the anemia in HHT requires iron replacement using either oral or parenteral (intravenous or intramuscular) iron therapy or red blood cell transfusion. Routine blood transfusion to correct iron deficiency is discouraged because of the potential to transmit viral infections, such as hepatitis C in blood products. Most patients with mild to moderate bleeding will respond to iron replacement therapy.

Patients with mild to moderate anemia [hematocrit in the 30 to 36 percent range (normal hematocrits are 37 to 45 percent)] can be initially treated with oral iron pills, such as ferrous sulfate, 325 mg three times a day with meals. It is recommended that oral iron be taken with food, starting once a day with a meal, slowly advancing to twice a day with two meals, then three times a day with each meal. This decreases the stomach irritation that oral iron may cause. Iron may also change the stool to a darker color, but this is an expected side effect.

For patients with mild to moderate iron-deficiency anemia who do not tolerate ferrous sulfate, for example, due to stomach irritation, other forms of oral iron pills are available, such as ferrous gluconate. These products usually cost more than ferrous sulfate, require higher doses, and are not more effective than ferrous sulfate. Patients should be aware that certain dietary components will affect iron absorption. For example, iron absorption is increased by the presence of orange juice, meat, poultry, and fish; iron absorption is decreased by cereals, milk, and tea. Since blood loss in HHT patients is usually lifelong, oral iron therapy in this disorder should be continued indefinitely. The best laboratory test to monitor a patient's iron stores is serum ferritin; levels less than 20 ng/ml usually indicate iron deficiency.

For patients who do not tolerate oral iron of any form, or who have severe anemia (hematocrit less than 30 percent), parenteral iron replacement should be considered. The preferred route of administration is intravenous. Parenteral iron can also be given by intramuscular injections, but this route of treatment causes staining of the skin, is uncomfortable, and may cause sterile abscesses.

Most patients do well with intravenous iron dextran. For the first intravenous iron treatment, a small amount is infused and the patient is observed for allergic reactions, which a small number of patients will exhibit. If no allergic signs occur (rash, shortness of breath), a large amount of iron can be infused over two to three hours. Intravenous administration of iron has the advantage of achieving more rapid replacement of deficient iron stores than oral iron. The intravenous infusions can be repeated at intervals (every one to three months) depending on the rate of clinical bleeding. This routine administration of intravenous iron may prevent recurrence of anemia in HHT patients, despite the fact that bleeding still occurs. Monitoring serum ferritin levels is useful to guide the frequency and dose of iron infusions. In patients who have pulmonary AVMs (or in patients who have not ruled out pulmonary AVMs), iron infusions, along with all other IVs, should be administered with a filter in the IV line, to prevent air embolization.

For the small number of patients with allergic reactions to iron dextran, an alternative intravenous iron product is available—iron gluconate. The availability of iron dextran and iron gluconate means that almost all HHT patients can have their iron-deficiency anemia treated without requiring transfusion of red blood cells. If transfusions are necessary, patients should be immunized with vaccines to prevent hepatitis A and B.

Other treatment issues

Recurrent epistaxis can be treated with laser treatments or with septal dermoplasty, in which the patient's abnormal nose tissue is replaced with normal donor tissue. Anti-fibrinolytic drugs such as Amicar® may improve nose or mouth bleeding. Female hormone therapy may also be useful. HHT patients with PAVM will benefit from procedures to "plug up" the abnormal lung vessels (embolotherapy). Brain telangiectasias may be treated by similar embolotherapy or surgery.

Although genetic screening is not necessary for the diagnosis, it may be clinically useful, since certain HHT complications (such as PAVM) are associated with certain genetic mutations.

The use of blood thinners (anticoagulants, aspirin, and nonsteroidal anti-inflammatory agents) should be avoided.

Because HHT patients present numerous medical issues requiring multiple medical subspecialties for treatment, some medical facilities have established comprehensive HHT clinics, with physicians who have interests and expertise in the disorder.

Resources
For a current listing of HHT centers:

HHT Foundation
P.O. 329
Monkton, MD 21111
Toll Free: 800-448-6389
Tel: 410-357-9932
Fax: 410-357-993
Email: hhtinfo@hht.org
www.hht.org.

The HHT Foundation provides newsletters and other information to interested patients. There are seven HHT centers in the United States: Yale University; University of Utah; Oregon

Health Sciences University; Washington University in St. Louis, Missouri; University of California, San Diego; Mayo Clinic in Rochester, Minnesota; and Medical College of Georgia in Augusta. Updated information on HHT centers in the United States and other countries is listed on their website.

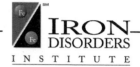

PART FIVE

Achieving Iron Balance

30

Oral, Injected, or Infused Iron

"The use of iron pills as a tonic for the treatment of an undiagnosed anemia can never be condoned."

—"Iron Deficiency: Misunderstood, Misdiagnosed and Mistreated."
C. K. Arthur & J. P. Isbistor, Drugs 33 (1987): 171–82

The underlying cause of anemia will dictate whether blood transfusion or oral, injected, or infused iron is used.

Moderately low iron reserves or mild anemia due to insufficient daily intake of iron might be corrected with oral iron in the form of pills. Ferrous sulfate, ferrous fumarate, or ferrous gluconate are common forms of iron in pills, which are usually inexpensive. Carbonyl iron, such as Feosol Caplet®, Ferra-Cap®, and Icar-C Plus™ is often used by physicians because it is less toxic to children who might take an accidental overdose.

The amount of iron contained in the various iron pills will vary. A 325 mg supplement is probably made of ferrous fumarate or gluconate and actually contains only 100 mg of iron per pill, the balance of the mass being the fumarate or gluconate counter ion (see the chart on next page).

Until 1999, in the United States, the vast majority of iron supplements were made with ferrous iron salts. That is, a positively charged iron and its counter ion (negatively charged counterpart). Popular and common counter ions are sulfate, gluconate, and fumarate. Fumarate and gluconate are carbon-containing carboxylic acids.

Typically, the way these compounds are made is that pure iron, usually as iron filings, is dissolved in sulfuric or hydrochloric

Compound	Formula Weight	Tablet Size	Iron Dose
Ferrous fumarate	169.9	300 mg*	97 mg
Ferrous fumarate	169.9	325 mg*	105.2 mg
Ferrous sulfate	278.0	300 mg*	59.4 mg
Ferrous gluconate	250.2	300 mg*	65.9 mg

* Pills contain "excipients" (binding and flow agents for tableting) as well as coatings of sugar or shellac, which contribute to pill size.

acid. Once dissolved, the counter ion is added and the pH is slowly adjusted back to neutrality. As this happens the iron is no longer soluble so it binds to the counter ion and drops out of solution. The slurry is then dehydrated and the remaining dry matter is the iron salt.

The manufacture of these products gives an important clue as to how they work in the body. Once ingested, it is imperative that the stomach contains acid to dissolve the iron salt. If a person is taking large doses of antacids, H2 blockers, or proton pump inhibitors, their stomach environment will become "hypo or achlorhydric"—reduced or no acid—and the iron salt will not dissolve. As such the person derives no benefit.

Currently iron salt supplements are available in a wide variety of doses. In the mid 1990s, the FDA made a ruling that required that iron supplements containing more than 30 milligrams of elemental iron per pill be packaged in "blister packs" to prevent child poisoning. Iron supplements are often sugar coated, so they are appealing to small children. At the time of the FDA ruling, poisoning from iron containing supplements was the leading cause of child poisoning. Additionally, besides the blister packing, all iron supplements must bear a warning prominently on the front label. Since then the packaging requirements have been repealed as a result of industry litigation.

Because of these FDA requirements, many manufacturers simply opted to make smaller iron dose products, so many of the over-the-counter iron supplements contain less than 30 milligrams of iron. Those that contain more may or may not be blister packed.

There are a few specialty manufacturers and pharmacies around the country that make special iron tonics or capsules. The tonics are made as solutions that keep the iron soluble so that people won't have to worry about whether the pills dissolve in their stomachs —it's already in solution. These present some danger, however, because if the whole bottle is consumed by a child, a very real risk of overdose exists. Because the manufacturers know this, they generally make them with very low iron concentrations.

Other manufacturers and pharmacies add things like "intrinsic factor" or liver extract. Liver extract contains ferritin (iron bound to protein) as well as some heme iron. The amount of iron in these preparations bound to heme is generally less than one-half milligram.

Intrinsic factor was so named because of its essential role in absorption of vitamin B_{12}. It is present in gastric juice and performs its duty by binding to B_{12}. Once bound, it changes its conformation, becoming less susceptible to digestion, and thereby protects B_{12} and allows for its absorption from gastric juice.

Most of us can get sufficient amounts of iron from daily diets that include a moderate amount of red meat, because meat contains heme, which is easily absorbed by the body. However, some people need supplemental iron. Finding the right type and dose is an individual decision made between the patient and the physician.

Proferrin® (Colorado Biolabs) contains heme iron, which is more readily absorbed by the body. Studies indicate that heme iron absorption rates are between 15 and 20 percent without erythropoietin (rHuEPO) therapy and as high as 30 percent with rHuEPO therapy even in patients with high serum ferritin values (>600 ng/ml). In one study, the change in serum iron from Proferrin® was nearly twenty-three times greater than from an identical dose of ferrous fumarate. Also, study participants were able to tolerate up to 60 mg per dose on an empty stomach with fewer gastrointestinal side effects; a common complaint from patients taking traditional oral iron preparations. An additional benefit of heme iron supplementation is that patients can take it with their meals, unlike ionic iron preparations, which must be taken on an empty stomach between meals.

The FDA allowed the marketing of Proferrin® in the United States in late 2000. It is available in both an over-the-counter and prescription form. Alaven Pharmaceuticals offers a form of Proferrin® in its oral iron supplement PreferaOB® for women who are pregnant.

Supplemental iron should not be taken unless a physician determines a real need. Our bodies regulate how much iron we absorb, so when iron is not absorbed, it will pass through the digestive tract with the feces. However, as excess iron passes through it may unnecessarily expose the colon to its uncontrolled oxidative properties, possibly leading to an increased risk of colon cancer.

Ionic iron supplements should only be taken two hours before or after meals or other medications. Iron can inhibit the effectiveness of thyroid medications, antibiotics, and some antidepressant drugs. Foods and substances that can interfere with the absorption of iron include chocolate, phytates from grains, calcium, tannins from coffee and tea, and polyphenolic compounds from grapes, red wine, and purple or red rice. As mentioned earlier, heme based supplements do not bind to these substances and can be taken with meals to minimize stomach upset.

Injected or infused (parenteral) iron

Parenteral iron, which is administered by infusion or injection, is given to patients who have problems of absorption or who have had portions of their stomach or small intestines removed.

Intramuscular injections are generally administered to the buttocks and can be somewhat painful and result in bleeding into the muscle. Intramuscular neoplasm (cancer) has been found at the injection site in some cases. Patients have also reported an orange discoloration at injection sites, which appears to be permanent. When iron is injected, it is properly done using a "Z technique" to prevent intramuscular bleeding or discoloration. Intravenous infusion is generally preferred by most hematologists over intramuscular injections (IM) because of these complications.

The intravenous iron or IV infusion procedure generally requires a series of doses that may take up to three to four hours to perform. The procedure is usually done at a hospital on an outpatient basis or at hemodialysis centers. Prior to an infusion, a test dose—25 mg of iron dextran—is given over period of five minutes. The patient is closely supervised to assure that he or she can tolerate the iron. If the patient develops no adverse reaction to the test dose, escalating doses are given over the next few days until 2 grams per infusion are tolerated. When IV iron is administered carefully, with close observation, patients usually tolerate the treatments well.

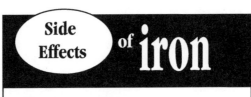

Nausea or vomiting
Stomach upset
Bowel changes
Anaphylactic shock
Low blood pressure
Fever
Joint pain (arthalgia)
Muscle pain (myalgia)
Swollen lymph nodes
Chest, back, or abdominal pain
Infection
Urticaria (rash/hives)
Severe itching
Seizures
Flushing
Headache
Phlebitis (inflammation of vein)
Rigors (sudden shivering)
Chronic pain at injection site
Skin staining
Local skin atrophy (wasting)
Abscess
Sarcoma (cancer)
Tissue iron overload
Increased risk of colon cancer

Side effects of iron toxicity can be acute, such as anaphylactic shock, or chronic, such as tissue iron overload. Unless a person takes an excessive amount of oral iron, acute symptoms with iron pills are generally isolated to gastrointestinal problems such as nausea, vomiting, or cramps.

There is a greater potential for acute side effects from injected or intravenous iron; for this reason the test dose and very slow infusion are used to lower the risk of a reaction.

IV iron preparations approved for use in end stage renal disease (ESRD) include: Venofer® (American Regent Labs, New York) and Ferrlecit® (Watson Pharmaceuticals, New York). These new preparations can be given much more quickly than Infed® and have an exceedingly low incidence of anaphylactoid reactions. Their development has been nothing less that revolutionary to the practice of nephrology.

31

Blood Transfusion

Patients with severe and chronic anemia, complicated or rare diseases often need blood transfusions to survive. The patient receiving the transfusion may receive whole blood or parts of blood such as:

- Red blood cells (erythrocytes) are cells that contain fats, proteins, and hemoglobin, which contains iron needed to carry oxygen to tissues and organs and carbon dioxide from tissues and organs.
- Platelets (thrombocytes) are cells that help in blood coagulation (clotting), which helps to control bleeding.
- Plasma is the liquid part of the blood.

Blood transfusion described

When a patient experiences a drop in red blood cells and cannot replace these cells normally or quickly enough, the physician might choose blood transfusion as part of the patient's therapy. Depending upon the underlying cause, the patient may only receive a few blood transfusions, such as for acute blood loss or surgery. Or the patient may require repeated transfusion as the only means of prolonging or saving the patient's life, such as to treat thalassemia, sickle cell anemia, some forms of hemolytic anemia,

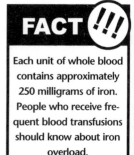

FACT

Each unit of whole blood contains approximately 250 milligrams of iron. People who receive frequent blood transfusions should know about iron overload.

some cancers, bone marrow failure, myelodysplasia, or some forms of leukemia.

A blood transfusion is administered in a hospital or infusion center as an outpatient. Prior to the transfusion some basic lab-work is done to determine hematocrit and blood type, also a physical exam is performed, which includes taking the recipient's temperature, pulse, respiration, and blood pressure. The infusion procedure requires inserting a needle into a vein in the hand or arm. The needle is connected to sterilized plastic tubing, which is attached to the blood product. During the transfusion, temperature and pulse are checked periodically to assure the patient is tolerating the procedure. A transfusion can take about thirty to forty minutes per unit of blood transfused.

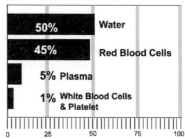

Contents of Blood

- 50% Water
- 45% Red Blood Cells
- 5% Plasma
- 1% White Blood Cells & Platelet

Source: American Association of Blood Banks

For sickle cell anemia (SCA) patients, the units of blood that are to be transfused must be checked for the anti-antibody to sickle cell disease. This process is very time consuming and expensive and requires advance notice of the need for transfusion for an SCA patient.

Each unit of blood contains about 500 cc, which is about two cups, and comprises red blood cells, white blood cells, platelets, nutrients, and water.

Blood used in transfusions is obtained from donations. Some donations are autologous, which means that the blood donor and transfusion recipient are the same. The purpose of autologous donation is for patients who are having surgery to be transfused with their own blood. Allogeneic blood donation is where the donor and the transfusion recipient are different. This type of donation represents the major portion of the blood supply.

Blood is collected at various establishments such as the American Red Cross, private blood centers, and hospitals. The

American Red Cross supplies approximately 43 percent of the nation's blood supply. ABC members supply about 50 percent and the balance is supplied by private centers or hospitals. Blood collection centers depend upon altruistic donors for their supply of blood.

In April of 1999, the FDA approved the use of blood taken from people with hemochromatosis safe for transfusion. Blood centers can apply for an FDA variance to use HHC blood. Variances are required for several reasons, but most notably, patients with hemochromatosis can give blood more often than other donors, though they are required to have a doctor's order to do so. Some HHC patients can donate up to twice a week without becoming anemic. Once excessive body iron stores are reduced to normal levels, donation frequency is reduced to several times a year to maintain healthy iron levels. Blood from HHC donors adds significant resources to the nation's blood supply.

Eighty-eight private blood centers and hospitals throughout the United States have obtained approval from the FDA to accept such frequent donations from hemochromatosis patients for use in blood transfusions. In 2008, the FDA proposed changes in the variance application process intended to further encourage the use of blood from HHC patients. If rule changes as proposed by the FDA are enacted, all licensed blood centers will be able to accept and use blood from HHC patients without obtaining one or more special variances.

A misconception about the blood obtained from people with hemochromatosis is that their blood contains more iron than other blood. This is not the case. Hemochromatosis is an inherited disorder of iron metabolism. It is not a blood disease. People with hemochromatosis absorb as much as four times the amount of dietary iron as do people with normal iron metabolism. Excess iron is stored in ferritin, an iron-containing protein, which is in every organ of the body. When a person with HHC donates blood, iron is released from ferritin to make new red blood cells.

A unit of blood from someone with HHC has the same amount of iron as any other donated blood: about 250 milligrams.

HHC blood is checked in exactly the same way as all other blood donated. Centers that provide this program report that the units of blood obtained from HHC patients are discarded at the same rate as non-HHC units of blood. This means that there is no greater risk associated with HHC blood.

Once blood is received, regardless of the donor, the blood cannot be used for transfusion until several things take place. Tests are done to assure the blood is safe for use. Each unit must be tested for:

- Antibodies to HIV-1 and HIV-2 (AIDS). An antibody is protein in the blood produced by the body in response to a foreign protein (antigen) such as the AIDS virus.
- Antibodies to HBc produced during and after infection with Hepatitis B virus
- Antibodies to HCV produced after infection with the Hepatitis C virus
- Antibodies to HTLV-I/II produced after infection with Human T-Lymphotropic virus (HTLV-I and HTLV-II)
- Antibodies to HBsAg produced after infection with Hepatitis B
- HIV-1 p24, a test for the HIV (AIDS) antigen
- Blood type (ABO) and Rh factor
- Hepatitis B Surface Antigen (HBsAg)
- Antibodies to the Hepatitis B Core (Anti-HBc)
- Antibodies to the Hepatitis C virus (Anti-HCV)
- Antibodies to the Human Immunodeficiency virus, Types 1 and 2 (Anti-HIV-1, -2)
- Antibodies to Human T-Lymphotropic virus, Types I and II (Anti-HTLV-I, -II)
- Syphilis
- Nucleic Acid Amplification Testing (NAT) (see Other tests below)
- Confirmatory Testing—to rule out donors who have tested with false positive results

A donor can have O+, A+, B+, AB+, O-, A-, B-, or AB- blood type. Knowing the type is critical in selecting compatible blood for a transfusion recipient. The positive or negative factor of the blood type is due to Rh factor.

According to the American Association of Blood Banks, though the exact percentage varies with race, 15 percent of the U.S. population is Rh-negative and 85 percent is Rh-positive. This factor is particularly important during pregnancy, where a mother can have Rh negative blood type while the offspring has inherited Rh positive blood type from the father. The mother may become sensitive to the baby's Rh positive blood and develop antibodies that begin to attack the blood of the developing fetus. The consequences can be Rh hemolytic anemia and this can be fatal to the newborn. In 1967 Rh immune globulin was commercially introduced to prevent Rh disease in the newborns of Rh negative women. This product can be given to pregnant women at 28 weeks into the pregnancy and to the child 72 hours after birth if an Rh problem is identified.

Other tests
ALT (Alanine-Aminotransferase) is a liver enzyme that when elevated may indicate liver inflammation, possibly caused by a hepatitis virus.

CMV is a test for the cytomegalovirus (performed on physician request).

NAT (Nucleic Acid Testing) is a new technology that can detect the genetic material of Hepatitis C and HIV. This technology can identify these viruses faster and more accurately than earlier testing methods that only checked for the development of human viral antibodies.

Cholesterol is measured by some centers as a benefit to donors.

About 70 percent of the blood products are filtered to remove leukocytes (white blood cells). White blood cells fight invaders such as bacteria; when these cells are present in donated blood, the person receiving the blood may have a reaction.

Processing and storing
Whole blood is separated into several components: red blood cells, plasma, platelets, and cryoprecipitated AHF (antihemophilic factor sometimes called CRYO). AHF is part of

the plasma clotting factors, which include von Willebrand factor, fibrogen, factor VIII, and factor XIII.

Red blood cells may be stored under refrigeration for a maximum of forty-two days, or they may be frozen for up to ten years.

Platelets are stored at room temperature and may be kept for a maximum of five days. Fresh frozen plasma, used to control bleeding due to low levels of some clotting factors, is usually kept in a frozen state for up to one year.

Cryoprecipitated AHF is made from fresh frozen plasma that is thawed slowly.

The risks of transfusion

Transfusion reactions can be fatal; therefore, the utmost care is taken to assure safety in the blood supply. As modern methods of detection and screening have reduced the rate of transfusion-associated infectious diseases, human errors such as blood product mislabeling persist and remain a serious factor even today.

Surveillance is a critical part of blood safety. As new infectious diseases such as Chagas or West Nile emerge, screening panels are amended to include these pathogens. Conditions that threaten the blood supply are also addressed. Transfusion Related Acute Lung Injury (TRALI) is a condition that has only recently been identified as a major risk factor in respiratory distress leading in some cases to fatalities. TRALI had been difficult to diagnose because it is often indistinguishable from other serious postoperative respiratory conditions. This condition is most often identified with plasma donated by females who have had multiply pregnancies (generally with more than one partner). The FDA has recently identified TRALI as the third most common cause of transfusion–related deaths.

As with any therapy, there are risks associated with blood transfusions. Recipients should be informed of these risks, such as disease transmission and adverse reactions to the blood product. The risk per unit transfused varies.

The safety of blood products is important for all people, especially those with hemophilia. The introduction of clotting factor concentrates in the 1970s greatly improved the

Risk per transfusion

Transfusion of red cells to the wrong patient	1 in 12,000 - 1 in 19,000
Transfusion of pre-deposited blood (autologous donation) to the wrong patient	1 in 16,000 - 1 in 25,000
Infection from unit of platelets	1 in 15,000
ABO incompatible transfusion	1 in 33,000 - 1 in 38,000
HTLV (Human T-Lymphotropic Virus)	1 in 641,000
Hepatitis B	1 in 140,000
Hepatitis C (without NAT testing)	1 in 225,000 - 1 in 790,000
(with NAT testing)	1 in 1,600,000
ABO incompatible related death	1 in 600,000
HIV (without NAT testing)	1 in 1,300,000
(with NAT testing)	1 in 1,900,000
Hepatitis A	1 in 1,000,000
Bacterial contamination of red blood cells	1 in 1,000,000
Malaria	1 in 1,000,000
Syphilis	1 in 1,000,000

Source: http://www.yoursurgery.com/, American Association of Blood Banks

treatment for hemophilia patients. Unfortunately, these products also introduced a new risk—the transmission of infectious diseases. While the risk of hepatitis from these products was recognized early on, the large number of persons with hemophilia who became infected with human immunodeficiency virus (HIV) in the early 1980s brought new questions to the safety of the blood supply.

In response, the U.S. Centers for Disease Control and Prevention (CDC), in cooperation with federally funded hemophilia treatment centers (HTCs), established the Universal Data Collection Project (UDC). Persons with bleeding disorders are eligible to enroll in UDC at their participating HTC. As part of the program, clinical data and a blood sample are collected from participants each year during their annual clinic visit. A portion of the blood sample is tested for viral hepatitis (hepatitis A virus [HAV], hepatitis B virus [HBV], hepatitis C virus [HCV]) and HIV, and the remainder is stored for possible use in future blood safety investigations.

Since the program began in May 1998, nearly 9,500

persons from 135 HTCs have been enrolled in UDC. As part of the program, each participant's annual test results are monitored for new infections with hepatitis or HIV. To date, no new cases of HAV, HBV, HCV, or HIV infection have been found among UDC participants. Additionally, the monitoring has revealed that more than 90 percent of UDC participants under the age of 20 have been vaccinated against HBV. Since UDC began, 191 participants who were not immune to either HAV or HBV when first enrolled have been vaccinated.

Learn more about UDC Project at www.cdc.gov/ncbddd/ hbd/blood_safety_facts.htm.

Content in this publication is not intended to be a substitute for professional medical advice, nor is it intended to replace the services of a medical professional or impair the patient– healthcare provider or caregiver relationship. Content in this publication should be used as information only and be discussed with a medical professional who is qualified to diagnose and treat your condition. Iron Disorders Institute, all contributors, and the publisher of this book are not responsible for the content on websites listed in the resources, nor do we endorse products promoted on such sites. We advise you to always seek the advice of a qualified health provider before making any changes to diet, supplementation, or starting any new treatment. Any application of the information or recommendations in this book is made at the reader's discretion.

Resources

For information about the blood supply or to find a private blood banking center in your area visit: www.americasblood.org.

To learn more about blood transfusion and centers that accept blood donations, visit the American Association of Blood Banks website: www.aabb.org or The National Library of Medicine link: www.nlm.nih.gov/medlineplus/blood transfusion-anddonation.html.

32

Bone Marrow Transplantation and Gene Therapy

Bone marrow transplantation (BMT) is also known as stem cell transplant or peripheral stem cell transplant.

Hematopoietic progenitor cells (derived from stem cells) are living human cells used in patient treatment. The American Association of Blood Banks (AABB) lists more than one hundred facilities in the United States that are accredited to engage in hematopoietic progenitor cell transplantation. Some of these cells are capable of regenerating cell growth in recipients and have proved effective in fighting some disease processes. These cells are usually derived from bone marrow from either an autologous or allogeneic donor. To increase compatibility in cases with different donors and recipients, the cells are generally processed to remove extraneous particles and incompatible donor plasma, red cells, and T-lymphocytes.

BMT has been used effectively to treat a number of potentially fatal diseases where anemia may be part of the treatment challenge, such as leukemias and lymphomas, multiple myeloma and other plasma cell disorders, myelodysplastic syndromes, severe aplastic anemia and other marrow failure states, and hemoglobinapathies such as thalassemia and sickle cell disease (SCD). In SCD bone marrow transplantation is the only known cure. Up to 90 percent of SCD patients who are recipients of BMT are cured of their disease.

BMT process described

A bone marrow or cord blood transplant (also called a BMT) replaces diseased blood-forming cells with healthy cells. Diseases that may be treated with a bone marrow or cord blood transplant include:

- Leukemias and lymphomas
- Multiple myeloma and other plasma cell disorders
- Severe aplastic anemia and other marrow failure states
- Sickle cell disease and thalassemia
- Inherited immune system disorders, such as severe combined immunodeficiency (SCID) and Wiskott-Aldrich syndrome
- Inherited metabolic disorders, such as Hurler's syndrome and leukodystrophies
- Myelodysplastic syndromes
- Familial erythrophagocytic lymphohistiocytosis and other histiocytic disorders

Cells used for transplant

The healthy cells for a transplant can come from three sources:

- Bone marrow
- Peripheral (circulating) blood that has an increased number of healthy blood-forming cells (also called peripheral blood stem cells or PBSC)
- Umbilical cord blood that is collected after a baby is born

If you need a transplant, your doctor will choose the source of the cells. Your doctor will also decide whether to use cells collected from you or another person.

- An **autologous transplant** uses cells collected from your body.
- An **allogeneic transplant** uses cells donated from a family member, unrelated marrow donor, or cord blood unit.

- A **syngeneic transplant** uses cells from an identical twin.

Your doctor decides on the cells used for transplant based on your disease, other treatments you have had, and your overall health.

Transplant as a treatment

When a bone marrow or cord blood transplant is being considered as a treatment option, it is helpful to understand the transplant process.

1) Your doctor searches for a marrow donor or cord blood unit. If you need an allogeneic transplant, your doctor will look for a marrow donor or cord blood unit that matches your HLA tissue type. HLA stands for human leukocyte antigen, a marker your immune system uses to recognize which cells belong in your body and which do not.

If a donor is not found in your family, your doctor can search for an unrelated donor through the Registry of the C.W. Bill Young Cell Transplantation Program. The program's registry lists potential donors who have agreed to donate their marrow and cord blood units donated by mothers.

As a contractor for the program, the National Marrow Donor Program® (NMDP) manages the registry. The registry has agreements with its global partners that provide access to 10 million potential marrow donors, including more than 190,000 cord blood units.

2) Your body is prepared for a transplant. Before and after your transplant, you will receive many medications. To make it easier for you to receive medication into your bloodstream, doctors often use a central line. A central line is inserted surgically into a large vein in your chest, just above the heart.

To prepare your body for the transplant, the diseased cells are destroyed. This is done using chemotherapy and sometimes radiation. (Chemotherapy is given through the central line.) The destroying of diseased cells is called a preparative regimen or a conditioning regimen.

3) You receive the cells for transplant. On the day of transplant, the cells from the marrow donor or cord blood unit are infused (flow) usually through the central line into your body. These healthy cells move into the spaces inside your bones where they create new marrow. They grow and make healthy new red blood cells, white blood cells, and platelets.

When your doctor may consider a transplant

Your doctor chooses your treatment based on several factors, including the status of your disease and your health. A disease can change over time. For example, when a disease is first diagnosed, it may be in a chronic (slow-moving), stable phase. Within weeks or months the disease can change to a crisis status. Or, after receiving one treatment, the disease can be in remission. Different treatments are better at different times for each disease.

Your health and risk factors must also be considered, and that, too, can change over time. For example, some treatments given before a transplant could damage your liver or kidneys, causing a risk factor you did not have before.

Your doctor will consider both your disease status and your current health when deciding on a treatment method. In general, results are better when the transplant is done:

- In the early process of the disease or when the disease is in remission
- When the disease responds to chemotherapy
- When you are as healthy as can be expected and your organs work well

Talking with your doctor

When you have a disease that may be treated with a bone marrow or cord blood transplant, talk to your doctor. Ask questions about your disease, your risk factors, and treatment options. Every question you have is important.

Some questions you may want to ask your doctor about treatment options are:

- What treatment do you recommend and why?
- Is the goal to cure my disease, or stop the disease progression, or control symptoms?

- What are other possible treatments?
- Will a bone marrow or cord blood transplant be an option at some point in my treatment?

Questions specific to a bone marrow or cord blood transplant might include:

- When do you recommend a transplant?
- When do you begin searching for a marrow donor or cord blood unit?
- What are the risks of waiting or trying other treatments first?
- What do you think the chances are that my transplant will be successful?

For more information about bone marrow transplantation, chemotherapy, and marrow donors, visit the National Marrow Donor Program® website: www.marrow.org.

Gene therapy

The Human Genome Project (HGP) successfully concluded in 2003 and generated many discoveries, including the genes for cystic fibrosis and neurofibromatosis (a common type of adult leukemia and Huntington's disease), as well as insights to the cause, diagnosis, and treatment of type II diabetes and Hutchinson-Gilford progeria, which is a rare disorder that causes a dramatic form of premature aging. Through the National Institutes (NIH) Intramural Research Program, founded by Dr. Collins, genome research continues in the exploration of molecular genetics of diseases such as breast cancer, prostate cancer, and adult-onset diabetes.

"We are 'beginning readers' of the 'genome book.'"
—*Francis Collins, MD, PhD, former Director of the National Human Genome Research Institute*

Rising also out of the successes of the HGP were new frontiers, challenges, and opportunities such as:

- Projects such as The Cancer Genome Atlas (TCGA)
- Services such as personalized medicine
- Professional coalitions such as the National Coalition for Health Professional Education and Genetics (NCHPEG) and the National Society of Genetic Counselors and The American Society of Gene Therapy
- Resources such as the statistical center of the Center for International Blood and Marrow Transplant Research (CIBMTR)
- Legislation such as GINA (Genetics Information Non-discrimination Act)
- Technology such as the DNA microarray
- Tests to determine metabolic responses such as AmpliChip™ CYP450

Research for cures with gene therapy is still highly experimental. Attempts to use this approach in humans have resulted in both successes and failures. These failures caused a pause in the pace of investigation; however, gene therapy offers hope for people with incurable or devastating diseases.

Gene therapy uses genes to treat or prevent disease. In the future, this technique may allow doctors to treat a disorder by inserting a gene into a patient's cells instead of using drugs or surgery. Researchers are testing several approaches to gene therapy, including:

- Replacing a mutated gene that causes disease with a healthy copy of the gene.
- Inactivating, or "knocking out," a mutated gene that is functioning improperly.
- Introducing a new gene into the body to help fight a disease.

In a National Heart, Lung, and Blood Institutes funded study, scientists successfully used gene therapy to cure sickle cell anemia in mice. However, this procedure is a long way from being approved for use in humans. According to Dr. Philippe Leboulch, principal investigator of the study and assistant professor of medicine at Harvard Medical School and the

Massachusetts Institute of Technology, "Gene expression continued for at least ten months in all mice in up to 99 percent of their circulating red blood cells. Up to 52 percent of the total hemoglobin incorporated the anti-sickling globin protein."

The process was done by using a virus called the lantivirus, which carried the newly engineered gene into the bone marrow. Initially, the marrow was removed from the bioengineered mice and genetically "corrected" by the addition of an anti-sickling human beta-hemoglobin gene. The new gene produces a beta chain of amino acids that, when incorporated into the hemoglobin molecule, gives rise to a modified normal hemoglobin molecule that prevents the sickling process.

After adding the anti-sickling gene, the corrected marrow was then transplanted into other mice with sickle cell disease whose bone marrow had been removed by radiation. Three months later blood samples from the transplanted mice showed a high level of expression of the anti-sickling beta-hemoglobin gene, verified by identifying high levels of anti-sickling hemoglobin protein in the blood cells.

Further analysis of the structure of the transplanted mice's red blood cells showed a dramatic reduction in the number of irreversibly sickled cells. For one of the mouse models transplanted, no irreversibly sickled cells could be detected. These mice also had changes in the density of the transplanted red blood cells that "showed a clear shift toward normal," according to the scientists.

The lantivirus appears to be the most powerful vehicle for incorporating genes into a genome, but there are drawbacks. This virus could become unpredictable and form new genes that could result in diseases. Also, currently this procedure would be toxic for humans.

Although there is much hope for gene therapy, it is still experimental. Oversight, ethics, and patient advocacy are crucial in the balance of use.

The Center for Biologics Evaluation and Research (CBER) regulates human gene therapy products—products that introduce genetic material into the body to replace faulty or missing genetic material, thus treating or curing a disease or abnormal medical condition. CBER uses both the Public Health Service Act and the Federal Food Drug and Cosmetic Act as enabling statutes for oversight.

The FDA has not yet approved any human gene therapy product for sale. However, the amount of gene-related research and development occurring in the United States continues to grow at a fast rate and the FDA is actively involved in overseeing this activity. The FDA has received many requests from medical researchers and manufacturers to study gene therapy and to develop gene therapy products. Such research could lead to gene-based treatments for cancer, cystic fibrosis, heart disease, hemophilia, wounds, infectious diseases such as AIDS, and graft-versus-host disease.

National Institutes of Health–Office of Biotechnology Activities

- Monitors scientific progress in human genetics research in order to anticipate future developments, including ethical, legal, and social concerns, in basic and clinical research involving recombinant DNA, genetic technologies, and xenotransplantation;
- Manages the operation of, and provides analytical support to, the NIH Recombinant DNA Advisory Committee, the DHHS Secretary's Advisory Committee on Genetics, Health, and Society, and the DHHS Secretary's Advisory Committee on Xenotransplantation;
- Coordinates and provides liaison with federal and non-federal national and international organizations concerned with recombinant DNA, human gene transfer, genetic technologies, and xenotransplantation;
- Provides advice to the NIH Director, other federal agencies, and state regulatory organizations concerning recombinant DNA research, human gene transfer, genetic technologies, and xenotransplantation;
- Responds to requests for information on highly technical matters and matters of public policy related to recombinant DNA, human gene transfer, genetic technologies, and xenotransplantation;
- Develops and implements NIH policies and procedures

for the safe conduct of recombinant DNA activities, and human gene transfer;

• Reviews and evaluates the composition of Institutional Biosafety Committees; and

• Develops registries of activities related to recombinant DNA research and human gene transfer.

Resources

Bone Marrow Transplantation:
www.nlm.nih.gov/medlineplus/bonemarrowtransplantation.html

American Society of Gene Therapy (ASGT)

555 East Wells Street
Suite 1100
Milwaukee, WI 53202
Voice: 414-278-1341
Fax: 414-276-3349
info@asgt.org
www.asgt.org

The Center for Biologics Evaluation and Research (CBER)

www.fda.gov/Cber/gene.htm
www.fda.gov/CBER/infosheets/genezn.htm
www.fda.gov/Fdac/features/2000/500_gene.html

Statistical Center of the Center for International Blood and Marrow Transplant Research (CIBMTR)

www.cibmtr.org/

The Human Genome Project and The Human Genome Research Institute

www.genome.gov

The Cancer Genome Atlas (TCGA)

cancergenome.nih.gov/

ghr.nlm.nih.gov/handbook/therapy/genetherapy

AmpliChip™ CYP450

www.amplichip.us

The National Society of Genetic Counselors

www.nsgc.org/

Genetic Alliance

www.geneticalliance.org/

National Coalition for Health Professional Education and Genetics (NCHPEG)

www.nchpeg.org/

Office of Biotechnology Activities (OBA)

www4.od.nih.gov/oba

National Marrow Donor Registry

www.marrow.org

33

Chelation Therapy

Patients who require repeated blood transfusions, such as those with sickle cell anemia, thalassemia major, and some forms of cancers, can develop transfusional iron overload. Each standard unit (about one pint) of blood used in transfusion contains approximately 250 milligrams of iron. The body cannot excrete iron, except in tiny amounts—about 1 milligram per day, which is sloughed off in skin or perspiration. Therefore the excess iron is trapped in the body. Over time the excess iron builds up in vital organs such as the pituitary, heart, liver, pancreas, bone marrow, and joints. Damage to these organs caused by the excess iron can result in organ failure and diseases such as diabetes, cirrhosis, liver cancer, osteoarthritis, osteoporosis, heart failure, and hormone imbalances. Hypothyroidism, infertility, hypogonadism, and sterility can result from these hormone imbalances.

In some cases the organ damage is irreversible; therefore, it is important to remove the unnecessary iron before damage can occur. For patients with anemia and iron overload, iron reduction is accomplished with chelation therapy, which is the removal of iron pharmacologically with an iron-chelating agent such as deferoxamine, brand name Desferal® or deferasirox, brand name Exjade®. These drugs are especially formulated to bind with iron so that the iron can be excreted.

The type of chelation therapy used to de-iron patients should not be confused with EDTA (ethylenediaminetetra-acetic acid), a method used by some alternative medicine practitioners. EDTA is a broad-spectrum chelator, meaning that it binds with and removes a wide number of minerals, including iron, but it is not specific. In contrast, deferoxamine, deferasirox, and deferiprone brand name Ferriprox®, are highly specific for iron.

Desferal® is not absorbed in the intestinal tract; therefore, this drug must be administered intravenously, which is done at an infusion center or hospital. Desferal® can also be administered subcutaneously using a portable battery-operated infusion pump designed for home use.

Generally, the pump is worn at night, where slow infusion of the iron chelating agent is administered over a period of about eight to twelve hours, for a duration of four to six nightly infusions per week. Patients are given a step-by-step demonstration of how to sterilize the skin, insert the needle, and operate the pump.

When a patient is prescribed iron chelation therapy, a test dose is given to be certain that there are no immediate reactions to the drug. Desferal® is administered slowly at first, beginning with 1 gram, three to four times per week, with monitoring of iron excretion in a cumulative 24-hour urine sample. If effective, the dose can then be adjusted upwards, one gram at a time, up to four times per week, until the patient reaches a tolerable level. The dose should not exceed 50 milligrams/kg weight, or about 3 grams per day. Periodic examination of the patient is necessary until positive response to treatment is confirmed.

Patients might be given an additional 2 grams of Desferal® intravenously for each unit of blood transfused. Desferal® is injected separately from blood transfusions.

Desferal® has been approved for use in the United States since the late 1970s. Deferiprone, also called L1 (brand name Ferriprox®), is different from Desferal® in that Ferriprox® can be taken orally but this drug is not yet approved for use in the USA. Another oral chelator deferasirox brand name Exjade® is approved for use in the US. This drug is dissolved in a juice and taken by mouth.

The primary role of iron-chelation therapy is to prevent premature death from heart attack due to myocardial iron overload. Statistically, 50 percent of patients with thalassemia major die of iron-related heart failure before the age of thirty-five.

Excessive iron can be detected in organs with technology such as specialized MRI (magnetic resonance imaging). The heart images pictured here demonstrate a normal heart and iron-laden heart of a thalassemic patient. Advances in imaging technology such as specialized MRI and FerriScan® allow for non-invasive ways to qualify and quantify iron in organs such as the heart, liver, and anterior-pituitary.

Side effects of iron chelators

Exjade®: The most frequently reported adverse side effects in the therapeutic studies of Exjade® were nausea, vomiting, diarrhea, stomach pain, fever, cough, headache, increases in kidney lab values, and skin rash. Some of these symptoms were dose related. Exjade® should not be chewed or swallowed

Normal heart and normal iron

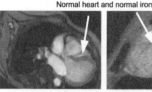
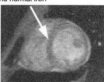

Severe iron-loaded heart

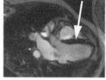
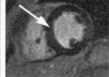

Images courtesy of Dr. D.J. Pennell, Cardiovascular Magnetic Resonance Unit, Royal Brompton Hospital, London

whole, and should not be taken at the same time as aluminum-containing antacids (for example, Maalox®).

Desferal®: Harmless side effects can include discolored urine. Immediate symptoms of adverse reaction to Desferal® chelation therapy might include: visual disturbances, blurred vision, rash or hives, itching, vomiting, diarrhea, stomach or leg cramps, fever, rapid heart beat, hypotension (low blood pressure), dizziness, anaphylactic shock, and pain or swelling at site of intravenous entry. Long-term problems might include kidney or liver damage, loss of hearing, or cataracts.

Limitations of iron chelators

Nursing mothers will need to talk with their physicians. It is not known how much of the drug gets into breast milk; thus, a mother who is receiving iron chelation treatment might consider low iron soy formula substitutes.

Patients who experience side effects such as those previously described should report such symptoms immediately to their physician, who can adjust the dosage. Further, physicians might examine patients' visual status with slit-lamp examination (means of examining the eye) and hearing status with audiometry or hearing test. Enzymes (ALT, AST, GGT, and ALP), a kidney function test such as BUN, serum ferritin, and transferrin iron saturation percentage might also be measured by the attending physician.

Pumps used for chelation therapy
A variety of pumps are available, such as the CADD Micro, the Grasby pump, the new, portable Crono ambulatory infusion pump, and the Eclipse C-Series Continuous Infusion System.

Also there are a number of needles available. Straight needles, butterfly, or thumbtack (also called button), or devices such as the MiniMed Sof-serter. The Sof-serter is a bit different from the other needles in that a spring-activated device inserts a tiny plastic catheter under the skin for infusion; the needle is removed after insertion.

Each patient is different and physicians can talk about the features and benefits of the various pumps and needles, such as size, portability, ease in operation, etc.

Tips
Patients should discuss the need for daily supplementation with vitamin C and E, selenium, B-complex, and other nutrients. Also, maintaining proper hydration is important for anyone on chelation therapy.

When to begin iron chelation therapy
Initiating chelation therapy depends upon several factors: the patient's overall health; hematologic values, especially hemoglobin and hematocrit; and the tissue iron levels.

Tissue iron is determined by measuring serum ferritin, and fasting serum iron and TIBC (total iron-binding capacity). These results help the physician to monitor iron buildup and to address the excess iron as soon as possible. Some physicians will begin chelation therapy

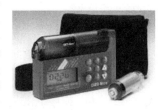

CADD Micro

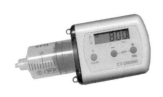

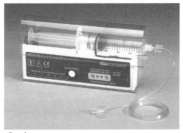

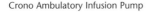

Crono Ambulatory Infusion Pump

Grasby pump

when serum ferritin is between 1,000 to 1,500 ng/mL. Serum ferritin should not be allowed to go above 2,500 ng/mL before beginning chelation.

Often patients become well informed about their disease and even their therapies—but many do not fully understand the impact of iron overload. The seriousness of removing excess iron cannot be stressed enough. If people are receiving blood transfusions or IVs or injected iron, it is critical that they learn about the dangers of excess iron and discuss with their physician the need for early intervention.

Resources
Product information:
The Eclipse C-Series Continuous Infusion System
I-Flow Corporation
20202 Windrow Drive
Lake Forest, CA 92630
Toll Free: 800-448-3569
Tel: 949-206-2700
Fax: 949-206-2600
Email: information@inflo.com

Grasby pump (sometimes called GRASB)
MarCal Medical, Inc.
1114 Benfield Blvd., Suite H
Millersville, MD 21108
Toll Free: 800-628-9214
Fax: 410-987-4004
www.marcalmedical.com

Crono Pump
Intra Pump Infusion Systems
900 Minters Chapel Road, Suite 200
Grapevine, TX 76051
Toll Free: 866-211-7867, Ext. 251
Toll Free Fax: 800-699-5936
www.intrapump.com

CADD Micro Pump
Sims Deltec, Inc.
1265 Grey Fox Road
St. Paul, MN 55112
Toll free: 800-426-2448
Tel: 612-633-2556
Fax: 612-628-7055

Chronimed, Inc.
10900 Red Circle Drive
Minnetonka, MN 55343
Toll Free: 800-444-5951
Tel: 952-979-3600
Fax: 952-979-3969
www.chronimed.com

Medtronic MiniMed
18000 Devonshire Street
Northridge, CA 91325-1219
Toll Free: 866-948-6633
Tel: 818-362-5958

FerriScan® Technology
www.ferriscan.com

Desferal® or Exjade® Novartis Pharmaceuticals
www.us.exjade.com
www.pharma.us.novartis.com/product/pi/pdf/desferal.pdf
www.askaboutiron.com
www.irontoxcity.com

For updates on chelators and other therapies for patients who have anemia complicated by iron overload, visit the following websites:

The Cooley's Anemia Foundation website, www.cooleys anemia.org, and the Children's Oakland Hospital website, www.thalassemia.com.

Iron Disorders Institute www.irondisorders.org

34

Erythropoietin Therapy

In light of the researched that has been released since the first edition of this book, perhaps the title of this chapter should be renamed "Erythropoiesis-stimulating Agent Therapy." While most medical professionals in this area of medicine immediately think of recombinant human erythropoietin (rHuEPO), other erythropoiesis-stimulating agents (ESAs) have been developed and are discussed in this chapter.

Erythropoietin (EPO) is an endogenous (i.e., naturally found in the body) hormone responsible for the regulation of red blood cell production. EPO is produced primarily (>90 percent) by the kidney, but smaller amounts of EPO are synthesized by the liver and by the brain.

An oxygen sensor within renal (kidney) cells detects how much oxygen is in the blood (oxygen is needed for vital cell functions). Oxygen content of the blood may be lower than normal because of anemia, a decrease in the amount of oxygen carried by the hemoglobin component of the red blood cells, or other factors. The kidneys regulate the amount of EPO released into the blood. The hormone acts on red blood cell precursor cells in the bone marrow to stimulate their proliferation and maturation and to increase the number of red blood cells in the circulation. The feedback loop is completed when kidney cells recognize the increase in oxygen content. Production of new red blood cells slows until the cells in the kidney once again recognize a need for more red blood cells.

Patients with chronic kidney disease are unable to produce adequate amounts of EPO to stimulate red blood cell production. Patients with cancer often have damaged bone marrow—with or without the insult of chemotherapy—that does not completely respond to the endogenous hormone. EPO concentrations may be low in patients with infection, inflammatory bowel disease, autoimmune diseases, arthritis, leukemia, myelodysplastic syndromes, or aplastic anemia.

Anemia is generally defined as a below-normal concentration of hemoglobin in red blood cells or insufficient number of red blood cells, and is typically determined by measuring hemoglobin concentration or hematocrit. Anemia is associated, of course, with low concentrations of EPO (as in patients with chronic kidney disease), but anemia can be caused by iron, vitamin B$_{12}$, or folic acid deficiency; thalassemia; lead poisoning; acute or chronic hemorrhage; parasitic infections; use of some drugs; exposure to some chemicals; or cirrhosis of the liver, among other conditions.

Before the introduction of rHuEPO as a therapeutic product, the traditional treatment for anemia and the fatigue associated with anemia was the use of red blood cell transfusion, androgen stimulation of red blood cell production, and/or iron supplementation, among other treatments. Transfusions and androgen therapy are effective in increasing red blood cell counts, but have inherent risks, albeit the risk of infection has decreased considerably with improvements in blood banking. Transfusions of red blood cells can be complicated by blood-borne pathogens, iron overload, immunologic consequences, and lack of or delayed hemoglobin response. Transfusions often improve but do not correct anemia and usually must be given frequently. Androgen therapy can cause viralization (i.e., appearance of masculine characteristics in women or children) or abnormal liver function. rHuEPO is an ideal therapy because it mimics the action of the endogenous hormone by stimulating the production of red blood cells, but recently has not been without some risks.

The cloning of the human EPO gene by Fu Kuen Lin and colleagues at Amgen in Thousand Oaks, California, was a difficult and frustrating endeavor. This milestone breakthrough and the subsequent creation and production of rHuEPO as a therapeutic option have enabled physicians to ameliorate anemia and its sequelae for numerous patients. Nearly all patients treated with rHuEPO report a return to more normal lives. rHuEPO is the standard of care for treatment of anemia in patients with chronic kidney failure, chemotherapy, and other disease settings.

Epoetin alfa, a type of rHuEPO manufactured by Amgen, has received marketing approval from the U.S. Food and Drug Administration (FDA) and is sold under the names of Epogen®- brand of epoetin alfa, marketed by Amgen; and Procrit®-brand of epoetin alfa, marketed by Ortho Biotech (Raritan, NJ). While both drugs are identical, Procrit® is marketed to patients with anemia associated with zidovudine (AZT) treatment of HIV infection, chemotherapy-induced anemia, or kidney disease not yet requiring dialysis, and for the reduction of allogeneic (i.e., donated) blood transfusion in patients undergoing elective sur- gery. Some patients use Procrit® to increase the number of red blood cells so that they can have their own blood collected to be used after surgery in a process called predonated autologous donation (PAD). Epogen® is marketed to patients with kidney disease who do require dialysis.

Epoetin alfa can be administered as either subcutaneous (under the skin) injection or as an intravenous (into a vein) transfusion. Physicians who prescribe epoetin alfa should con- sult the current package inserts as the dosing paradigm and warnings have been changed as of July 2008.

Epoetin alfa is not known to have any interaction with other drugs a patient may be receiving. Patients with uncon- trolled hypertension (i.e., high blood pressure), history of seizure disorders, and/or cardiovascular disease should not receive epoetin alfa. Patients with known hypersensitivity to mammalian-derived recombinant human products or human albumin-containing products should not receive epoetin alfa. Other causes of anemia, such as low iron concentration, infec- tion, and bleeding, should be discounted before epoetin alfa therapy is started.

Blood counts should be monitored at regular intervals dur- ing therapy with epoetin alfa (more frequently at beginning of treatment and after a dose adjustment). The dose may be increased in patients in whom the response is not satisfactory (i.e., transfusion requirement not reduced or hematocrit not increased), but if patients do not respond after the dose has been increased, higher doses are not likely to be beneficial. Increases in hemoglobin concentration and hematocrit values are usually seen within 7 days of therapy in patients with renal disease, but may require 3 to 4 weeks to be apparent. Patients with cancer often do not respond to therapy with epoetin alfa for reasons that are not entirely clear. All patients require adequate amounts of iron, measured as serum ferritin values and transferrin saturation, and some patients may benefit from concomitant treatment with iron supplementation. Iron may be given as an intravenously administered solution or as an oral supplement.

Some patients receiving dialysis who can not tolerate IV or injected epoetin alfa may need to have intraperitoneal administration of the drug. Intraperitoneal delivery is done by placing a shunt in the abdomen. The dose may need to be increased when this method is used.

As with any medication there can be side effects with epoetin alfa. The most common side effects reported include fever, diarrhea, nausea and vomiting, edema (water retention), asthenia (weakness), fatigue, and dyspnea (shortness of breath) that may be associated with the underlying disease, such as cancer and its treatment. Again, the current package inserts for Epogen® and Procrit® should be consulted before administration.

Epoetin beta is another rHuEPO available in countries other than the United States (i.e., it is available in Europe). Epoetin alfa and epoetin beta have identical amino-acid sequences, half lives, and per-unit efficacy, but they differ in the number of sugar molecules (called glycosylation).

Darbepoetin alfa, trade name Aranesp® (manufactured by Amgen), is a recombinant human ESA that stimulates the production of red blood cells. Darbepoetin alfa was produced by modifying the human EPO gene and by adding two additional glycosylation sites. Darbepoetin alfa, like epoetin alfa, can be administered either as a subcutaneous injection or an intravenous infusion. Darbepoetin alfa has a threefold longer half-life in the blood than epoetin alfa because of its increased glycosylation, which means that it does not need to be injected as often as epoetin alfa.

Side Effects: E P O

Adverse event reported in patients	% of 1,598 taking Aranesp	% of 600 taking rHuEPO
Hypertension (high blood pressure)	23	26
Hypotension (low blood pressure)	22	24
Myalgia (muscle pain)	21	27
Headache	16	18
Diarrhea	16	21
Vomiting	15	20
Upper respiratory infection	14	23
Nausea	14	24
Dyspnea (shortness of breath)	12	18
Abdominal pain	12	17
Peripheral edema (fluid)	11	17
Arthralgia (joint pain)	11	14

Source: Allen R. Nissenson, MD, *American Journal of Kidney Disease*, Vol 38, 2001, p.1395

Darbepoetin alfa is approved for use in patients with chemotherapy-induced anemia and the anemia associated with chronic renal failure (including patients requiring and not yet requiring dialysis). The package insert should be consulted for current prescribing information.

No formal drug interaction studies have been done with darbepoetin alfa. Darbepoetin alfa should not be administered to patients with uncontrolled hypertension (high blood pressure). ESA therapies may increase the risk of thrombotic and other serious events; dose reductions are recommended if the hemoglobin concentration increases more than 1.0 g/dL in any two-week period. The most common side effects reported during clinical trials with darbepoetin alfa for the treatment of chemotherapy-induced anemia were fatigue, edema (water retention), nausea, vomiting, diarrhea, fever, and dyspnea (shortness of breath). The most common side effects reported during clinical trials with darbepoetin alfa for the treatment of chronic renal insufficiency were infection, hypertension (high blood pressure), hypotension (low blood pressure), myalgia (muscle pain), headache, and diarrhea.

Starting in 1998 until approximately 2002, an area of concern with ESA therapy was the appearance of a very rare, but serious, complication of treating anemia with ESAs—pure red cell aplasia (PRCA). PRCA occurs when patients who are treated with ESAs develop antibodies to the ESA that also attack endogenous EPO. A severe, transfusion-dependent anemia results. The cases of PRCA were almost entirely confined to Europe and were thought to have been associated with the subcutaneous administration of epoetin alfa produced by a single drug manufacturer after a change in formulation.

Recently (2005–2008), much work has been done concerning the controversy about how best to use ESAs in patients with cancer. Studies suggested that certain groups of patients with cancer who were administered ESAs had shorter survival compared with similar patients who were not administered ESAs. Interpretation of these studies is complicated by a variety of factors, such as the degree to which anemia was to be corrected, the point at which ESA therapy was started, and specific patient characteristics. Other studies suggest that use of ESAs to correct the anemia of renal failure to entirely normal values (as opposed to the usually recommended 12 g/dL upper limit for correction) is associated with decreased survival.

For these reasons, physicians considering ESA therapy for their patients should review the most current guidelines for the proposed indication and discuss the risks and benefits with the patient.

Many other ESAs are in clinical development or are available in countries outside the United States. A novel peptide, hematide, works the same way as rHuEPO and endogenous EPO, but has no structural homology (i.e., it has a different amino-acid sequence) than rHuEPO. Hematide was used to "rescue" ten patients who had developed PRCA.

Resources

For Product information:

Epogen® or Aranesp®

Amgen Inc. (Headquarters) Amgen Center
One Amgen Center Drive
Thousand Oaks, CA 91320-1799
Tel: 805-447-1000
Fax: 805-447-1010
www.amgen.com

Procrit®

Ortho Biotech Products, L.P.
430 Route 22 East
P.O. Box 6914
Bridgewater, NJ 08807-0914
Toll Free: 800-325-7504 (prompt #2)
Tel: 908-541-4000
www.orthobiotech.com

We greatly appreciate the contributions to this chapter made by Dr. MaryAnn Foote, a consultant to the biopharma industry.

35

Diet Plan

For those with anemia, the ability to achieve iron balance through diet depends upon many factors: the cause and severity of anemia, general health, age, weight, gender, and ethnicity, as well as the patient's healthcare provider recommendations, access to certain foods, bioavailability of iron, and the type of iron consumed.

Humans consume two types of iron: heme iron and nonheme iron. Heme iron is derived from organic sources such as the blood proteins, hemoglobin and myoglobin contained in meat. This type of iron is in a form more easily absorbed by the body. About 10 percent or less of dietary iron consumed in American diets is heme iron, even though meat consumption in the United States is high. For persons with normal iron metabolism only 20 to 25 percent of the heme iron consumed is actually absorbed. For example, a four-ounce hamburger contains about 3 milligrams of iron; about 1.2 milligrams are heme and about 1.8 milligrams are nonheme. The amount of heme iron absorbed from that four-ounce hamburger would be approximately a third of a milligram.

About 40 to 45 percent of the iron contained in meat is heme; the other 55 to 60 percent is nonheme. Iron contained in plants is almost entirely nonheme iron, although some rare types of plants can contain minute traces of heme iron. Nonheme iron represents the majority of dietary iron humans consume. Nonheme iron is derived from grains, nuts, fruits, vegetables, fortificants, or contaminant iron such as from water, soil, or cooking utensils. Except for heme iron, the iron from all these sources must be changed before absorption can take place.

When nonheme iron is ingested it is in a form called ferric iron. Ferric iron cannot be absorbed by humans; it must be united with oxygen to become ferric oxide. Ferric oxide cannot be absorbed by the body either, but when ferric oxide reaches the stomach, it mixes with stomach acid (hydrochloric acid) and is changed into ferrous iron. Ferrous iron is the form of iron that can be absorbed. Ferrous iron moves out of the stomach into the first part of the intestine called the duodenum. This is the point where the majority of nutrient absorption takes place. Some scientists believe that there is another absorption site further down in the intestinal tract where minute amounts of iron can be absorbed.

Iron bioavailability

Bioavailability is the extent to which a nutrient or drug is accessible to the body for its intended use. In the case of iron, heme iron is highly bioavailable to the body, whereas nonheme iron is not. Certain substances can interfere with the absorption of iron; knowing what these are and avoiding or including these substances with main meals can help an individual improve iron absorption through improved bioavailability. According to Dr. Janet Hunt, Agricultural Research Team, Grand Forks Human Nutrition Research Center, "Iron absorption from food can vary up to ten-fold depending on the bioavailability of iron."

Regardless of the type of iron one consumes, there are foods and substances that can affect bioavailability by impairing or improving the absorption of iron.

Substances that increase iron absorption

Ascorbic acid or vitamin C occurs naturally in vegetables and fruits, especially citrus; it can also be synthesized for use in supplements. Ascorbic acid enhances the absorption of nutrients such as iron. In studies about effects of ascorbic acid on iron absorption, 100 milligrams of ascorbic acid increased iron absorption from a specific meal by 4.14 times. In a standard meal of meat, potatoes, and milk, 100 milligrams (mg) of ascorbic acid increased absorption of iron by 67 percent. The addition of 100 mg of ascorbic acid to a specially formulated liquid meal containing 85 mg of phytate increased absorption of iron by 3.14.

Alcohol

Although alcohol can enhance the absorption of iron, no one is encouraged to drink alcohol as a means of improving iron status. Moderate consumption of alcohol has known health benefits, but heavy or abusive drinking, especially when in combination with high body iron levels, increases the risk for liver damage, liver cancer, and abnormal blood cell production. Approximately 20 to 30 percent of those who are heavy consumers of alcohol acquire up to twice the amount of dietary iron as do moderate or light drinkers, but alcohol abuse increases the risk of liver disease such as cirrhosis. Patients who have developed cirrhosis increase their chance of developing liver cancer by 20–200-fold. A standard drink is defined as 13.5 grams of alcohol (e.g., 12 ounces of beer, 5 ounces of wine, or 1.5 ounces of distilled spirits). Moderate consumption is defined as two drinks per day for an adult male; one drink per day for females or those older than 65 regardless of gender. Alternatives to consider are nonalcoholic or low-alcohol-content beer and wine. For more about alcohol consumption and blood cell production, see chapter 15.

Beta-carotene is one of more than 100 carotenoids that occur naturally in plants and animals. Carotenoids are yellow to red pigments that are contained in foods such as apricots, beets and beet greens, carrots, collard greens, corn, red grapes, oranges, peaches, prunes, red peppers, spinach, sweet potatoes, tomatoes, turnip greens, and yellow squash. Beta-carotene enables the body to produce vitamin A. In studies of the effects of vitamin A and beta-carotene on absorption of iron, vitamin A did not significantly increase iron absorption under the experimental conditions employed. However, beta-carotene significantly increased absorption of the metal. Moreover, in the presence of phytates or tannic acid, beta-carotene generally overcame the inhibitory effects of both compounds depending on their concentrations. Like vitamin E, beta-carotene is an excellent antioxidant, but one should take

FOODS HIGH IN

BETA-CAROTENE

micrograms/100 grams edible portion

Apricots	2,554
Asparagus	493
Beets	2,560
Broccoli	1,042
Brussels sprouts	465
Butter with salt	158
Carrots	8,836
Chard	3,954
Cilantro	3,440
Collards	4,418
Endive	960
Grape leaves (canned)	2,838
Grapefruit (pink)	603
Kale (cooked)	6,202
Lettuce (Romaine)	1,272
Lettuce (iceberg)	192
Mangos (fresh)	445
Margarine spread	721
Melon (cantaloupe)	1,595
Okra	170
Orange (fresh)	122
Papayas (fresh)	276
Peaches (fresh)	97
Peas	320
Peppers green	22
Peppers red	2,220
Peppers yellow	120
Spinach (cooked)	5,242
Spinach (raw)	5,597
Squash (yellow)	90
Squash (zucchini)	410
Sweet potato	9,488
Tomatoes (paste)	1,242
Tomatoes (fresh)	393

Beta-Carotene is one of the carotenoids, which are the the red, green, yellow, and orange pigments found in fruits and vegetables. Beta-Carotene enables the body to produce vitamin A and is highly effective as an antioxidant.

chart created from carotenoid values database USDA

any of these judiciously. Studies have shown that taking vitamin A habitually in amounts of 25,000 IU can cause liver problems, and that taking supplemental beta-carotene can enhance the progression of some cancers. The best source of these nutrients is whole foods.

EDTA+fe and Ferrochel are additive iron compounds and are emerging as candidates for fortification by major food manufacturers. Both additives were found to exceed absorption capabilities of the commonly used fortificant ferrous sulfate.

Ferrochel is an iron bis-glycine chelate. Glycine is a nonessential amino acid used as a chelate. This chelate has a 2:1 ratio to the mineral—hence, "bis," meaning two, glycines to one iron atom. Albion Laboratories, Salt Lake City, Utah, owns the patent rights to produce this type of chelate, which is much more effective at delivering a high bioavailable form of iron than ferrous sulfate.

Fe-EDTA is a compound of iron salts and EDTA (ethylenediaminetetra-acetic acid), which is a broad-spectrum chelate, which means it binds with many minerals. It too performed well in the same absorption studies. Both EDTA and bis-glycine chelated iron were absorbed at the rate of two to three times that of ferrous sulfate. When combined with phytase, the enzyme that breaks down phytates in fiber, Ferrochel and EDTA increase the bioavailability of iron even more.

Hydrochloric acid

Hydrochloric acid (HCl), present in the stomach, frees nutrients from foods so that they can be absorbed. In the case of iron, stomach acid and other acidic foods change ferric iron, which cannot be absorbed, into ferrous iron, which can. People who do not have adequate amounts of HCl have problems of absorption. Inadequate levels of HCl is called hypochlorhydria. People who take medications to reduce the amount of acid in the stomach or who chronically ingest antacids can experience hypochlorhydria. Achlorhydria is the complete absence of stomach acid.

Meat, especially red meat, increases the absorption of nonheme iron. Beef, lamb, and venison contain the highest amounts of heme as compared to pork and chicken, which contain low amounts of heme. It has been calculated that one gram of meat (about 20 percent protein) has an enhancing effect on nonheme iron absorption equivalent to that of 1 milligram of ascorbic acid. A Latin American–type meal (maize, rice, and black beans) with a low iron bioavailability had the same improved bioavailability when either 75 g of meat or 50 mg of ascorbic acid was added.

Sugar

As part of the Framingham Heart Study, a National Institutes of Health project, investigators looked at the factors that increased iron stores such as diet and iron supplementation. Participants included more than six hundred elderly patients. Those who took supplemental iron along with fruit had higher iron stores, some as much as three times. No one is encouraged to consume sugar to improve iron absorption. Too much sugar can lead to other health problems, such as obesity and diabetes. Refined white sugar has no nutritional value except calories.

Comparing Nutritional Values

	Vitamin A	Vitamin B6	Folic acid	Zinc	Iron
White sugar 1 oz.	none	none	none	none	none
Blackstrap Molasses 1 tablespoon	none	0.14 mg	none	0.20 mg	3.50 mg
Dried Fruit (apricots) 10 halves	2534 IU	0.06 mg	4.0 mcg	0.26 mg	1.65 mg

Source: http://www.nal.usda.gov/fnic/foodcomp/Data/SR14/wtrank/wt_rank.html

However, eating fruits or adding honey or blackstrap molasses to foods such as cereals can boost iron absorption and add nutrients that are lacking in refined sugar.

Substances that inhibit absorption of iron

Calcium, like iron, is an essential mineral, which means the body gets this nutrient from diet. Calcium is found in foods such as milk, yogurt, cheese, sardines, canned salmon, tofu, broccoli, almonds, figs, turnip greens, and rhubarb and is the only known substance to inhibit absorption of both nonheme and heme iron. Whereas 50 milligrams or less of calcium has little, if any, effect on iron absorption, calcium in amounts 300 to 600 milligrams inhibit the absorption of heme iron similarly to nonheme iron. One cup of skim milk contains about 300 milligrams of calcium. When calcium is recommended by a healthcare provider, as is often the case for women trying to prevent bone loss, these supplements can be taken at bedtime. Calcium supplements are best taken with vitamin D and in a citrate rather than carbonate form.

Eggs, which are often recommended for their high-iron content, actually contain a compound that impairs absorption of iron. Phosphoprotein, called phosvitin, is a protein with an iron-binding capacity that may be responsible for the low bioavailability of iron from eggs. This iron-inhibiting characteristic of eggs is called the "egg factor." The egg factor has been observed in several separate studies. One boiled egg can reduce absorption of iron in a meal by as much as 28 percent.

Oxalates impair the absorption of nonheme iron. Oxalates are compounds derived from oxalic acid and found in foods such as spinach, kale, beets, nuts, chocolate, tea, wheat bran, rhubarb, and strawberries, as well as in herbs such as oregano, basil, and parsley. The presence of oxalates in spinach explains why the iron in spinach is not absorbed. In fact, it is reported that the iron from spinach that does get absorbed is probably from the minute particles of sand or dirt clinging to the plant rather than the iron contained in the plant.

Polyphenols are major inhibitors of iron absorption. Polyphenols or phenolic compounds include chlorogenic acid found in cocoa, coffee, and some herbs. Phenolic acid found in apples, peppermint, and some herbal teas, and tannins found in black teas, coffee, cocoa, spices, walnuts, and fruits such as apples, blackberries, raspberries, and blueberries all have the ability to inhibit iron absorption. Of the polyphenols, Swedish cocoa and certain teas demonstrate the most powerful iron absorption inhibiting capabilities, in some cases up to 90 percent.

Coffee is high in tannin and chlorogenic acid; one cup of certain types of coffee can inhibit iron absorption by as much as 60 percent. These foods or substances should not be consumed within two hours prior to and following your main iron-rich meal.

Phytate is a compound contained in soy protein and fiber. Even low levels of phytate (about 5 percent of the amounts in cereal whole flours) have a strong inhibitory effect on iron bioavailability. Phytate is found in walnuts, almonds, sesame, dried beans, lentils and peas, and cereals and whole grains. Phytate compounds can reduce iron absorption by 50 to 65 percent.

Zinc is an essential mineral found in meat, eggs, seafood, and to some degree in grains. High doses of supplemental zinc can interfere with copper utilization, which can lead to impaired metabolism of iron. Supplemental zinc can be taken in doses of 20 milligrams or less, between meals, without interfering with iron absorption.

Fats are important to metabolism, but certain fats are better for us than others. Omega-3 fatty acids are highly beneficial to health; cold-water salmon is an excellent source of this type of fat. Monounsaturated fats are also beneficial; this type of fat is derived from plant sources such as olive, canola (rapeseed), and peanut oil, as well as avocados and certain nuts. Monounsaturated fats do not increase serum cholesterol or LDL levels; there is evidence that this type of fat may lower the risk of cardiovascular disease and breast cancer. Unhealthier fats can be united with free iron and increase free-radical activity and oxidative stress on vital organs.

Eating plan to improve iron levels

Often mild iron-deficiency anemia can be corrected with either a diet that includes eating red meat or modest iron supplementation, while abstaining from or including certain foods or substances with a meal. Consuming red meat may eventually replenish iron stores, although this approach singularly takes a bit longer than oral iron supplementation. Sometimes a combination approach of supplemental iron and diet changes will replenish iron stores and improve hemoglobin values sooner than dietary changes alone.

When anemia is complicated by iron overload or other

diseases, an experienced nutritionist should be consulted to create an eating plan that is customized for the patient's individual needs. Most agree that a properly balanced diet is a good foundation on which a nutrition plan can be based.

Variety without too much redundancy is the key to any good diet plan. Certain foods might be allowed occasionally, but occasionally must be defined. For some, "occasionally" means every three days, while to others, it may mean once a week, once a month, etc. Discuss diet with your healthcare provider or nutritionist to determine when and how often certain foods or substances may be consumed.

When planning meals, a few thoughtful steps can be helpful:

- Use the food composition charts provided in this book to calculate the amount of iron in foods you intend to use in your weekly meal plan. Visit www.irondisorders.org and click on the links for diet and iron content in foods.
- Incorporate foods and substances that improve absorption of iron, such as foods high in vitamin C and beta-carotene. Avoid foods and substances (or take between meals) that impair iron absorption: tea, coffee, dairy, fiber, and supplemental calcium.
- Do not eat raw shellfish and take precaution when walking barefoot on beaches if your anemia is complicated with iron overload. Oysters especially can be contaminated with Vibrio vunulficus; when consumed by a person with high iron, the result may be death by septicemia if emergency medical attention is not received.
- Freely eat the low-sugar fruits and high-fiber vegetables. Fruits such as berries, apples, and kiwi versus ripe or high-sugar fruits are the best choices. Eventually you can begin to mix in some of the riper, higher-sugar fruits (e.g., bananas and pineapple). Fruits and vegetables contain antioxidants, which help control oxidative stress that can be triggered by excess iron in patients whose anemia is complicated by high body iron levels.
- Consume good fats. Use olive oil for cooking and salad dressings. Enjoy avocados and coconuts, which are rich in nutrients known to lower the risk for some cancers.

- Cook in cast iron skillets.
- Be compliant with therapy. Iron chelation therapy is sometimes challenging, especially for youths. Compliance with therapy reduces the risk for many unpleasant or even life-threatening consequences and gives the healthcare provider opportunities to assess disease status and adjust therapies as needed.
- Keep hydrated. Your body can get some water from foods but most people tend not to eat adequate amounts of foods with high water content such as fruits and vegetables. Investigators have demonstrated that a sodium-coconut water mixture hydrates better than sports drinks.
- Don't smoke. Tobacco smoking robs the body of precious oxygen. A little known fact is that tobacco leaves contain a great deal of iron. Inhaled iron collects in lung cells called alveolar macrophages. These are the cells that help fight against infections and cancers in the lungs. When heavily burdened with iron, these cells cannot protect a person against opportunistic disease, such as pneumonia or cancer. Chewing tobacco increases the risk of gum, throat, and esophageal cancer. Nicotine-containing gum will elevate serum ferritin levels.
- Plan ahead. Deciding what meals will be consumed during a week helps save money and reduces the temptation to eat what is handy, which is often fast food or foods that are not nutritious. Planning ahead also offers opportunities for "reward meals," such as an occasional lean cut of steak or glass of red wine.

For copies of blank forms, worksheets, and sample menu planners, visit our website: www.irondisorders.org.

Foods high in phytate, tannins, etc., inhibit iron absorption.

FOOD	PHYTATE AND IRON BINDING POLYPHENOLS			TOTAL
	phytate phosphorus	tannin equivalents	chlorogenic acid	tannin equivalents
	mg/100 g dry matter			

CEREALS, CRACKERS, BRAN AND GRAINS

Cereals:				
Corn flakes	12.0	-	-	-
Millet	217.0	-	-	-
Oats, rolled	282.0	0	-	0
Semolina	19.0	-	-	-
Sorghum				
Red	279.0	480	-	480
White	389	15	-	15
Wheat germ	467	0	-	0
Flours:				
Barley	185	-	-	-
Oat	399-628	0	-	-
Rice	27	-	-	-
Wheat	680-1189	0	58	28
Crackers:				
Rye, thin	72-86	-	-	-
Rye, fiber	114-193	-	-	-
Graham	192	-	-	-
Oat	166	-	-	-
Rice cakes	113	-	-	-
Rice				
Long grain	53-64	-	-	-
Wild, brown	181-215	0	-	0
Spaghetti				
Barilla brand	71	-	-	-
Buitoni brand	6	-	-	-

FOOD	phytate phosphorus	tannin equivalents	chlorogenic acid	TOTAL tannin equivalents
PHYTATE AND IRON BINDING POLYPHENOLS				

Fruits and Berries

FOOD	phytate phosphorus	tannin equivalents	chlorogenic acid	TOTAL tannin equivalents
Apple	0.1	160	-	0
Apricot	-	0	-	0
Avocado	1.0	0	-	0
Banana	0.4	40	-	40
Blackberry	4.0	390	-	390
Blueberry	6.0	80	-	80
Currants				
Black	78.0	-	-	-
Red	55.0	-	-	-
Dates	-	5	-	5
Figs	-	0	-	5
Kiwi	10.0	0	0	0
Cowberry	5.0	3	250	122
Mango	1.0	-	-	-
Melon, honeydew	0.6	-	-	-
Orange	2.0	0	-	0
Pear	0.2	4	70	37
Raspberry	4.0	70	61	99
Rhubarb	0.2	0	16	8
Strawberry	4.0	-	-	-

PHYTATE AND IRON BINDING POLYPHENOLS

FOOD	phytate phosphorus	tannin equivalents	chlorogenic acid	TOTAL tannin equivalents
		mg/100 g dry matter		

VEGETABLES

Asparagus				
Green	2	-	-	-
White	3	-	-	-
Beans				
Black	262	0	-	0
Brown	195	0	-	0
Green	15	-	-	-
Mung	188	140	-	140
Red	271	1	-	1
White	269	0	-	0
Beets	2	3	-	3
Broccoli	10	1	40	20
Brussels sprouts	11	0	-	0
Cabbage				
Chinese	2	-	-	-
White	1	0	-	0
Carrot	4	0	28	13
Cauliflower	3	0	-	0
Celery	5	0	-	0
Chicory	2	0	-	0
Corn	24	-	-	-
Cucumber	1	0	0	0
Eggplant	3	7	51	31
Garden cress	7	-	-	-
Garlic	4	0	7	3
Horseradish	13	-	-	-
Leeks	4	0	11	5
Lentils				
Brown	142	190	-	190
Red	122	0	-	0
Lettuce, iceberg	0.5	-	-	-
Mushroom	13	1	-	1
Olives, black	3	-	-	-
Onion				
Red	5	10	-	10
Yellow	16	6	-	6

PHYTATE AND IRON BINDING POLYPHENOLS				
FOOD	phytate phosphorus	tannin equivalents	chlorogenic acid	TOTAL tannin equivalents
		mg/100 g dry matter		

SPICES

Food	phytate phosphorus	tannin equivalents	chlorogenic acid	TOTAL tannin equivalents
Allspice	-	0.0	-	0.0
Basil	-	2.7	7.9	6.5
Caraway	-	2.8	6.4	5.8
Cardamom	-	0.3	-	0.3
Chervil	-	0.4	2.0	1.4
Cinnamon	-	43.0	14.3	50.0
Clove	-	95.0	-	95.0
Cumin	-	2.8	6.4	5.8
Curry	-	6.2	9.9	10.9
Fennel	-	0.3	-	0.3
Ginger	-	0.2	-	0.2
Marjoram	-	6.4	9.9	11.1
Oregano	0.2	21.0	6.0	24.0
Pepper				
Black -	2.0	-	2.0	-
Green -	1.4	-	1.4	-
Red -	0.4	0.8	0.8	-
White -	0.4	-	0.4	-
Thyme	-	12.0	4.4	14.1
Turmeric	-	34.0	0.7	34.0
Vanilla	-	0.7	-	0.7

NUTS AND SEEDS

Food	phytate phosphorus	tannin equivalents	chlorogenic acid	TOTAL tannin equivalents
Almonds	296.0	43.0	-	43.0
Brazil nuts	-	10.0	-	10.0
Cashews	-	0.0	-	0.0
Hazelnuts	-	256.0	-	256.0
Peanuts	-	0.0	-	0.0
Walnuts	303.0	1400.0	-	1400.0
Linseeds	296.0	14.0	-	14.0
Sesame seeds	576.0	-	-	-

PHYTATE AND IRON BINDING POLYPHENOLS

FOOD	phytate phosphorus	tannin equivalents	chlorogenic acid	TOTAL tannin equivalents
		mg/100 g dry matter		
*serving sizes**				
Coffee	-	21	71	55
Tea				
English Brkfst	-	53	14	60
Green	26	17	35	
Herb	-	18	-	18
Cocoa				
Marabou	504	4400	520	4648
Dutch	513	-	-	-
Swiss	481	-	-	-
Beer				
Light lager	-	0.4	-	0.4
Whiskey, scotch	-	2.9	-	2.9
Wine				
White	-	0	4	2
Red	-	0.2 to 2.3	20-40	10-21

*serving sizes**
coffee: 3.3 grams/100 mL water or approx. 1oz:3.5
tea: 1 gram /100 mL water
Note: 1 milligram of phytate phosphorus= 3.5 milligrams phytic acid

The previous five charts provided lists of foods high in phytate, tannins, etc., which inhibit iron absorption. The next series of charts list the iron content (heme and nonheme) of foods along with other key nutrients.

food item	serving size	IRON* MILLIGRAMS		VITAMIN C MILLIGRAMS	FAT GRAMS	CARBOS GRAMS	FIBER GRAMS	PROTEIN GRAMS	CALORIES
		heme	nonheme						
Beverages									
Beer 8 oz		0.0	-	-	10.8	-	-	1.4	101
Whiskey									
(scotch) 1 oz		0.0	0.0	-	-	t	-	-	70
Wine 4 oz *									
Red dry		0.0	0.5	-	-	1 to 5	-	-	120
White dry		0.0	0.5	-	-	1 to 5	-	-	120
Sweet wines		0.0	0.5	-	-	8 to 9	-	-	120
Soft drinks 12 oz									
Lemon		0.0	0.2	-	-	36.2	-	-	144
Cola		0.0	0.1	-	-	40.0	-	-	154
Ginger ale		0.0	0.7	-	-	33.0	-	-	120
Root beer		0.0	0.2	-	-	42.0	-	-	154
Coffee		0.0	0.1	-	-	0.8	-	-	4
Tea		0.0	0.1	-	-	0.9	-	-	2

*due to the great variety of wines these numbers represent typical amounts. Consult a more detailed food value composition reference list for specific wines.

*EXCEPT FOR KNOWN PERCENTAGES: iron content values for meat is expressed as 40% heme and 60% nonheme

food item serving size	IRON*		VITAMIN C	FAT	per serving FOOD VALUES CARBOS	FIBER	PROTEIN	CALORIES
	MILLIGRAMS		MILLIGRAMS	GRAMS	GRAMS	GRAMS	GRAMS	
	heme	nonheme						

serving size is one slice or piece unless otherwise specified

Breads:

	heme	nonheme						
Biscuit (2X2 in.)	0.0	0.2	0.0	6.5	17.0	-	3.0	138
Cinnamon	0.0	0.7	0.0	3.0	15.0	2.0	2.0	90
Cornbread	0.0	1.2	0.0	7.0	29.0	1.7	4.0	200
English muffin	0.0	1.4	0.0	1.0	26.0	2.0	4.0	134
French bread	0.0	0.4	0.0	0.6	11.0	-	1.8	55
Pita pocket	0.0	1.4	0.0	2.0	33.0	-	6.0	165
Pumpernickel	0.0	0.8	0.0	4.0	17.0	-	2.9	79
Raisin	0.0	0.3	0.0	0.6	12.0	-	1.5	60
Rye	0.0	0.4	0.0	0.3	12.0	-	2.1	56
Taco shell	0.0	0.3	0.0	2.0	7.0	0.2	1.0	50
Tortilla, corn	0.0	1.4	0.0	1.0	13.0	0.3	2.0	65
White	0.0	0.7	0.0	1.0	12.0	0.5	2.0	65
Whole wheat	0.0	1.0	-	1.0	13.0	1.4	3.0	70
Cereal: basic								
Bran flakes	0.0	12.4	12.0	1.0	28.0	1.0	4.0	105
Corn flakes	0.0	1.8	15.0	-	24.0	0.4	2.0	110
Shredded wheat	0.0	1.2	-	1.0	23.0	3.3	3.0	100
Rice (puffed)	0.0	0.3	0.0	0.1	12.5	0.2	1.0	54
Cream of wheat	0.0	8.2	-	-	22.0	0.6	3.0	105
Oatmeal	0.0	1.6	-	2.0	25.0	4.0	6.0	145
Cornmeal	0.0	4.2	0.0	2.0	43.0	6.8	4.0	210
Cornstarch, 1 tbsp	0.0			0.0	7.0	-	0.0	30
Crackers								
Graham	0.0	0.4	-	1.0	11.0	2.8	1.0	60
Melba	0.0	0.1	-	-	4.0	-	1.0	20
Rye								
Saltine	0.0	0.5	-	1.0	9.0	0.5	1.0	50
Flour:								
Barley	0.0	6.6	0.0	4.0	135.0	32.0	23.0	651
Buckwheat	0.0	4.8	0.0	1.0	41.0	7.1	7.0	190
Oat	0.0	1.6	0.0	2.0	25.0	4.0	6.0	145
Rice	0.0	1.0	0.0	2.0	46.0	4.0	5.0	218
Rye	0.0	2.9	0.0	1.9	79.0		13.0	385
Wheat	0.0	4.6	0.0	2.2	87.1	15.1	16.4	407
Soy	0.0	5.7	0.0	2.4	33.4	3.7	40.9	287
Macaroni	0.0	2.1	0.0	1.0	39.0	1.2	7.0	190
Popcorn	0.0	0.3	-	3.0	6.0	-	1.0	55
Pretzels	0.0	0.3	-	1.0	13.0	-	2.0	65
Rice								
Brown	0.0	0.5	0.0	1.0	25.0	2.4	2.0	115
White	0.0	0.9	0.0	-	25.0	0.1	2.0	110
Wild	0.0	1.0	0.0	0.6	35.0	0.5	6.5	166

*EXCEPT FOR KNOWN PERCENTAGES: iron content values for meat is expressed as 40% heme and 60% nonheme

food item serving size	IRON* MILLIGRAMS		VITAMIN C MILLIGRAMS	FAT GRAMS	per serving FOOD VALUES CARBOS GRAMS	FIBER GRAMS	PROTEIN GRAMS	CALORIES
	heme	nonheme						

1 oz servings unless otherwise specified

Dairy
(milk, cheese, eggs)
Cheese

American	0.0	0.1	0.0	9.0	0.0	0.0	6.0	105
Bleu	0.0	0.2	0.0	9.0	1.0	0.0	6.0	103
Brie	0.0	0.1	0.0	7.0	0.0	0.0	6.0	85
Cheddar	0.0	0.2	0.0	9.0	0.0	0.0	7.0	113
Cottage								
1 cup	0.0	0.3	0.0	1.0	3.0	0.0	25.0	123
Cream								
1 tbsp	0.0	0.2	0.0	5.0	0.0	0.0	1.0	51
Feta	0.0	0.1	0.0	6.0	1.1	0.0	4.0	75
Fontina	0.0	t	0.0	8.8	0.4	0.0	7.6	110
Gouda	0.0	t	0.0	7.8	0.6	0.0	8.5	101
Gruyere	0.0	0.3	0.0	8.9	0.5	0.0	8.1	115
Havarti								
Monterey								
Jack	0.0	0.2	0.0	8.5	0.2	0.0	6.9	106
Mozzarella	0.0	t	0.0	4.5	0.7	0.0	6.9	72
Muenster	0.0	t	0.0			0.3	6.6	104
Neufchatel	0.0	t	0.0	6.6	0.8	0.0	2.8	74
Parmesan	0.0	0.1	0.0	7.3	0.8	0.0	10.0	110
Provolone	0.0	0.1	0.0	7.5	0.6	0.0	7.3	100
Ricotta (C)	0.0	1.0	0.0	19.4	12.6	0.0	28.0	340
Swiss	0.0	0.2	0.0	7.9	0.5	0.0	7.8	99
Velveeta								
Cream 1 cup								
Light	0.0	0.0	0.0	28.0	11.1	0.0	7.7	240
Heavy	0.0	0.0	0.0	90.0	7.4	0.0	5.2	861
Sour	0.0	0.0	0.0	43.2	8.0	0.0	6.4	456
Egg (1 lg)								
Yolk only	0.0	0.9	0.0	5.6	t	0.0	2.8	63
White only	0.0	0.1	0.0	0.0	0.4	0.0	3.3	16
Substitute								
1 oz	0.0	0.6	0.0	3.1	0.9	0.0	3.2	45
Ice cream ½ cup								
plain	0.0	0.6	0.0	7.9	15.9	0.0	2.4	134
Ice milk	0.0	0.9	0.0	4.0	18.0	0.0	3.0	120
Frozen yogurt	0.0	0.1	0.0	1.0	23.0	0.0	3.0	120

*EXCEPT FOR KNOWN PERCENTAGES: iron content values for meat is expressed as 40% heme and 60% nonheme

food item serving size	IRON* MILLIGRAMS		VITAMIN C MILLIGRAMS	FAT GRAMS	*per serving* FOOD VALUES CARBOS GRAMS	FIBER GRAMS	PROTEIN GRAMS	CALORIES
	heme	nonheme						
Milk 1 cup								
Chocolate	0.0	0.6	0.0	8.5	25.9	0.2	7.9	208
Whole	0.0	0.1	0.0	8.2	11.4	0.0	8.0	150
2%	0.0	0.1	0.0	4.7	11.7	0.0	8.1	121
1%								
Skim	0.0	0.1	0.0	0.1	11.8	0.0	8.4	86
Buttermilk	0.0	0.1	0.0	2.2	11.7	0.0	8.1	99
Canned								
sweetened	0.0	0.5	0.0	26.6	166.5	0.0	24.2	982
condensed	0.0	0.6	0.0	19.1	25.3	0.0	17.2	338
Soy	0.0	1.3	0.0	4.6	4.3	2.6	7.0	79
Yogurt lowfat								
vanilla	0.0	t	t	2.8	31.3	0.0	11.2	194
Fats (I tbsp.)								
Butter	-	t	0.0	11.5	-	-	0.1	101
Margarine		0.0	0.0	11.4	-	-	-	101
Mayonnaise	-	0.1	0.0	11.0	0.4	-	0.2	99
Oils								
Canola	-	-	0.0	14.0	-	-	-	124
Corn	-	-	0.0	13.6	-	-	-	115
Olive	-	-	0.0	13.5	-	-	-	120
Salad Dressings								
Bleu cheese	-	-	0.0	7.7	1.1	-	0.7	77
French	-	0.1	0.0	6.1	2.7	0.1	0.1	67
Italian	-	-	0.0	6.8	1.5	-	0.1	68
Ranch	-	0.1	0.0	5.0	1.0	-	0.0	50
Thousand	-	0.1	0.0	5.3	2.4	0.3	0.1	59

*EXCEPT FOR KNOWN PERCENTAGES: iron content values for meat is expressed as 40% heme and 60% nonheme

food item serving size	IRON* MILLIGRAMS heme	nonheme	VITAMIN C MILLIGRAMS	FAT GRAMS	*per serving* FOOD VALUES CARBOS GRAMS	FIBER GRAMS	PROTEIN GRAMS	CALORIES

serving size is one cup unless otherwise specified

FRUITS

food item	heme	nonheme	VITAMIN C	FAT	CARBOS	FIBER	PROTEIN	CALORIES
Apple	0.0	0.25	8	0.5	21.0	1.0	0.2	81
Applesauce	0.0	0.29	2	0.1	27.5	1.3	0.4	106
Apricot	0.0							
Fresh	0.0	0.58	11	0.4	11.7	0.6	1.4	51
Dried (10 halves)	0.0	1.65	1	0.1	21.6	1.0	1.2	83
Avocado	0.0	2.05	24	30.8	14.8	4.2	4.0	324
Banana	0.0	0.35	10	0.5	26.7	0.5	1.2	105
Blackberries	0.0	0.24	15	0.5	20.5	1.8	0.9	82
Blueberries	0.0	1.12	9	0.3	16.0	3.5	1.4	66
Cherries	0.0	0.56	5	1.4	24.0	0.6	1.7	104
Cranberries	0.0	0.19	13	0.2	12.0	1.1	0.3	46
Dates (10)	0.0	0.96	-	0.3	61.0	1.8	1.6	228
Grapefruit (½)	0.0	0.10	41	0.1	9.7	0.2	0.7	38
Grapes	0.0	0.30	5	0.3	15.7	0.7	0.5	58
Kiwi (1)	0.0	0.30	74	0.3	11.3	0.8	0.7	46
Lime (1 oz)	0.0	0.01	9	-	2.8	-	0.1	8
Mango	0.0	0.20	57	0.5	35.0	1.7	1.0	135
Melon (½)	0.0	0.50	58	0.7	22.0	0.9	2.3	94
Orange	0.0	0.6	96	0.1	15.4	0.5	1.2	62
Peach	0.0	0.1	12	-	9.6	0.5	0.6	37
Pear	0.0	0.2	7	0.6	25.0	2.3	0.6	98
Pineapple	0.0	0.6	24	0.6	19.2	0.8	0.6	77
Plum	0.0	0.1	12	0.4	8.6	0.4	0.5	36
Prunes (10)	0.0	2.0	4	-	52.7	1.7	2.1	201
Raisins	0.0	4.3	4	0.9	12.9	1.1	4.2	488
Raspberries	0.0	0.7	50	0.7	14.2	3.7	1.1	61
Strawberries	0.0	0.5	85	0.5	10.4	0.8	0.9	45
Watermelon	0.0	0.3	15	0.6	11.5	0.48	1.0	50

*EXCEPT FOR KNOWN PERCENTAGES: iron content values for meat is expressed as 40% heme and 60% nonheme

food item serving size	IRON* MILLIGRAMS	VITAMIN C MILLIGRAMS	FAT GRAMS	CARBOS GRAMS	FIBER GRAMS	PROTEIN GRAMS	CALORIES
serving size 3 oz unless otherwise specified							
Beef							
Brisket	0.55	1.6	0.0	14.2	0.1	0.0	21.8	222
Chuck roast	1.18	1.2	0.0	22.5	0.0	0.0	20.7	291
Dried beef (1 oz)	0.64	0.6	0.0	1.1	4.4	0.0	8.2	47
Flank steak	0.55	1.6	0.0	14.2	0.1	0.0	21.8	222
Ground (lean)	0.8	1.2	0.0	9.7	0.0	0.0	5.0	224
Liver	3.0	4.6	0.0	4.3	6.5	0.0	22.6	161
Prime rib	0.95	0.9	0.0	33.0	0.0	0.0	18.2	375
Round steak	1.05	1.0	0.0	19.8	0.0	0.0	22.0	273
Sirloin	1.25	1.2	0.0	22.8	0.0	0.0	20.6	294
Tenderloin	1.35	1.3	0.0	20.4	0.0	0.0	21.0	275
Poultry							
Chicken (3.2 oz)							
Breast	0.4	0.7	0.0	4.2	0.0	0.0	27.0	154
Dark meat	0.5	0.8	0.0	10.0	0.0	0.0	27.0	203
Turkey							
Breast	0.4	0.7	0.0	3.5	0.0	0.0	29.8	91
Dark meat	0.5	0.8	0.0	4.0	0.0	0.0	16.0	104
Pork							
Bacon (1)	0.15	0.5	0.0	14.7	0.0	0.0	2.4	157
Canadian							
bacon	0.18	0.6	0.0	19.8	0.0	0.0	23.4	178
Ham	0.25	0.8	0.0	25.0	0.0	0.0	19.9	206
Pork							
chop (5 oz)	0.18	0.6	0.0	43.0	0.0	0.0	20.0	345
Shoulder	0.25	0.8	0.0	25.7	0.0	0.0	18.2	312
Tenderloin	0.2	0.7	0.0	5.0	0.0	0.0	17.0	186
Roast	0.18	0.6	0.0	34.2	0.0	0.0	25.5	422
Spareribs	0.15	0.5	0.0	33.0	0.0	0.0	12.0	201
Venison							
(3.2 oz)	2.3	2.2	0.0	3.6	0.0	0.0	19.0	114
Veal (3 oz)							
breast	0.3	0.5	0.0	5.0	0.0	0.0	22.0	143
roast	0.3	0.5	0.0	8.0	0.0	0.0	29.0	192

per serving **FOOD VALUES**

food item serving size	IRON* MILLIGRAMS		VITAMIN C MILLIGRAMS	FAT GRAMS	per serving FOOD VALUES CARBOS GRAMS	FIBER GRAMS	PROTEIN GRAMS	CALORIES
	heme	nonheme						

serving size 1 oz unless otherwise specified

Luncheon meat

food item	heme	nonheme	Vit C	FAT	CARBOS	FIBER	PROTEIN	CALORIES
Beef Bologna	0.1	0.2	-	9.1	0.4	0.5	3.3	89
Pork Bologna	t	0.1	-	9.1	0.6	0.2	4.3	70
Italian Sausage	0.4	0.6	-	8.9	0.2	0.0	4.0	98
Pepperoni	t	t	-	13.0	0.0	0.0	6.0	140
Polish Sausage	0.1	0.2	-	8.1	0.5	0.0	4.0	92
Pork Sausage	t	0.1	-	8.8	0.3	0.0	5.6	105
Pork Salami	t	t	-	9.6	0.2	0.0	6.4	115
Turkey Hot Dog	t	0.1	-	5.0	0.4	0.0	4.1	64

*EXCEPT FOR KNOWN PERCENTAGES: iron content values for meat is expressed as 40% heme and 60% nonheme

food item serving size	IRON* MILLIGRAMS		VITAMIN C MILLIGRAMS	FAT GRAMS	FOOD VALUES CARBOS GRAMS	FIBER GRAMS	PROTEIN GRAMS	CALORIES
	heme	nonheme						

serving size is 3 oz unless otherwise specified

Seafood

food item	heme	nonheme	Vit C	FAT	CARBOS	FIBER	PROTEIN	CALORIES
Anchovies (5)	0.37	0.5	0	1.9	0.0	0	5.8	42
Catfish	0.4	0.6	0	3.6	0.0	0	15.5	99
Caviar (1T)	0.7	1.0	0	2.8	0.6	0	3.9	40
Clams (9)	10.0	15.0	0	0.6	4.6	0	23.0	130
Cod	t	0.1	0	0.6	0.0	0	15.0	70
Crab	0.2	0.3	0	0.5	0.0	0	15.6	71
Haddock	0.4	0.6	0	0.6	0.0	0	16.0	70
Halibut	0.3	0.4	0	2.0	0.0	0	17.7	93
Herring	0.4	0.5	0	7.7	0.0	0	15.0	134
Lobster (3 oz)	0.2	0.3	0	0.7	0.4	0	16.0	77
Mackerel	0.5	0.8	0	2.8	0.0	0	22.8	114
Oysters (6)	2.2	3.3	0	2.1	0.0	0	5.9	58
Perch	0.3	0.5	0	1.4	0.0	0	15.8	80
Pollack	0.2	0.2	0	0.8	0.0	0	16.4	75
Salmon	0.3	0.4	0	6.0	0.0	0	17.0	121
Sardines (2)	0.3	0.4	0	2.7	0.0	0	5.9	50
Scallops (3 oz)	t	0.1	0	0.6	0.0	0	14.3	75
Shrimp	0.8	1.2	0	1.5	0.0	0	17.3	90
Snails (escargot)	1.7	2.6	0	0.3	0.0	0	6.6	20
Snapper	t	t	0	1.0	0.0	0	17.4	85
Swordfish	0.3	0.4	0	3.4	0.0	0	16.8	103
Trout	0.5	0.8	0	5.6	0.0	0	17.7	126
Tuna	1.1	1.7	0	0.6	0.0	0	20.0	94
Whitefish	0.1	0.1	0	5.0	0.0	0	16.0	114

*EXCEPT FOR KNOWN PERCENTAGES: iron content values for meat is expressed as 40% heme and 60% nonheme

food item serving size	IRON*		FOOD VALUES					
	MILLIGRAMS		VITAMIN C MILLIGRAMS	FAT GRAMS	CARBOS GRAMS	FIBER GRAMS	PROTEIN GRAMS	CALORIES
	heme	nonheme						

serving size 1 oz unless otherwise specified

Nuts and Seeds

	heme	nonheme	VITAMIN C	FAT	CARBOS	FIBER	PROTEIN	CALORIES
Almonds	0.0	6.7	0.0	77	27.7	3.8	26.4	849
Cashews	0.0	5.3	0.0	64	41.0	1.9	24.1	785
Coconut	0.0	1.4	0.0	28.2	7.5	2.7	2.8	277
Hazelnut	0.0	4.6	0.0	84.2	22.5	1.1	17.0	856
Macadamia	0.0	3.2	0.0	98.8	18.4	7.1	11.0	940
Peanut	0.0	3.2	0.0	70.1	29.7	3.9	37.7	838
Pecan	0.0	2.6	0.0	76.9	15.8	2.3	9.9	742
Pistachio	0.0	8.6	0.0	61.9	31.7	2.4	26.0	739
Pumpkin	0.0	15.7	0.0	65.4	21.0	2.7	40.6	774
Sesame	0.0	3.6	0.0	80	26.4	3.6	27.3	873
Sunflower	0.0	10.3	0.0	68.6	28.9	5.5	34.8	812
Walnut	0.0	3.1	0.0	64	15.8	2.1	14.8	651
Peanut Butter	0.0	0.3	0.0	8.1	3.2	0.3	3.9	86

*EXCEPT FOR KNOWN PERCENTAGES: iron content values for meat is expressed as 40% heme and 60% nonheme

food item* serving size	IRON MILLIGRAMS		VITAMIN C MILLIGRAMS	FAT GRAMS	CARBOS GRAMS	FIBER GRAMS	PROTEIN GRAMS	CALORIES
	heme	nonheme						
Condiments/misc 1 tbsp								
Bacon								
bits ¼ oz	0.0	0.1	0.0	0.3	0.4	-	0.6	7
Barbecue								
Sauce	0.0	0.1	0.7	0.3	5.0	-	0.2	15
Bouillon 1 cube								
Beef	t	t	-	-	1.0	-	-	10
Chicken	t	t	-	-	1.0	-	-	10
Catsup	0.0	0.1	2.5	0.1	4.3	-	0.3	19
Garbanzo								
beans 1 oz	0.0	0.6	t	1.7	17.2	1.8	5.5	103
Horseradish		t	-	t	0.5	-	0.1	2
Mustard .	0.0	0.1	-	0.8	0.5	-	t	11
Olives 1 lg								
Black	0.0	-	-	0.8*	1.0	-	-	10
Green	0.0	-	-	0.8*	1.0	-	-	10
Pimento	0.0	0.2	10	t	0.6	0.1	0.1	3
Pickle								
Dill 2 oz	0.0	0.3	-	t	0.3	0.1	t	1
Sweet 2 oz	0.0	0.4	-	-	10.0	-	-	36
Soy sauce	0.0	0.5	-	-	0.9	-	-	10
Vinegar cider	0.0	0.1	-	-	1.0	-	-	2
Worcestershire	0.3	-	t	t	-	0.1	4	

*olives and olive oil are high in monounsaturated fat, which is beneficial to ones health.

t=trace

*EXCEPT FOR KNOWN PERCENTAGES: Iron content values for meat is expressed as 40% heme and 60% nonheme

food item serving size	IRON* MILLIGRAMS	FOOD VALUES					
		VITAMIN C MILLIGRAMS	FAT GRAMS	CARBOS GRAMS	FIBER GRAMS	PROTEIN GRAMS	CALORIES
	heme nonheme						

serving size ½ cup unless otherwise specified   t=trace

Vegetables

food item	heme / nonheme	VITAMIN C	FAT	CARBOS	FIBER	PROTEIN	CALORIES
Artichoke	0.0 | 1.1	8.0	0.2	9.9	6.0	2.8	44
Asparagus							
(1 spear)	0.0 | 0.1	5.3	0.6	0.6	-	0.3	16
Beans (1 cup)							
Black	0.0 | 5.2	0.0	1.0	40.8	7.2	15.2	226
Green	0.0 | 0.7	0.2	8.9	10.0	4.0	2.0	44
Kidney	0.0 | 5.2	2.0	1.0	40.0	13.0	15.0	225
Lima	0.0 | 4.4	0.0	1.0	42.0	14.0	15.0	229
Navy	0.0 | 2.5	0.0	0.0	19.0	4.0	7.0	109
Pinto	0.0 | 2.2	2.0	0.4	43.6	6.8	14.0	234
Beets	0.0 | 0.5	5.0	t	5.7	0.7	0.9	26
Broccoli	0.0 | 0.6	58.0	0.2	3.9	2.0	2.3	22
Brussels							
sprouts	0.0 | 0.5	0.5	0.4	6.8	3.4	2.0	30
Cabbage	0.0 | 0.2	18.0	0.1	1.9	0.4	0.4	8
Carrots	0.0 | 0.2	2.0	0.1	5.6	1.8	0.6	24
Cauliflower	0.0 | 0.2	36.0	0.1	2.9	1.4	1.2	15
Celery	0.0 | 0.2	4.0	0.1	2.2	1.0	0.5	10
Collards	0.0 | 0.1	8.0	t	1.3	0.1	0.3	6
Corn	0.0 | 0.5	5.0	1.1	20.6	3.0	2.7	89
Cucumber	0.0 | 0.1	2.0	0.1	1.5	0.5	0.3	7
Eggplant	0.0 | 0.2	1.0	0.1	3.2	0.5	0.4	13
Garlic 1 clove	0.0 | t	1.0	t	1.0	0.1	0.2	4
Kale	0.0 | 0.6	27.0	0.3	3.7	0.5	1.2	21
Kohlrabi	0.0 | 0.3	44.0	0.1	5.5	0.9	1.5	24
Leeks	0.0 | 0.6	2.0	0.2	7.4	0.6	0.8	32
Lettuce							
Bibb	0.0 | 0.5	13.0	0.1	0.7	0.3	0.4	4
Iceberg	0.0 | 0.3	1.0	0.1	0.6	0.3	0.3	4
Leaf	0.0 | 0.4	5.0	0.1	1.0	0.2	0.4	5
Romaine	0.0 | 0.3	7.0	0.1	0.7	0.5	0.5	4
Mushrooms	0.0 | 0.4	1.0	0.2	1.6	0.5	0.7	9
Mustard greens	0.0 | 0.5	10.0	0.1	1.4	0.2	0.8	7
Okra	0.0 | 0.4	13.0	0.1	3.8	0.5	1.0	25
Onions	0.0 | 0.2	5.0	0.1	6.9	1.3	0.9	30
Parsley	0.0 | 1.8	27.0	0.1	2.1	1.3	0.7	10
Parsnips	0.0 | 0.4	10.0	0.2	15.2	2.1	1.0	63
Peas	0.0 | 1.2	11.0	0.2	12.5	3.0	4.3	67
Peppers							
Green	0.0 | 0.2	45.0	0.1	3.2	0.8	0.4	13
Red	0.0 | 0.2	95.0	0.1	3.2	0.8	0.4	13
Potato							
Sweet	0.0 | 0.7	25.0	0.1	24.3	3.0	1.7	103
White	0.0 | 0.8	26.0	0.1	24.4	1.0	2.2	105
w/skin	0.0 | 2.7	15.0	0.2	51.0	5.3	4.7	220
Pumpkin	0.0 | 0.7	6.0	0.1	6.0	1.0	0.9	24
Radishes (10)	0.0 | 0.1	10.0	0.2	1.6	0.2	0.3	7
Sauerkraut	0.0 | 1.7	17.0	0.2	5.1	1.3	1.0	22
Spinach	0.0 | 0.7	8.0	0.1	1.0	0.7	0.8	6
Squash	0.0 | 0.6	8.0	t	8.0	3.0	1.0	29
Tomato	0.0 | 0.4	17.0	0.3	4.2	1.2	0.8	19
Zucchini	0.0 | 0.3	4.0	0.1	1.9	0.3	0.8	9

*EXCEPT FOR KNOWN PERCENTAGES: iron content values for meat is expressed as 40% heme and 60% nonheme

Glossary

absolute neutrophil count: a measure of the actual number of neutrophils present in the blood per unit volume.

acidosis: a condition resulting from accumulation of too much acid in the body due to excess carbon dioxide. Acidic individuals may sigh frequently, have insomnia, or suffer from migraines. Neutral pH is 7.0—above 7.0 is alkaline, below 7.0 is acidic. Ideal body pH is around 7.4.

acquired nonreversible sideroblastic anemias: forms of SA that occur later in life and for which the cause cannot be reversed. Also called acquired idiopathic SA.

acquired reversible sideroblastic anemias: forms of SA that can be reversed by eliminating the cause, such as nutritional deficiencies or use of certain drugs.

ACTH (adrenocorticotropic hormone): hormone secreted by the anterior pituitary gland that stimulates adrenal glands to secrete the hormones such as cortisone, the body's natural pain-reliever. ACTH is secreted in during moments of stress, trauma, major surgery, and fever.

ACTH (adrenocorticotropic hormone) deficiency: too little ACTH produced by the pituitary gland.

acute: occurring suddenly and severely but of short duration, can define pain as sharp.

Addison's disease or syndrome (adrenal insufficiency): inactive or underactive adrenal function.

adrenal cortex: the outer part of the adrenal gland.

adrenal glands: glands that secrete hormones, including adrenaline (from the adrenal medulla) and cortisol, aldosterone, and adrenal androgens (from the adrenal cortex).

adrenal medulla: the inner part of the adrenal gland.

advance directive: written instructions, as in a living will, whereby all hospitalized patients have a form on file indicating their desires.

AFP (alpha-fetoprotein): a protein that is produced by fetal liver and yolk sac during the first trimester. Increased maternal serum levels may indicate neural tube or abdominal wall defects in the fetus. Increased non-maternal AFP may indicate tumor development in the breast, ovaries/testes, kidney, or liver.

AIDS (Acquired Immune Deficiency Syndrome): usually fatal condition whereby the immune system loses the ability to fight infection because of the human immunodeficiency virus (HIV), which can be contracted from sexual contact with an infected person, using a syringe used by infected person, or from an infected mother who passes the virus to a fetus.

aldosterone: a hormone excreted by the adrenal cortex; indirectly regulates blood levels of potassium and chloride, bicarbonate, as well as pH, blood volume, and blood pressure.

alkalosis: abnormal condition in which body fluids are more alkaline than normal.

allele: any one of a series of two or more different genes that occupy the same position (locus) on a chromosome. Since autosomal chromosomes are paired, each autosomal locus is represented twice. If both chromosomes have the same allele occupying the same locus, the condition is referred to as homozygous for this allele. If the alleles at the two loci are different, the individual or cell is referred to as heterozygous for both alleles.

allergen: a substance that causes an allergic reaction.

allogeneic bone marrow transplantation: process in which bone marrow cells from a donor are infused into a patient.

ALP (alkaline phosphatase): an enzyme that is concentrated in developing bone, plasma, and kidney and is excreted by the liver. Increased levels may indicate biliary obstruction or diseases of the pancreas, lung, liver, or bone. ALP can also be naturally elevated in youths who are experiencing bone growth.

ALT (alanine aminotransferase): an enzyme (*see also* SGPT) that can concentrate in muscles, liver, and brain. Increased levels indicate cell death or disease in these tissues.

alveolus (alveoli, pl.): tiny air sacs in the lungs where the exchange of carbon dioxide and oxygen occur.

Alzheimer's disease: Named for Alois Alzheimer, neurologist, 1864–1915. A chronic, progressive disorder that accounts for more than 50 percent of all cases of dementia.

amenorrhea: cessation of menstruation for at least three months in a woman who has previously menstruated.

amino acids: organic compounds mostly made of proteins. The body contains at least twenty amino acids. Ten are essential, which means that the body does not make or form these, so they must be acquired through diet.

amyloidosis: disorder in which starch-like glycoproteins (amyloids) accumulate in tissues, impairing function.

ANA (anti-nuclear antibody): used to diagnose various autoimmune diseases, such as rheumatoid arthritis, scleroderma, or systemic lupus erythematosus.

anaphylaxis: also called anaphylactic shock, it is a severe allergic reaction to a foreign substance that the patient has had contact with. Infused or injected iron can cause anaphylaxis in some patients.

androgens: hormones that stimulate pubic and underarm hair growth in both males and females, but that are produced in much greater quantities (especially testosterone from the testes) and are more important in stimulating and maintaining secondary sexual characteristics in males.

anemia: reduced red blood cell mass.

anemia, aplastic: complete failure of the bone marrow to produce blood cells.

anemia, Cooley's: (also known as thalassemia) inherited disorder where a recessive trait is responsible for interference with hemoglobin synthesis.

anemia, Diamond Blackfan: a rare inherited hypoplastic condition characterized by age of onset.

anemia, Fanconi: (also known as Fanconi's syndrome) a rare inherited hypoplastic anemia characterized by reduced production of all types of blood cells in the body. Fanconi is sometimes called a "chromosome breakage" condition.

anemia, hemolytic: inherited disorder where premature destruction of mature red blood cells occurs.

anemia, hypoplastic: failure of the bone marrow to produce one or several blood cells or an overall reduction of all blood cells. In hypoplastic anemias one or more types of blood cells are affected as compared with aplastic anemia where all types of cells are affected.

anemia, iron-deficiency: anemia caused by blood loss, dietary insufficiencies, or rapid growth where iron demands exceed intake and stores.

anemia of chronic disease: mild anemia that accompanies inflammation due to chronic disease.

anemia, megaloblastic: a type of anemia where red blood cells are larger than normal, usually resulting from a deficiency of folic acid or vitamin B$_{12}$.

anemia, pernicious: anemia caused by inadequate absorption of vitamin B$_{12}$ due to the absence of intrinsic factor, a substance secreted by the mucous membranes of the stomach.

anemia, pyridoxine-responsive: an anemia that responds to pyridoxine (**B$_6$**) treatment.

anemia, renal disease: anemia associated with acute and chronic renal failure.

anemia, sickle cell: anemia in sickle cell disease patients resulting from chronic hemolysis caused by a sickling crisis.

anemia, sideroblastic: type of anemia in which the bone marrow deposits iron prematurely into red blood cells.

anemia, thalassemia major: *see* anemia, Cooley's.

anesthesiologist: *see* physicians, types of.

angina: chest pain or pressure usually beneath the sternum (breastbone). Caused by inadequate blood supply to the heart. Often brought on by exercise, emotional upset, or heavy meals in someone who has heart disease.

angiocardiography: cardiac catheterization used to visualize the heart chambers, arteries, and veins.

angiography: (also called arteriography) an X ray technique used to determine blood flow abnormalities and some tumors, and to pinpoint internal bleeding.

angiomas: benign tumors, usually congenital, made up of mostly blood vessels or lymph vessels.

angioplasty: the use of surgery to make a damaged blood vessel function properly again; may involve widening or reconstructing the blood vessel.

angiotension-converting enzyme (ACE) inhibitor: a drug used to treat high blood pressure.

anisocytosis: excessive variation in red cell size.

antibody: a protein made by white blood cells that reacts with a specific foreign protein as part of the immune response; fights infection or harmful foreign substances (antigens).

anti-diuretic: substance that controls the amount of water reabsorbed by the kidney.

antigen: a marker on the surface of cells that identifies what type of cell it is.

apheresis: a procedure where whole blood is removed from the patient or donor and blood components such as red cells, leukocytes, or plasma are separated.

aplastic: failure of an organ or tissue to develop normally.

APTT; partial thromboplastin time; activated partial thromboplastin time: a test that measures the intrinsic clotting time in plasma.

arrhythmia: an irregular heartbeat.

arthritis: inflammatory condition of the joints, characterized by pain, stiffness, and swelling.

arthrography/arthrogram: X ray of a joint with contrast dye.

arthropathy: disease of a joint.

arthroscopy: a procedure that allows direct examination of the interior of a joint using an endoscope.

ascites: accumulation of fluid in the abdomen.

aspiration: withdrawal by suction of fluids, air, or foreign bodies.

AST (aspartate aminotransferase): an enzyme concentrated in the muscle, liver, and brain. Increased levels may indicate disease within these tissues.

ataxia: defective muscular coordination, as in unsteadiness of gait.

atherosclerosis: common disorder of the arteries characterized by thickening, loss of elasticity, and calcification of artery walls.

atrophy: wasting away of a tissue or organ.

autoantibody: an antibody made by a person that reacts with their own tissues.

autoimmune disease: a disorder in which the body's immune system attacks itself; sometimes referred to as autoimmune response.

autoimmune hemolytic anemia: a condition where antibodies attack the red blood cells, causing them to be prematurely destroyed.

autoimmune thyroiditis: chronic inflammation that can lead to Graves' disease (hyperthyroidism) or hypothyroidism if the thyroid gland diminishes in size. *See* Hashimoto's thyroiditis, hypothyroidism.

autosomal dominant: a pattern of inheritance in which the dominant gene on any non-sex chromosome carries the defect.

autosomal recessive: non-sex chromosome in which two defective gene copies must be inherited, one from each parent, for the disease to manifest itself.

autosomal gene: located on a non-sex chromosome.

bacterium (bacteria, pl.): a tiny, single-celled microorganism; some are naturally present in the intestinal tract; some are pathogenic and can cause disease.

bacteriuria: the presence of bacteria in the urine.

basophils: a type of white blood cell responsible for controlling inflammation and damage of tissues in the body.

benign: non-cancerous tumor or growth that does not interfere with normal function.

beta-blocker: a drug used to treat hypertension (high blood pressure), heart arrhythmia, circulation, and sometimes angina or migraine.

bile duct: passages that convey bile from the liver to the hepatic duct, which joins the duct from the gall bladder to form the common bile duct, which enters the duodenum.

bilirubin: red blood cell waste product in bile; blood carries it to the liver. Orange-yellowish in color, it contributes to the yellow color of urine. Abnormal accumulation of bilirubin in the blood and skin results in jaundice.

biopsy: removal of a small amount of tissue or fluid, usually by needle, for laboratory examination; aids in diagnosis.

blast cells: immature cells that mature into various blood cells.

bleeding, gastrointestinal: condition of internal blood loss occurring somewhere in the digestive system: esophagus, stomach, small and large intestine.

bleeding time: lab test performed to determine the time for blood flow to cease (normal 2–8 minutes).

blood: liquid pumped by the heart through arteries, veins, and capillaries. Blood consists of a pale yellow fluid called plasma, red blood cells (erythrocytes), white blood cells (leukocytes), platelets (thrombocyte-essential blood clotting element), and suspended chemicals, hormones, proteins, fats, and carbohydrates.

blood pressure: measure of tension caused by blood pressing against the walls of the arteries as it flows through the body.

blood sugar: measure of glucose in the blood.

blood test: a lab procedure where blood is drawn from the arm, a port, or obtained by finger prick to examine for specific values such as blood cell size, shape, color, and volume or the presence of specific abnormalities or disease.

bone marrow: specialized soft tissue that fills the core of bones, especially the sternum and long bones. Yellow marrow consists primarily of fats and does not participate in hematopoiesis (blood cell production). Red marrow produces all the types of blood cells.

bone marrow aspiration: removal of a portion of the soft organic material filling the cavities of the bone. Used to evaluate and diagnose many blood diseases such as anemia, leukemia, iron storage deficiency, bone marrow deficiencies, or identification of tumors.

bone marrow transplant: procedure in which bone marrow filled with disease is destroyed by radiation or chemotherapy and then replaced with healthy cells from a donor.

brain infarctions: localized area of brain tissue death resulting from lack of oxygen to that area because of an interruption in blood supply.

BUN (blood urea nitrogen): a blood test that measures the amount of urea nitrogen in the blood; used to determine liver and kidney function.

calcification: a process in which organic tissue becomes hardened by the deposition of minerals such as calcium.

calcitonin: a hormone produced by the parathyroid glands that affects levels of calcium in the blood.

calcium: mineral contained in the blood that helps regulate the heartbeat, transmit nerve impulses, contract muscles, and form bones and teeth.

calcium channel blocker (CCB): a drug used to relax the blood vessels and heart muscle, causing pressure inside blood vessels to drop. CCB drugs can be used to regulate heart rhythm.

cancer: abnormal and malignant growth of cells.

Candida (C. albicans): a genus of yeasts (fungi) that is part of the normal body flora found in the mouth, skin, intestinal tract, and vagina. Abnormal growth of Candida results in a yeast infection called candidiasis.

cardiac arrest: a sudden stop of heart function; "sudden death."

cardiac catheterization: a procedure in which a thin hollow tube is inserted into a blood vessel. The tube is then advanced through the vessel into the heart, enabling a physician to study the heart and its pumping activity.

cardiac enzymes: various enzymes that are indicative of injury to the heart, such as creatine kinase (CK), aspartate aminotransferase (AST), and lactate dehydrogenase (LDH), which are of variable specificity to cardiac muscle.

cardiologist: *see* physicians, types of.

cardiomyopathy: disease involving the heart muscle.

catabolize: to break down complex chemical compounds into simpler ones.

celiac disease: (also called celiac sprue) a malabsorption disease caused by an intolerance for gluten, a protein present in most grains, which affects the jejunal portion of the small intestine.

cerebrospinal fluid: a clear, normally colorless and blood-free fluid that cushions and nourishes the brain and spinal cord.

ceruloplasmin (Cp): a blood glycoprotein that binds with copper but is also essential to the transport of iron.

chelators, chemical: agents that bind with metals to remove them from the body.

chemotherapy: treatment of cancer with medication intended to kill cancer cells without harming healthy tissue.

cholesterol: complex chemical produced by the liver and contained in dietary fats that is transported through the bloodstream attached to lipoproteins. Low-density lipoproteins (LDL) carry cholesterol that builds up plaque; high-density lipoproteins (HDL) carry cholesterol to the liver where the body can get rid of it.

chromosome: structures inside the nucleus of living cells that contain hereditary information (DNA).

chronic: long-term; continuing.

cirrhosis: a chronic disease of the liver where scar tissue replaces normal, healthy tissue, causing loss of function of liver cells and decreased blood flow through the liver.

coagulation, blood: the process of lumping together blood cells to form a clot.

colitis: inflammation of the colon.

colonoscopy: investigation of the inside of the colon using a long, flexible fiberoptic tube called an endoscope.

complement: a system of serum proteins that work to help antibodies destroy antigens.

complete blood count (CBC): usually includes hemoglobin, hematocrit, the number of red and white cells, mean corpuscular volume (MCV), MCH (mean corpuscular hemoglobin), and the MCHC (mean corpuscular hemoglobin concentration).

computed tomography (CT): sometimes called a CAT scan. A type of X ray where the X ray beams pass through the body and are detected by sensors. Information from sensors is computer processed and then displayed as an image on a television-like screen. Sometimes contrast agents are used to block certain tissue from the X ray. Tumors, primary and metastatic, will show up as bright white spots on the film.

congenital: present at, and existing from, the time of birth.

congestive heart failure: life-threatening condition where the heart loses its full pumping capacity and fluid accumulates in the lungs.

connective-tissue disease (collagen disease): any one of many abnormal conditions characterized by inflammatory changes in small blood vessels and connective tissue. Some collagen diseases include systemic lupus erythematosus (chronic inflammation resulting in arthritis), scleroderma (autoimmune disease resulting in hardening of the skin), polymyositis (muscle inflammation), and rheumatic fever (resulting in heart valve damage).

Coombs' (direct): test used to identify hemolysis due to autoimmune reaction.

Coombs' (indirect): test used to detect circulating antibodies to red blood cells.

coronary thrombosis: presence of blood clot obstructing the flow of blood to the heart.

corticosteroids: hormones produced by the adrenal cortex that regulate sexual function, salt and water balance, the body's response to stress, metabolism, and immune system function.

corticotropin: a hormone released by the pituitary gland that stimulates the adrenal glands' production of hormones.

cortisol: (also called hydrocortisone) a hormone released by the adrenal cortex that affects the metablolism of fats, carbohydrates, and proteins.

creatine phosphokinase (CPK, CP, or CK): an enzyme found predominantly in the heart muscle, skeletal muscle, and the brain. Elevated levels indicate damage to these organs.

creatinine: compound found in the blood, urine, and muscle tissue. Elevated creatinine in the blood usually indicates the presence of kidney disease.

Crohn's disease: chronic inflammatory condition primarily involving the colon and the terminal portion of the small intestines, but can be present in the mouth, esophagus, stomach, duodenum, appendix, rectum, and anus.

cross match: type and cross; test in which the blood cells of a donor and a recipient are mixed together to determine if they are compatible.

culture: procedure used to identify the source of infection; specimen of blood, urine, sputum, or stool is taken and tested to determine the type of infection and the appropriate antibiotic.

cytokines: chemicals made by the cells that act on other cells to stimulate or inhibit their function; hormone-like proteins secreted by many different cell types that regulate cell proliferation and function, for example: cytokines that stimulate growth are called "growth factors."

cytopenia: a deficiency of cells in the blood.

cytotoxic: destructive to cells.

deferasirox: an oral iron chelator drug; brand name Exjade®.

deferiprone: an oral iron chelator drug, brand name Ferriprox®.

deferoxamine: (also sometimes spelled *desferrioxamine*) a drug used in iron chelation therapy; brand name Desferal®

depression: a condition accompanied by feelings of hopelessness, sadness, or discouragement often with inability to function or participate in activities.

dermatitis herpetiformis: a chronic disease of the skin marked by a symmetric itching eruption of vesicles and papules that occur in groups; relapses are common; associated with gluten-sensitive enter-opathy and IgA immune complexes beneath the epidermis of lesioned and normal-appearing skin.

Desmopressin (DDAVP): synthetic drug that resembles vasopressin. It is used in nonreplacement treatment of von Willebrand disease.

diabetes: either of two disorders, diabetes insipidus or diabetes mellitus. *Diabetes insipidus:* metabolic disorder of the hormone system caused by a deficiency of antidiuretic hormone (ADH) normally secreted by the pituitary gland. Usually a temporary condition. *Diabetes mellitus:* chronic metabolic disorder due to insufficient or ineffective insulin. Two forms of diabetes mellitus are Type I or juvenile-onset diabetes and Type II or adult-onset diabetes. Insulin dependent: those with an inability to produce enough insulin to process carbohydrates, fat, and protein efficiently will require insulin injections. Non-insulin dependent: most prevalent among obese adults. Often controlled with weight loss, exercise, and diet.

dialysis: medical procedure for filtering waste products from the blood of some patients with kidney disease.

differential: percent of different types of blood cells in the blood.

differentiate: in diagnosis, a particular test or procedure that helps to narrow the possible causes of an illness.

digitalis: a drug used to increase the force of the heart's contraction and to regulate specific irregularities of heart rhythm.

dilated cardiomyopathy: enlargement of the heart's chambers, causing the heart to lose its pumping ability.

diuretic: a drug that helps eliminate excess body fluid; usually used in the treatment of high blood pressure and heart failure.

diverticulosis: refers to a condition in which the inner, lining layer of the large intestine (colon) bulges out (herniates) through the outer, muscular layer.

doppler studies: named after Johann Christian Doppler, Austrian scientist (1803–53), Doppler studies are measurements of systolic blood pressure using sound waves. Doppler studies are also used to measure fetal heart rate in expectant mothers.

dyserythropoiesis: abnormal RBC synthesis, characterized by nuclear abnormalities, including abnormal chromatin pattern, bizarre shapes, and nuclear fragmentation.

dyspnea: shortness of breath.

E. coli (Escherichia coli): bacteria that normally live in the digestive tract of of humans and animals.

The bacteria are passed on to others when infected feces contaminate food, water, or any other substance that people or animals might ingest. Some strains of *E. coli* can cause diarrhea and other digestive system (gastrointestinal) problems. A few strains of *E. coli* bacteria, including the O157:H7 strain, can produce poisons (toxins) that can harm the intestines, blood, and kidneys.

eculizumab: a drug to treat patients with PNH; brand name Soliris®.

echocardiogram: the record of a procedure (echocardiography) using ultrasound waves to visualize internal heart structure.

echocardiography (EEG or EKG): a test that bounces sound waves off the heart to produce pictures of its internal structures.

edema: abnormal accumulation of fluid in body tissues.

electrocardiogram (EKG or ECG): the most common test used to diagnose a heart attack.

elliptocytosis: inherited, usually benign form of hemolytic anemia characterized by elongated or elliptical shaped red blood cells.

embolism: sudden blockage of a blood vessel by a embolus (blood clot).

embolotherapy: a procedure to occlude ("plug in") abnormal blood vessels. This is used to treat PAVM and brain telangiectasias.

endocarditis: serious bacterial infection of the membrane lining of the heart and valves or heart muscle.

endocrine gland: an organ containing a group of cells that produce and secrete hormones into the bloodstream.

endocrinologist: *See* physicians, types of.

endoglin: a protein that is deficient in HHT.

endoscope/endoscopy: an endoscope as used in the field of gastroenterology is a thin flexible tube that uses a lens or miniature camera to view various areas of the gastrointestinal tract.

endothelial cells: cells in the tissue layer that line blood vessels.

enzyme: a chemical (protein), originating in a cell that can act outside the cell and regulate reactions in the body; acts as a catalyst to induce chemical changes in other substances.

eosinophils: a type of white blood cell that reacts to allergies and can destroy parasites.

epinephrine: the principal blood pressure and heart rate raising hormone secreted by the adrenal medulla; also called adrenaline.

epistaxis: nose bleeds.

erythroblastosis fetalis: refers to two potentially disabling or fatal blood disorders in infants: Rh incompatibility disease and ABO incompatibility disease. Either disease may be apparent before birth and can cause fetal death in some cases. The disorder is caused by incompatibility between a mother's blood and her unborn baby's blood.

erythrocyte: a mature red blood cell.

erythropoiesis: synthesis (creation) of red blood cells.

erythropoietin (EPO): a hormone produced in the kidneys that stimulates the production of red blood cells in the bone marrow.

esophageal varices: enlarged veins on the lining of the esophagus subject to severe bleeding; often they appear in patients with chronic alcoholism and other forms of liver disease.

esophagitis: inflammation of the mucous-membrane lining of the esophagus.

ESRD: end-stage renal disease.

estrogen: the female sex hormone; a hormone produced primarily by the ovaries in women that stimulates breast development, menstruation, and other female secondary sexual changes.

ethanol: a form of alcohol contained in beverages.

exocrine gland: a gland (like a salivary gland or the digestive enzyme-producing part of the pancreas) that releases a secretion external to or at the surface of an organ, often through a canal or duct.

Factor VIII: clotting factor in human blood that can be measured to help diagnose von Willebrand disease.

familial adenomatous polyps (FAP): an inherited condition in which hundreds of polyps develop in the colon and rectum.

Fanconi anemia: an inherited form of aplastic anemia.

fasting: going without food for a period of time, such as twelve-hour fasting prior to bloodwork.

Fe: symbol for the element iron.

febrile: an elevated body temperature.

fecal: pertaining to body waste, matter discharged from the bowel.

fecal occult blood test: test in which a stool sample is chemically tested for hidden blood.

ferritin: a complex protein formed in the intestine, containing about 23 percent iron. The amount found in serum is directly related to iron storage in the body. Increased ferritin levels may indicate iron loading and conditions such as hemochromatosis; when low, iron deficiency anemia exists.

ferrous sulfate/gluconate: common forms of oral iron.

fertility: capability to reproduce.

fetal: pertaining to the fetus.

fibrocystic breast disease: presence of benign cysts in the breasts; common condition that should be monitored; reduced consumption of caffeine is recommended.

fibroids: abnormal growth of cells in the muscular wall of the uterus; uterine fibroids are composed of abnormal muscle cells and are almost always benign.

fibromas: non-malignant (benign) tumor of the connective tissue.

fibrosis: abnormal formation of connective or scar tissue.

fifth disease: a mild childhood illness caused by the human parvovirus B19 that causes flu-like symptoms and a rash. It is called fifth disease because it was fifth on a list of common childhood illnesses that are accompanied by a rash, including measles, rubella or German measles, scarlet fever (or scarlatina), and scarlatinella, a variant of scarlet fever. Latin name for the disease is *erythema infectiosum*, meaning "infectious redness." It is also called "slapped cheek disease."

folate (also called folic acid): folate and folic acid are forms of a water-soluble B vitamin. Folate is found in foods, where folic acid is the synthetic form found in supplements and fortified foods.

folic acid anemia: a shortage of red blood cells due to lack of folic acid in the diet.

FT3 (triiodothyronine): free T3; one form of thyroid hormone that occurs when T4 is converted.

FT4 (free thyroxine): one form of thyroid hormone in response to TSH (thyroid stimulating hormone).

fungi: a yeast, mold, or mushroom.

fulminating infection: infection that occurs suddenly and with great intensity.

G-CSF: a hormone that stimulates growth of white blood cells and may increase the effectiveness of erythropoietin among people with acquired nonreversible SA.

G-lamblia (Giardia lamblia): a parasite that can live and reproduce in human or animal intestines. Once in the intestines, they attach to the inside of the intestinal wall, where they can damage or disrupt the normal function of the intestines and compete for important nutrients. This leads to the symptoms of giardiasis.

gallbladder disease: any disease involving the gallbladder or biliary tract. The gallbladder is a reservoir for bile; the biliary tract is the passageway that transports bile to the small intestine.

gallstones: calculus or stones formed in the gallbladder.

gastrectomy (total): surgical removal (excision) of the entire stomach.

gastrin: hormone that stimulates the production of gastric acid or stomach acid.

gastrinoma: benign or malignant gastrin-secreting islet-cell tumor of the pancreas.

gastritis: irritation, inflammation, or infection of the stomach lining.

gastroenteritis: inflammation of the stomach and intestines accompanying many digestive-tract disorders.

gastroenterologist: *see* physicians, types of.

gastrointestinal disease: any disorder of the gastrointestinal tract, which includes the mouth, esophagus, stomach, duodenum, small intestine, cecum, appendix, the ascending colon, transverse colon, descending colon, sigmoid colon, rectum, and anus.

gastrointestinal symptoms (GI symptoms): any symptoms relating to the stomach or intestine, such as vomiting, diarrhea, constipation, bloating, flatulence, ascites, abdominal pain, or heartburn.

gastrointestinal tract: the entire length of the digestive system, running from the stomach, through the small intestine, large intestine, and out the rectum and anus.

genetic mutation: (also called a genetic variation) any abnormal change in the makeup of a gene.

GGT (gamma glutamyl transpeptidase): an enzyme found mainly in the liver but also in many other parts of the body. Increased GGT levels are involved in hepatitis, cirrhosis, jaundice, and other chronic diseases.

globin: one of the six proteins associated with the hemoglobin molecule.

glucagon: a hormone that works with insulin to regulate glucose levels in the blood.

glucose: simple sugar that is the body's major source of energy.

glucose tolerance test: useful in the diagnosis of diabetes or hypoglycemia.

glucose-6-phosphate dehydrogenase (G6PD): an enzyme, G6PD deficiency is an inherited X-linked autosomal recessive disorder that can result in hemolytic anemia when an individual consumes fava beans or alcoholic beverages or is given certain drugs such as antimalarial, or sulfa, drugs. The constant hemolysis (destruction of red blood cells) leads to siderosis/iron overload.

gluten: the insoluble protein (prolamines) constituent of wheat and other grains; a mixture of gliadin, glutenin, and other proteins; the presence of gluten allows flour to rise.

gluten enteropathy: hereditary malabsorption disorder caused by sensitivity to gluten, a protein found in wheat, rye, barley, and oats. Also called non-tropical sprue or celiac disease.

glycogen: substance formed from glucose, stored chiefly in the liver. When the blood-sugar level is too low, glycogen is converted back to glucose for the body to use as energy.

gonadotropin: hormone that stimulates function of the gonads.

gonads: parts of the reproductive system that produce and release eggs (ovaries in the female) or sperm (testes in the male).

granulocyte: one of the three types of white blood cells (the others being monocytes and lymphocytes), so called because they have granules that contain enzymes that help fight infection.

granulomas: nodule of firm tissue formed as a reaction to chronic inflammation, such as from foreign bodies or bacteria.

growth hormone (GH): a hormone regulating cell division and protein synthesis needed for normal growth.

H. pylori (Helicobacter pylori): a bacterium found in the stomach lining that can be a risk factor for some gastric diseases, especially ulcer and carcinoma.

HAA (hepatitis-associated antigen): a protein used to detect hepatitis A and/or B virus.

Ham's test: an acid serum test for paroxysmal nocturnal hemoglobinuria (PNH).

haptoglobin: a complex protein to which hemoglobin released from lysed red blood cells is bound. The serum haptoglobin test is used to detect intravascular destruction of red blood cells (hemolysis).

Hashimoto's thyroiditis: a form of autoimmune thyroiditis that results in inflammation of the thyroid gland and hypothyroidism.

HbA1c: a monitor of the rise and fall of blood sugar over a period of time. If the blood glucose level has been carefully controlled and regulated over a period of five to six weeks, the HbA1c level will be normal; if it is elevated, it is an indication that the blood glucose level has not been controlled and has also been elevated.

HBV: hepatitis B virus.

HCV: hepatitis C virus.

HDL (high-density lipoprotein): a lipoprotein produced mainly in the liver but also in the intestine; carries cholesterol to the sites where it is needed. Also called "good cholesterol."

heart failure: loss of pumping ability by the heart.

Heinz bodies: granular deposits in red blood cells that can be seen in premature infants, inherited hemolytic anemias, and drug sensitivities.

hematocrit (Hct): the percentage of total blood volume consisting of red blood cells, found by centrifuging the whole blood and measuring the volume of red cells in a given volume of blood.

hematologist: a physician specializing in the study of blood and in the diagnosis and treatment of disorders of the blood and blood-forming tissues, including bleeding disorders and blood diseases.

hematopoiesis: the production of blood cells.

hematuria: abnormal presence of blood in the urine.

heme: the iron-containing portion of the hemoglobin molecule.

hemodialysis: a method of removing waste products from the blood; used in the treatment of kidney failure patients.

heme synthesis: a process where iron accumulates in the mitochondria (the functional portion of the cell) waiting to be inserted into the heme ring of a red blood cell.

hemochromatosis: inherited metabolic disorder in which excessive iron may accumulate in the liver, pancreas, heart, brain, joints, and skin, resulting in liver disease, diabetes mellitus, heart attack, hormonal imbalances, depression, impotence, and a bronze or ashen gray-green skin color.

hemoglobin (Hgb): the red blood cell protein-iron compound responsible for transporting oxygen from the lungs to the cells, and carbon dioxide from the cells to the lungs.

Hemoglobin A: normal adult hemoglobin that contains a heme molecule, two alpha-globin molecules, and two beta-globin molecules.

hemoglobin electrophoresis: a test that identifies blood diseases such as sickle cell disease, hemoglobin C and H disease, and thalassemia, both major and minor forms.

Hemoglobin F: fetal hemoglobin present in babies.

Hemoglobin S: produced in association with the sickle cell trait; the beta-globin molecules of hemoglobin S are defective.

hemoglobinopathy: diseases associated with abnormal hemoglobin.

hemoglobinuria: the presence of hemoglobin in the urine. Causes can include burns, hemolysis, kidney disease including cancer, reaction to blood transfusion, diseases such as thrombotic thrombocytic purpura (TTP) or paroxysmal nocturnal hemoglobinuria (PNH), constant marching or foot pounding (exercise or marathon running). With hemoglobinuria the urine can be dark yellowish-rusty color. Normal urine is straw colored.

hemolysis: process by which red blood cells break down and hemoglobin is released.

hemolytic anemia: a disorder characterized by chronic premature destruction of red blood cells.

hemolytic episode: separation of hemoglobin from red blood cells.

hemophilia: a blood clotting disorder due to Factor VIII Deficiency.

Hemophilia A and B: X-linked recessive bleeding disorders caused by deficiency of either factor VIII (hemophilia A) or factor IX (hemophilia B).

hemoptysis: coughing up blood.

hemorrhage: a severe internal or external bleeding.

hemosiderosis: a condition marked by excessive iron in the tissues, especially in the liver and spleen, also called siderosis.

hemostasis: the arrest of bleeding.

heparin: an anticoagulant used in the prevention and treatment of blood clots and in the management of heart attacks.

hepatic disease: any disease involving the liver, including many types of hepatitis and cirrhosis.

hepatic dysfunction: poor liver function.

hepatitis: inflammatory liver condition.

hepatitis A: form of viral hepatitis caused by the hepatitis-A virus that is contracted through contaminated food or water, usually because of unsanitary conditions (improper hand washing after restroom use) or contaminated shellfish. A is usually mild, although it can be severe; the acute stage being about two weeks in duration. There is a hepatitis A vaccination.

hepatitis B: form of viral hepatitis caused by the hepatitis-B virus that can enter the body through blood transfusions contaminated with the virus or by the use of contaminated needles or instruments. Infection may be very severe and result in prolonged illness, cirrhosis or death. There is a hepatitis B vaccination. *See* cirrhosis.

hepatitis C: form of viral hepatitis caused by the hepatitis-C virus spread through blood or sexual contact; there is no vaccine.

hepatitis, acute viral: characterized by rapid onset of symptoms, loss of appetite, vomiting, fever, joint pain, and itchy skin with some forms of hepatitis, jaundice, flu-like symptoms, enlarged liver, loss of appetite, upper right quadrant abdominal pain, abnormal liver function, dark urine, and clay-colored stool. Acute hepatitis can occur in all forms of viral hepatitis infection but is most common in B and C.

hepatitis, chronic: inflammation of the liver lasting more than six months, can be due to hepatitis B or C, alcohol, drugs, medications, toxic chemicals, or autoimmune conditions.

hepatocellular injury: injury of liver cells.

hepatologist: *see* physicians, types of.

hepatomas: malignant tumor that begins in the liver (primary site of cancer), as opposed to liver cancer that has spread from another site.

hepatotoxicity: destructive effect on the liver usually caused by a medication or alcohol.

hereditary: inherited, transmitted genetically from generation to generation.

hereditary hemorrhagic telangiectasia (HHT): (also known as Osler-Weber-Rendu syndrome) an inherited bleeding disorder where abnormally dilated blood vessels (telangiectasias) rupture, causing significant blood loss.

HFE: first identified in 1996, the first hemochromatosis-associated gene, located on chromosome 6. Two mutations were reported Cys282Tyr (C282Y) and His63Asp (H63D). Of these the C282Y mutation is considered to be a major cause of iron loading.

histocompatibility antigens: *see* HLA.

histology: science dealing with the microscopic identification of cells and tissue.

HLA (human lymphocyte antigen): a "genetic fingerprint" existing on the surface of a specific type of white blood cell, this antigen is determined genetically and is therefore useful in paternity investigation and compatibility with tissue transplantation.

hormone: a chemical produced by a specific gland or tissue that is released into the bloodstream to a target organ.

human growth hormone (HGH): hormone needed for normal growth and sexual maturity from birth until the end of puberty; secreted by cells in the pituitary gland.

hyper-: a prefix meaning excessive, above, or beyond.

hyperglycemia: too much sugar in the blood, as in diabetes.

hyperinsulinemia: an excessive amount of insulin in the blood.

hyperplastic: involving an increased number of cells.

hypersplenism: a type of disorder that causes the spleen to rapidly and prematurely destroy blood cells.

hypertension: high blood pressure.

hyperthyroidism: overactivity of the thyroid.

hyperviscosity: blood that is too thick.

hypo: a prefix meaning deficient, beneath, or under.

hypochromasia: decrease in hemoglobin concentration per red cell. Morphologically, this is reflected by

436

increased size of the central pallor of the RBC when observed on a peripheral blood smear.

hypochromic: refers to a red blood cell with a decreased concentration of hemoglobin.

hypoglycemia: a condition of low blood sugar.

hypogonadism: gonads with deficient secretion and that are small in size.

hypokalemia: a condition of low level of potassium.

hypopituitarism: a condition resulting from diminished secretion of pituitary hormone; *see* human growth hormone.

hypoplastic: involving a decreased number of blood cells.

hypothalamus: a centrally located structure in the brain that regulates the pituitary gland.

hypothyroidism: underactive thyroid gland, which results in decreased metabolic rate.

hypoxia: an oxygen deficiency.

idiopathic: refers to a disease or condition of unknown cause.

Idiopathic thrombocytopenic purpura (ITP or ITTP): a bleeding disorder caused by an abnormally low level of platelets in the patient's blood. An autoimmune disorder characterized by the production of anti-platelet antibodies.

IG: or immunoglobulins, IgG, IgA, IgM are tests that measure immune status. Examples:
IgA: increases in chronic nonalcoholic disease, primary biliary cirrhosis.
IgG: increases in infections of all types, liver disease, myeloma, and rheumatoid arthritis.

IgM: increases in malaria, infectious mononucleosis, and rheumatoid arthritis.

immune system: body system responsible for producing various cells and chemicals that fight infection by viruses, bacteria, fungi, and other foreign invaders.

immunocompromised: state in which the immune system is weakened or is not functioning properly due to chronic disease.

immunologic therapy: the treatment of disease using medicines that boost the body's natural immune response.

immunosuppressed: state in which the immune system is suppressed by medications during the treatment of other disorders, like cancer, or following an organ transplantation.

infarction: an infarct or area of tissue that undergoes necrosis (cell death) as a result of loss of blood supply due to an occlusion (blockage) or stenosis (narrowing or constriction of blood vessels).

infection: presence and growth of a microorganism that produces tissue damage.

inflammation/inflammatory: a nonspecific immune response that occurs in reaction to any type of bodily injury.

inflammatory bowel disease: a group of disorders that cause the intestines to become inflamed (red and swollen).

insulin: a hormone secreted by the beta cells of the islets of Langerhans of the pancreas that regulates blood glucose levels; works with glucagon to regulate glucose levels in the blood and supply fuel to the body's cells for the production of energy.

internist: *see* physicians, types of.

interstitial: occupies space between tissues, such as interstitial fluid.

intestines: also known as the bowels, they are divided into the large and small intestines.

intravenously (IV): administered through a vein.

intrinsic factor: a hormone produced in the stomach; essential for the absorption of vitamin B_{12}.

iron: an essential micronutrient.

iron chelation therapy: the removal of iron from the tissues using a drug such as Desferal®, which is formulated to specifically bind with iron.

iron-deficiency anemia: a type of anemia due to blood loss, insufficient iron in the diet, or when demands for iron exceed stores, such as during a growth spurt.

iron overload: a potentially fatal condition where iron accumulates in tissues of the body, seen with some hemolytic anemias, hemochromatosis, and a common side effect of numerous blood transfusions.

iron panel: series of tests that measure levels of iron actively in the body such as amount of circulating (functional), stored, or bound to proteins and in transport such as serum iron, transferrin, total iron binding capacity (TIBC), transferrin-iron saturation percentage, serum ferritin, unbound or unsaturated iron-binding-capacity (UIBC), hemoglobin, and hematocrit.

ischemia: decreased blood supply to a body organ or part.

IV: intravenous.

jaundice: condition of yellow skin, yellow whites of the eyes, dark urine, and light-colored stools. It is a symptom of diseases of the liver and blood caused by abnormally elevated amounts of bilirubin in the blood.

juvenile: youths generally aged three to ten, or between weaned from the breast and puberty.

koilonychia: (also known as spoon nails) a malformation of the nails in which the outer surface is concave;

often associated with iron deficiency or softening by occupational contact with oils.

Kupffer cell: a type of macrophage found in the liver and a part of the reticuloendothelial system (RES).

lactoferrin: a protein found in human secretions such as tears, seminal and vaginal fluids, saliva, and mother's milk that binds with iron to withhold the iron from harmful germs.

lamina: a thin flat layer or membrane.

LDL: low density lipoprotein, *see* cholesterol.

leukemia, myeloblastic: malignancy of blood cells in which the predominant cells are myeloblasts (early stage of white blood cell).

leukocyte: white blood cells, important in defending against infection and clearing the body of harmful material, of which there are several types: granulocytes, monocytes, and lymphocytes.

libido: sexual drive or urge.

lipase: a fat-splitting enzyme found in the blood, pancreatic secretion, and tissues.

liver biopsy: procedure where a tiny sample of the liver is removed using a needle inserted into the liver so that a tissue sample can be examined for liver damage or malignancy (liver cancer).

liver function tests: include: alanine aminotransferase (ALT), also known as serum glutamic pyruvic transminase (SGPT); aspartate aminotransferase (AST), also known as serum glutamic-oxaloacetic transaminase (SGOT); gamma-glutamine transferase (GGT); and alkaline phosphatase (ALP).

lymph: a clear, transparent filtrate of plasma that is collected from tissues throughout the body and eventually flows to the lymphatic system.

lymphatic system: an important aspect of the body's immune system, consisting of vessels that carry lymph fluid from tissues throughout the body through the lymph nodes to the venous blood circulation.

lymphocyte: one of three types of white blood cells (the others being granulocytes and monocytes), and the primary cell of the immune response, responsible for attacking antigens; divided into two forms, B-cells and T-cells.

lymphoma: cancer of the lymph glands.

macro-: combining form meaning large or long.

macrocytic: descriptive term applied to a larger than normal red blood cell.

macrocytosis: a condition where cells are abnormally large.

macrophage: a monocyte (a type of white blood cell) that has left the bloodstream and settled in a tissue. Macrophages are found in large quantities in the spleen, lymph nodes, alveoli, and tonsils and are one of the major cells of the immune system. About 50 percent of all macrophages are found in the liver as Kupffer cells.

magnetic resonance imaging (MRI): a diagnostic procedure where a large magnet surrounds a person; radio frequencies interact with the magnet, providing information to the computer.

malabsorption: inadequate absorption of nutrients from the intestinal tract, especially the duodenal portion of the small intestine.

malaise: vague feeling of body discomfort generally prior to onset of illness.

malignant: capable of causing destruction of normal tissue; may lead to death. Usually refers to cancer growth.

maternal: pertaining to, or inherited from, the mother.

MDS: myelodysplastic syndromes.

mean corpuscular hemoglobin (MCH): is the measure of the amount or weight of hemoglobin within a red blood cell.

mean corpuscular hemoglobin concentration (MCHC): the measure of the average concentration or percentage of hemoglobin with a single red blood cell.

mean corpuscular volume (MCV): the measure of the average volume or size of a single red blood cell.

megakaryocyte: multinucleated cell in the bone marrow that gives rise to platelets.

megaloblast: an abnormally large immature erythrocyte that develops in the large numbers in the bone marrow; a large abnormal red blood corpuscle found in the blood in cases of certain anemias (megaloblastic).

megaloblastic anemia: a type of anemia where red blood cells are larger than normal, usually resulting from a deficiency of folic acid or vitamin B_{12}.

melanoma: any of a group of malignant tumors, primarily of the skin. The most severe form of skin cancer.

menorrhagia: excessive or prolonged menstrual bleeding. It is defined as blood loss exceeding 80 milliliters per cycle.

metabolism: combined chemical and physical processes that take place in the body. Involves distribution of nutrients, growth, energy production, elimination of wastes, and other body functions. There are two phases of metabolism: *anabolism,* the constructive phase formation of tissues and organs, and *catabolism,* the breaking down phase during which molecules are broken down.

metastasis: process by which cancerous cells or infectious germs spread from their original location to other parts of the body.

MI: myocardial infarction (heart attack).

micro-: denotes small size or extent.

microbes: microorganism (small, living organism) many are capable of producing disease.

microcytic: red blood cells that are abnormally small.

microcytosis: blood disorder characterized by abnormally small (microcytic) red blood cells often associated with iron deficiency anemia, lead poisoning, or thalassemia.

mitochondria: self-replicating portion of the cell where metabolic and respiratory functions provide a cell's energy source.

mitral valve: valve located in the heart between the left atrium and left ventricle.

mitral valve prolapse: condition in which the mitral valve becomes floppy, resulting in mitral regurgitation.

monocyte: one of three types of white blood cells (the others being granulocytes and lymphocytes), normally constituting 3 to 7 percent of the blood.

morphism: in blood production, morphism has to do with the structure and formation of a blood cell.

MPV (mean platelet volume): measures the average volume (size) of platelets.

multiple myeloma (primary bone marrow cancer): malignancy beginning in the plasma cells of the bone marrow. Plasma cells normally produce antibodies to help destroy germs and protect against infection. With myeloma, this function becomes impaired, and the body cannot deal effectively with infection.

myeloid: pertaining to, derived from, or resembling bone marrow.

myelodysplastic syndrome: a condition of abnormalities in the bone marrow characterized by a defect in the development of one of the marrow cell lines, limiting the release of functioning cells.

myelofibrosis: a disorder in which bone marrow is replaced by fibrous tissue.

myoglobin: iron containing pigment that provides the red color in muscles; it also contains oxygen needed by the muscles for proper function.

neoplasm/neoplastic: a new and abnormal formation of tissue, as a tumor or growth. It serves no useful function, but grows at the expense of the healthy organism.

nephrosis: conditions in which there are degenerative changes in the kidneys or kidney disease.

neurological: pertaining to the nervous system.

neutropenia: low neutrophil (poly) count; a deficiency of neutrophils in the blood.

neutrophil: the most numerous of the white blood cells, important for helping the body fight infections.

normo-: denotes normal or usual.

normochromic: refers to a red blood cell with a normal concentration of hemoglobin.

normocytic: refers to a red blood cell of normal size.

obstruction: a blockage.

orthopedist: *see* physicians, types of.

osmotic fragility: a test to detect abnormal fragility of red blood cells.

osteoporosis: a general term describing any disease process that results in reduction in bone mass.

ovaries: female reproductive organs (gonads) that release eggs and female sex hormones.

packed cells: red blood cells that have been separated from the plasma and used for conditions that require red blood cells but not the liquid components of whole blood.

pancreas: an exocrine and endocrine organ. The exocrine portion secretes digestive enzymes into the duodenum; the endocrine portion secretes insulin, which regulates blood sugar; glucagon, which stimulates the liver to convert glycogen to glucose; and somatostatin, which inhibits the release of insulin, glucagon, growth hormone, and gastrin so that levels of these hormones do not exceed normal (negative feedback system).

pancreatitis: inflammation of the pancreas.

pancytopenia: low number of blood cells; a deficiency of all types of blood cells.

parathyroids: four glands located on the corners of the thyroid gland that release parathyroid hormone and calcitonin, which affects fluid balance and the levels of calcium in the blood.

paroxysmal nocturnal hemoglobinuria (PNH): a rare, acquired bleeding disorder where the hemolysis is intermittent, occurring during sleep.

paternal: pertaining to, or inherited from, the father.

PAVM: pulmonary arteriovenous malformations. These are large lung telangiectasias seen in some HHT patients.

pediatric: concerning the treatment of children.

pericarditis: an inflammation of the two layers of the thin, sac-like membrane that surrounds the heart.

percutaneous: effected through the skin, such as a medication applied by rubbing, or to inject a fluid through the skin with a needle.

peripheral blood smear test: a blood test; the examination of the edge, sometimes called the "feather edge" of a blood sample where most of the red cells are almost, but not quite, touching.

pernicious anemia: chronic anemia that occurs as a result of B_{12} deficiency due to the lack of intrinsic factor, a substance secreted by the mucous membranes of the stomach that is essential for absorption of B_{12}.

petechiae: tiny red dots on the skin due to bleeding under the skin.

phagocytize: to engulf and destroy microorganisms or cells, a function performed by certain white blood cells.

phlebotomy: therapeutic withdrawal of blood from the vein.

phosphates: form of inorganic phosphorus found in the body.

physicians, types of:
anesthesiologist: specialist in administering an anesthetic agent, usually for surgical procedures.

cardiologist: specialist in care of disorders of the heart.

emergency care physician: those treating conditions requiring immediate care.

endocrinologist: specialist in care and treatment of all types of disorders of the ductless glands.

family practitioner: one who cares for the entire range of diseases affecting persons of all ages and sexes and not limited to a particular organ system or disease; a general practitioner.

gastroenterologist: a physician whose practice covers disorders of the stomach, intestines, and related structures such as the esophagus, liver, gall bladder, and pancreas.

hematologist: specialist in the study of blood and in the diagnosis and treatment of disorders of the blood and blood-forming tissues, including bleeding disorders and blood diseases.

hepatologist: specialist in diseases of the liver.

internist: specialist in the treatment of diseases of the internal organs by other than surgical means.

nephrologist: one who is concerned with the structure and function of the kidneys.

neurologist: specialist in diseases of the nervous system and the brain.

ob-gyn: specialist in pregnancy, childbirth, and gynecology (female reproductive system).

oncologist: specialist in cancer; often hematologists are oncologists.

orthopedist: specialist in prevention and correction of musculoskeletal disorders.

pathologist: specialist in analyzing tissue for disease.

pediatrician: physician treating children and children's diseases.

psychiatrist: specialist in the study, treatment, and prevention of mental disorders.

pulmonologist: a physician whose practice is concerned or involved with the lungs.

radiologist: a physician trained in the diagnostic and/or therapeutic use of X rays, CT scans, MRIs, and ultrasounds.

rheumatologist: specialist in rheumatic diseases of the joints.

surgeon: specialist who does surgery; general or specific, such as head-neck surgeon, cancer surgeon, heart surgeon, etc.

urologist: a physician whose practice is concerned with disorders of the urinary tract.

phytates: compounds found in whole grains.

pica: an appetite or craving for substances not fit as food or of no nutritional value, such as clay, dried paint, ice, hair, coins, dirt, paper, starch.

plasma: the liquid part of the blood and of the lymph; the fluid (non-cellular) portion of the circulating blood.

platelet: non-nucleated cells essential for blood clotting.

platelet adhesion: the process by which platelets adhere to the basement membrane at sites of vascular injury. Von Willebrand factor functions as the glue that sticks the platelet to the basement membrane collagen. Platelet adhesion is defective in von Willebrand disease.

platelet aggregation: the process by which platelets stick to each other at the site of vascular injury, forming a platelet plug. Platelet aggregation is abnormal with the use of certain drugs (e.g., aspirin, ibuprofen), and in disseminated intravascular coagulation and renal failure.

platelet count: an actual count of the number of platelets (thrombocytes) in a given volume of blood.

poikilocytosis: variation in red blood cell shape.

polycythemia vera: (also called myeloproliferative disorder) abnormal increased production of red blood cells and hemoglobin concentration.

polydipsia: excessive thirst.

polyp: an abnormal growth that develops on the inside of a hollow organ such as the colon, stomach, or nose.

polyuria: excessive production of urine.

porphyria: excretion of porphyrins into the urine.

porphyrins: any number of pigments widely distributed in hemoglobin, myoglobin, and cytochromes.

posthemorrhagic anemia: loss of red blood cells due to massive or prolonged bleeding.

progesterone: a female hormone involved in the menstrual cycle.

prolactin: a hormone that stimulates milk production in women who are breast-feeding.

proliferation: growth by reproduction of similar cells.

protein: one of a class or kind of complex compound synthesized by all living things, which provide the amino acids essential for growth and repair of tissue.

prothrombin: test to measure the activity of factor II (one of the substances used for coagulation) in the blood. Typically it is prolonged in liver disease, vitamin K deficiency, disseminated intravascular coagulation, and coumarin therapy.

pruritus: itching.

PSA (prostate-specific antigen): an antigen found in all males, greatly increased in cases of prostate cancer.

pulmonary: concerning or involving the lungs.

pulmonologist: *see* physicians, types of.

pulse oximeter: a clip placed on the tip of the ear, finger, or toe and connected to a machine that measures the oxygen in the blood.

pure red cell aplasia: a condition in which there is a near absence of red blood cell precursors in bone marrow.

pyelonephritis: infection of the kidney.

pyridoxine: vitamin B_6.

pyruvate kinase deficiency (PK): an inherited hemolytic anemia due to a deficiency of the enzyme pyruvate kinase (PK).

q-wave: the downward or negative wave of an electrocardiogram (EKG) that follows the p-wave. Abnormal or elogated q-wave is an indication of problems with the conduction system of the heart.

radiation therapy: treatment using high-energy radiation from X ray machines, cobalt, radium, or other sources.

RBC: red blood cell.

RDW (red blood cell distribution width): an indication of the variation in red blood cell size.

recessive trait: an inherited trait that is outwardly obvious only when two copies of the gene for that trait are present, as opposed to a dominant trait where one copy of the gene for the dominant trait is sufficient to display the trait.

red cell indices: aids in the classification of anemias. Indices include mean corpuscular volume (MCV), mean corpuscular hemoglobin (MCH), and mean corpuscular hemoglobin concentration (MCHC). MCV expresses the average size of many cells and indicates whether most red blood cells are undersized (microcytic), oversized (macrocytic), or normal sized (normocytic). MCH is the hemoglobin-to-red-blood-cell ratio and gives the weight (concentration) of hemoglobin in an average red blood cell. MCHC defines the volume of hemoglobin in an average red cell and helps distinguish normally colored (normochromic) red blood cells from pale (hypochromic) red cells.

renal: pertaining to the kidneys.

restless legs syndrome: uncontrollable jumpiness or twitching in the legs.

reticulocyte count: the number of reticulocytes, usually expressed as the percentage of red blood cells.

reticulocytes: young, immature red blood cells. The normal reticulocyte count in the peripheral blood is 1 percent. The reticulocyte count is a measure of effective erythropoiesis.

reticulocytosis: excess amount of reticulocytes in the blood.

reticuloendothelial system (RES): the system of the body that includes the function of defense against infection and disposal of the products resulting from the breakdown of cells. The RES includes the macrophages, Kupffer cells of the liver, the bone marrow, spleen, and lymph system.

rheumatologist: *see* physicians, types of.

ringed sideroblast: an immature red blood cell that has a ring of iron surrounding the nucleus.

rouleaux: red blood cells appear stuck together like stacks of coins when observed on a peripheral smear.

schistocyte: fragmented red blood cell, which may be irregular in shape with pointed ends.

sex chromosomes: the pair of chromosomes responsible for sex determination. In humans and most animals, the sex chromosomes are designated X and Y; females have two X chromosomes, males have one X and one Y chromosome.

SGOT (serum glutamic-oxalo-acetic transaminase): a test used in cases of suspected coronary occlusive heart diseases or liver diseases such as hepatitis or cirrhosis.

SGPT (serum glutamic-pyruvic transaminase): an enzyme released into the bloodstream by injury or disease affecting the liver.

short bowel syndrome (small intestine insufficiency): a condition of malabsorption related to the surgical removal or disease of a large portion of the small intestine.

sickle cell disease: an inherited condition of anemia characterized by red blood cells that are sickle shaped.

sideroblasts: young red blood cells that contain excess iron.

sigmoid colon: the final portion of the large intestine, which empties into the rectum.

Sjogren's or Sjögren's syndrome: an autoimmune disorder characterized by dryness of the eyes and mouth and recurrent salivary gland enlargement.

sleep apnea: the stopping of breathing during sleep for a duration of at least ten seconds.

spherocytosis: a hereditary disorder where the red blood cells (RBCs) are spherically shaped and lack the light centers seen in normal, round RBCs.

splenomegaly: an enlargement of the spleen beyond its normal size.

steatohepatitis: fatty and inflamed liver.

steatorrhea: passage of fat in large amounts in the feces due to failure to digest and absorb it; occurs in pancreatic disease and the malabsorption syndromes; an absence of bile acids will increase steatorrhea.

stem cell: also called pluripotent because these cells have the potential to develop into any type of blood cell.

stool occult blood: a measure of the presence of more than minimal amounts of blood in a stool sample; may indicate abnormalities in the gastrointestinal tract.

subcutaneous: beneath the skin.

sugar-water hemolysis test: a test to detect increased fragility of red blood cells by swelling in low ionic (low salt) solution. Also known as sucrose hemolysis test.

synovial: pertaining to the synovia, the lubricating fluid of the joints.

synovium: synovial membrane.

synthesis: a building up, putting together, or composition.

systemic lupus erythematosus (SLE): a chronic, inflammatory autoimmune disorder that may affect many organ systems including the skin, joints, and internal organs.

T3: triiodothyronine, one of two forms of thyroid hormone.

T4: thyroxine, one of the principal hormones secreted by the thyroid gland.

T-lymphocyte: a lymphocyte that is important in the immune response, but which in aplastic anemia suppresses the stem cells; also known as a T-cell lymphocyte.

tachycardia: rapid heartbeat.

target cell: abnormal red blood cell that has an excess amount of membrane resulting in hemoglobin accumulation in the center of the cell. Target cells have an area of staining in the center of the cell and look like a bull's eye.

teardrop RBC: abnormal red blood cell that is shaped like a teardrop.

telangiectasia: abnormal blood vessels, seen in disorders such as HHT, which may bleed easily.

testes: male reproductive glands (gonads) in the scrotum that produce sperm and the hormone testosterone.

testosterone: a hormone, produced primarily in the testes, that stimulates the development of secondary sexual characteristics and supports the production of sperm in males; principal male hormone.

thalassemia: name for a complex of hereditary anemias that occur in populations bordering the Mediterranean and in Southeast Asia.

therapeutic: a healing agent or results obtained from treatment.

thiamine: one of the B vitamins, a group of water-soluble vitamins that participate in many of the chemical reactions in the body.

thrombocyte: platelet.

thrombocytopenia: a deficiency in the number of platelets.

thrombosis: abnormal blood clots.

thyroid gland: large endocrine gland located in the throat area, which produces a hormone that helps to regulate metabolism.

thyroiditis: inflammation of the thyroid gland.

thyroxine: a hormone produced by the thyroid gland.

total iron binding capacity (TIBC): a measurement of all proteins available for binding free iron in the body; an indirect but accurate measure of transferrin, *see* transferrin.

transferrin: protein that transports iron from the intestine into the blood.

TRH (thyrotropin-releasing factor): substance secreted by the hypothalamus that controls the release of thyroid-stimulating hormone (TSH) from the anterior pituitary gland.

triglycerides (TGs): a form of fat in the bloodstream, produced in the liver.

triiodothyronine (T3): a hormone produced by the thyroid gland.

TSH (thyroid-stimulating hormone): substance secreted by the anterior pituitary gland that controls the release of thyroid hormone from the thyroid gland.

tumor: a spontaneous new growth of tissue that forms an abnormal mass and that does not follow normal laws of growth; may be malignant or non-malignant.

tumor marker: a substance in blood serum whose presence may indicate a possible malignancy.

ulcer/ulceration: an open sore on the skin or on a mucous membrane.

ultrasound: the use of very high frequency sound waves to produce an image or photograph of an organ or tissue.

unbound or unsaturated iron-binding capacity (UIBC): the difference between the TIBC and the serum iron.

urea: a substance formed in the liver and found in blood, lymph, and urine; the end product of protein metabolism in the body.

urologist: *see* physicians, types of.

vascular: pertaining to blood vessels.

ventricles: the two lower chambers of the heart. The left ventricle is the main pumping chamber in the heart.

ventricular fibrillation: rapid, irregular quivering of the heart's ventricles, with no effective heartbeat.

vibrio: a member of a genus of gram-negative bacilli that can be found in raw shellfish or contaminated water; these can be deadly to someone with high iron levels.

villi: tiny, finger-like projections that enable the small intestine to absorb nutrients from food.

viral: caused by a virus.

vitiligo: a skin condition in which there is loss of pigment from areas of skin, resulting in irregular white patches with normal skin texture.

von Willebrand factor (vWF): a glue-like blood protein that helps platelets stick to each other and to the blood vessel wall at the site of injury and stabilizes factor VIII and transports it through the bloodstream.

WBC: white blood cells.

Wilson's disease: inherited disorder of copper metabolism in which copper accumulates in the liver, red blood cells, and brain, leading to anemia, tremors, liver dysfunction, and dementia.

X chromosome: one of the two types of sex chromosomes, present twice in female cells and once in male cells.

X ray: a name for a machine using the energy of electromagnetic waves to visualize hard tissues such as bone, or a treatment with such a machine.

Y chromosome: one of the two types of sex chromosomes; males have one X and one Y chromosome.

zinc: a metallic element and an essential element in the diet of all animals, including humans. Lack of zinc in the diet can cause to slow down growth or healing of wounds among other things, and during pregnancy may cause developmental disorders in the child.

Bibliography

Allen, L. H. "Pregnancy and Iron Deficiency: Unresolved Issues." *Nutrition Reviews* 55 (1997): 99–101.

Al-Rimawa, H. S., M. F. Jallard, Z. O. Amarin, and B. R. Obeidat. "Hypothalamic-Pituitary-Gonadal Function in Adolescent Females with Beta-Thalassemia Major." *International Journal of Gynecology & Obstetrics* 90 (2005): 44–47.

American Academy of Pediatrics Work Group on Breast-feeding. "Breast-feeding and the Use of Human Milk." *Pediatrics* 100 (1997): 1035–39.

Anderson, G. H., N. L. Catherine, D. M. Woodend, and T. M. Wolever. "Inverse Association between the Effect of Carbohydrates on Blood Glucose and Subsequent Short-Term Food Intake in Young Men." *American Journal of Clinical Nutrition* 76 (2002): 1023–30.

Angulo-Kinzler, R. M., P. Peirano, E. Lin, M. Garrido, and B. Lozoff. "Motor Activity in Human Infants with Iron-Deficiency Anemia." *Early Human Development* 66 (2002): 67–79.

Annibale, B., G. Capurso, and G. Delle Fave. "Consequences of Helicobacter Pylori Infection on the Absorption of Micronutrients." *Digestive and Liver Disease* 2 (2002): S72–77.

Arthur, C. K., and Isbister, J. P. "Iron Deficiency: Misunderstood, Misdiagnosed and Mistreated." *Drugs* 33 (1987): 171–82.

Au, W. Y., W. M. Lam, W. C. Chu, S. Tam, W. K. Wong, D. J. Pennell, A. K. Lie, and R. Liang. "A Magnetic Resonance Imaging Study of Iron Overload in Hemopoietic Stem Cell Transplant Recipients with Increased Ferritin Levels." Unbound Medline/Transplant Proc journal articles 39 (2007): 3369–74.

Aul, C., D. T. Bowen, and Y. Yoshida. "Pathogenesis, Etiology and Epidemiology of Myelodysplastic Syndromes." *Haematologica* 83 (1998): 71–86.

Ayas, M., A. Al-Jefr, M. M. Mustafa, M. Al-Mahr, L. Shalaby, and H. Solh. "Congenital Sideroblastic Anaemia Successfully Treated Using Allogeneic Stem Cell Transplantation." *British Journal of Haematology* 113 (2001): 938–39.

Ballew, C., S. Kuester, and C. Gillespie. "Beverage Choices Affect Adequacy of Children's Nutrient Intakes." *Archives of Pediatrics and Adolescent Medicine* 154 (2000): 1148–52.

Barisani, D., S. Ceroni, S. Del Bianco, R. Meneveri, and M. T. Bardella. "Hemochromatosis Gene Mutations and Iron Metabolism in Celiac Disease." *Haematologica* 89 (2004): 1299–1305.

Beard, J. L. "Iron Biology in Immune Function, Muscle Metabolism and Neuronal Functioning." *Journal of Nutrition* 72 (2001): S568–79.

Beard, J., and B. Tobin. "Iron Status and Exercise." *American Journal of Clinical Nutrition* 72 (2001): S594–97.

Bendich, A. "Calcium Supplementation and Iron Status of Females." *Nutrition* 17 (2001): 46–51.

Beutler, E., and T. Gelbart. "Estimating the Prevalence of Puruvate Kinase Deficiency from the Gene Frequency in the General White Population." *Blood* 11 (2000): 3585–88.

Bjork, J., M. Albin, N. Mauritzson, U. Stromberg, B. Johansson, and L. Hagmar. "Smoking and Melodysplastic Syndromes." *Zeitschrift fur Emahrungswissenschaft* 29 (1990): 54–73.

Bodnar, L. M., K. S. Scanlon, M. E. Cogswell, D. S. Freedman, and A. M. Siega-Riz. "High Prevalence of Postpartum Anemia Among Low-Income Women in the United States." *American Journal of Obstetrics and Gynecology* 185 (2001): 438–43.

Boelaert, J. R., M. Locht, J. Van Cutsem, V. Kerrels, B. Cantineaux, A. Verdonck, N. W. Landuyt, and Y. J. Schneider. "Mucomycosis during Deferoxamine Therapy Is a Siderophore-Mediated Infection in In Vitro and In Vivo Animal Studies." *Journal of Clinical Investigation* 91 (1993): 1979–86.

Boelaert, J. R., J. Van Cutsem, M. de Locht, Y. J. Schneider, and R. R. Critchton. "Deferoxamine Augments Growth and Pathogenicity of Rhizopus, while Hydroxypyridinone Chelators Have No Effect." *Kidney International* 45 (1994): 667–71.

Borel, M. J., S. M. Smith, J. Derr, and J. L. Beard. "Day-to-Day Variations in Iron-Status Indices in Healthy Men and Women." *American Journal of Clinical Nutrition* 54 (1999): 729–35.

Bothwell, T. H. "Overview and Mechanisms of Iron Regulation." *Nutrition Reviews* 53 (1995): 237–45.

Bothwell, T. H., R. D. Baynes, B. J. MacFarlane, and A. P. MacPhail. "Nutritional Iron Requirements and Food Iron Absorption." *Journal of Internal Medicine* 226 (1989): 357–65.

Bottomly, S. S. "Secondary Iron Overload Disorders." *Seminars in Hematology* 35 (1998): 77–86.

————. "Sideroblastic Anemias." *Wintrobe's Clinical Hematology*, 10th ed. (1998): 1022–45.

Bravo, L. "Polyphenols: Chemistry, Dietary Sources, Metabolism, and Nutritional Significance." *Nutrition Reviews* 56 (1998): 317–33.

Bridges, K. R. "Sideroblastic Anemia: A Mitochondrial Disorder." *Journal of Pediatric Hematology/Oncology* 19 (1997): 274–78.

Brigham, D., and J. Beard. "Iron and Thermoregulation: A Review." *Critical Reviews in Food Science and Nutrition* 35 (1996): 747–63.

Brill, J. R., and D. J. Baumgardner. "Normocytic Anemia." *American Family Physician* 62 (2000): 2255–64.

Brown, N. W. "Medical Consequences of Eating Disorders." *Southern Medical Journal* 78 (1985): 403–5.

Brugnara, C., B. Schiller, and J. Moran. "Reticulocyte Hemoglobin Equivalent (Ret He) and Assessment of Iron-Deficient States." *Clinical & Laboratory Haematology* 28 (2006): 303–8.

Bunevicius, R., N. R. Jakubonien, J. Jurkevicius, J. Cernicat, L. Lasas, and A. J. Prange Jr. "Thyroxine vs. Thyroxine Plus Triodothyronine in Treatment of Hypothyroidism after Thyroidectomy for Graves' Disease." *Endocrine* 18 (2002): 129–33.

Burke, M. D. "Liver Function: Test Selection and Interpretation of Results." *Clinical Laboratory Medicine* 22 (2002): 377–90.

Burns, R. W., and T. W. Burns. "Pancytopenia Due to Vitamin B_{12} Deficiency Associated with Grave's Disease." *Missouri Medicine* 93 (1996): 368–72.

Butterworth, J. R., B. T. Cooper, W. M. Rosenberg, M. Purkiss, S. Jobson, M. Hathaway, D. Briggs, W. M. Howell, G. M. Wood, D. H. Adams, and T. H. Iqbal. "The Role of Hemochromatosis Susceptibility Gene Mutations in Protecting against Iron Deficiency in Celiac Disease." *Gastroenterology* 123 (2002): 444–49.

Centanni, M., M. Marignani, L. Gargano, V. Corleto, A. Casini, G. Delle Fave, and B. Annaballe. "Atrophic Body Gastritis in Patients with Autoimmune Thyroid Disease: An Underdiagnosed Association." *Archives of Internal Medicine* 160 (2000): 1573–75.

Centers for Disease Control and Prevention. "Centers for Disease Control and Prevention Criteria for Anemia in Children and Childbearing-aged Women." *Morbidity and Mortality Weekly Report* 38 (1989): 400–404.

Chanty, C. J., C. R. Howard, and P. Auinger. "Full Breast-feeding Duration and Risk for Iron Deficiency in U. S. Infants." *Breast-feeding Medicine* 2 (2007): 63–73.

Chaparro, C. M., R. Fornes, L. M. Neufeld, G. Tena Alavez, R. Eguia-Liz Cedillo, and K. G. Dewey. "Early Umbilical Cord Clamping Contributes to Elevated Blood Lead Levels Among Infants with Higher Lead Exposure." *The Journal of Pediatrics* 151 (2007): 506–12.

Cheson, B. D. "Standard and Low-Dose Chemotherapy for the Treatment of Myelodysplastic Syndromes." *Leukemia Research* 22 (1998): S17–21.

Christian, P., and K. P. West. "Interactions between Zinc and Vitamin A: An Update." *American Journal of Clinical Nutrition* 68 (1998): S435–41.

Cook, J. D., and C. A. Finch. "Assessing Iron Status of a Population." *American Journal of Clinical Nutrition* 32 (1979): 2115–19.

Cook, J. D., and E. R. Monsen. "Comparison of the Effect of Animal Proteins on Nonheme Iron Absorption." *American Journal of Clinical Nutrition* 29 (1976): 859–67.

Cook, J. D., and M. B. Reddy. "Ascorbic Acid Has a Pronounced Enhancing Effect on the Absorption of Dietary Nonheme Iron When Assessed by Feeding Single Meals to Fasting Subjects." *American Journal of Clinical Nutrition* 73 (2001): 93–98.

Cook, J. D., B. S. Skikne, S. R. Lynch, and M. E. Reusser. "Estimates of Iron Deficiency: The Global Perspective." *Advances in Experimental Medicine and Biology* 356 (1994): 219–28.

———. "Estimates of Iron Sufficiency in the U.S. Population." *Blood* 68 (1986): 726–31.

Cooper, M. J., and S. H. Ziotkin. "Day-to-Day Variation of Transferrin Receptors and Ferritin in Healthy Men and Women." *American Journal of Clinical Nutrition* 64 (1996): 738–42.

Cotter, P. D., A. May, L. Li, A. I. Al-Sabah, E. J. Fitzsimons, M. Caxzzola, and D. F. Bishop. "Four New Mutations in the Erythroid-Specific 5-Aminolevulinate Synthase (ALAS2) Gene Causing X-Linked Sideroblastic Anemia: Increased Pyridoxine Responsiveness After Removal of Iron Overload by Phlebotomy and Coinheritance of Hereditary Hemochromatosis." *Blood* 5 (1999): 1757–69.

Craddock, C. "Nonmyeloablative Stem Cell Transplants." *Current Opinion in Hematology* 6 (1999): 383–87.

Dallman, P. R., M. A. Simes, and A. Stekel. "Iron Deficiency in Infancy and Childhood." *American Journal of Clinical Nutrition* 33 (1980): 86–118.

Dallman, P. R., R. Yip, and C. Johnson. "Prevalence and Causes of Anemia in the United States, 1976 to 1880." *American Journal of Clinical Nutrition* 39 (1984): 437–45.

Damianaki, A., E. Bakogeorgou, M. Kampa, A. Hartzoglou, S. Panagiotou, C. Gemetzi, E. Kouromalis, P. M. Martin, and E. Castanas. *Journal of Cellular Biochemistry* 78 (2000): 429–41.

Davidsson, L. T., Walcyk, N. Zavaleta, and R. F. Hurrell. "Improving Iron Absorption from a Peruvian School Breakfast Meal by Adding Ascorbic Acid or Na (2)EDTA." *American Journal of Clinical Nutrition* 73 (2001): 283–87.

Dawe, S. A., T. J. Peters, A. DuVivier, and J. D. Creamer. "Congenital Erythropoietic Porphyria: Dilemmas in Present Day Management." *Clinical and Experimental Dermatology* 27 (2002): 680–83.

De Laere, E., A. Louwagie, and A. Creil. "Congenital Dyserythropoietic Anemia Type II: A Case Study." *Acta Clinica Belgica* 57 (2002): 85–89.

De Vries, C., M. Wieringa-de Ward, C. L. Vervoort, W. M. Ankum, and P. J. Bindels. "Abnormal Vaginal Bleeding in Women of Reproductive Age: A Descriptive Study of Initial Management in General Practice." *BioMed Central Women's Health Ltd.* 8 (2008).

Dorronsoro de Cattoni, S. T., L. S. Cornejo, S. Lopez de Blanc, S. Calamari, F. Femopasse, A. I. Azcurra, and L. J. Battelino. "Abstract: Evaluation of Serum and Saliva Components in Candiasis Patients." *Acta Odontol Latinoamericano* 10 (1997): 133–48.

Dubsky, P., P. Sevelda, R. Jakesz, H. Haumaninger, H. Samonigg, M. Seifert, U. Denison, et al. (Austrian Breast and Colorectal Cancer Study Group, Collaborators). "Anemia Is a Significant Prognostic Factor in Local Relapse-free Survival of Premenopausal Primary Breast Cancer Patients Receiving Adjuvant Cyclophosphamide/Methotrexate/5-Fluorouracil Chemotherapy." *Clinical Cancer Research* 14 (2008): 2082–87.

Dugbartey, A. T. "Neurocognitive Aspects of Hypothyroidism." *Archives of Internal Medicine* 158 (1998): 1413–18.

Duntas, L. H. "Thyroid Disease and Lipids." *Thyroid* 12 (2002): 287–93.

Earley, C. J., R. P. Allen, J. L. Beard, and J. R. Connor. "Insight into the Pathophysiology of Restless Legs Syndrome." *Journal of Neuroscience Research* 62 (2000): 623–28.

Eberman, L. E., and M. A. Cleary. "Celiac Disease in an Elite Female Collegiate Volleyball Athlete: A Case Report." *Journal of Athletic Training* 40 (2005): 360–64.

Eden, A. N., and M. A. Mir. "Iron Deficiency in 1- to 3-Year-Old Children: A Pediatric Failure?" *Archives of Pediatric Adolescent Medicine* 15 (1997): 986–88.

Eknoyan, G., et al. "DOQI Update." *American Journal of Kidney Diseases* 37 (2001): S190–222.

Enns, C. W., J. Goldman, and A. Cook. "Trends in Food and Nutrient Intakes by Adult NFC1977–1978, CSFII1989–91 1994–1995." *Family Economics and Nutritional Review* 10 (1997): 1–15.

Erikson, K. M., D. J. Pinero, J. R. Conor, and J. L. Beard. "Regional Brain Iron, Ferritin and Transferrin Concentrations During Iron Deficiency and Iron Repletion in Developing Rats." *Journal of Nutrition* 127 (1997): 2030–38.

Farrell R. J., and C. P. Kelly. "Diagnosis of Celiac Sprue." *American Journal of Gastroenterology* 96 (2001): 3237–46.

Fasano, A., M. Araya, S. Bhatnagar, D. Cameron, C. Catassi, M. Dirks, M. L. Mearin, L. Ortigosa, A. Phillips, Celiac Disease Working Group. "Federation of International Societies of Pediatric Gastroenterology, Hepatology, and Nutrition Consensus Report on Celiac Disease." *Journal of Pediatric Gastroenterology and Nutrition* 47 (2008): 214–19.

Fasano, A., I. Berti, T. Gerarduzzi, T. Not, R. Colletti, S. Drago, Y. Elitsur, et al. "Prevalence of Celiac Disease in At-Risk and Not-At-Risk Groups in the United States." *Archives of Internal Medicine* 163 (2003): 286–92.

Finch, C. A., and J. D. Cook. "Iron Deficiency." *American Journal of Clinical Nutrition* 39 (1994): 471–77.

Fleming, D. J., P. F. Jacques, K. L. Tucker, J. M. Massaro, R. B. D'Agostino Sr., P. W. Wilson, and R. J. Wood. "Iron Status of the Free-Living, Elderly Framingham Heart Study Cohort: An Iron-Replete Population with a High Prevalence of Elevated Iron Stores." *American Journal of Clinical Nutrition* 73 (2001): 638–46.

Fleming, D. J., K. L. Tucker, P. F. Jacques, G. E. Dallal, P. W. Wilson, and R. J. Wood. "Dietary Factors Associated with the Risk of High Iron Stores in the Elderly Framingham Heart Study Cohort." *American Journal of Clinical Nutrition* 76 (2002): 1375–84.

Fratti, R. A., P. H. Belanger, M. A. Ghannoum, J. E. Edwards Jr., and S. G. Filler. "Endothelial Cell Injury Caused by Candida Albicans Is Dependent on Iron." *Infectious Immunity* 66 (1998): 191–96.

Freeman, H. J. "Pearls and Pitfalls in the Diagnosis of Adult Celiac Disease." *Canadian Journal of Gastroenterology* 22 (2008): 273–80.

Ganz, T. "Hepcidin: A Key Regulator of Iron Metabolism and Mediator of Anemia of Inflammation." *Journal of the American Society of Hematology, Blood* 102 (2003): 783–88.

Garcia-Casal, M. N., I. Leets, and M. Layrisse. "Beta-Carotene and Inhibitors of Iron Absorption Modify Iron Uptake by Caco-2 Cell." *Journal of Nutrition* 130 (2000): 724–28.

Geier, A., C. Gartung, I. Theurl, G. Weiss, F. Lammert, C. G. Dietrich, R. Weiskirchen, H. Zoller, B. Hermanns, and S. Matern. "Occult Celiac Disease Prevents Penetrance of Hemochromatosis." *World Journal of Gastroenterology* 11 (2005): 3323–26.

Geming, U., N. Gattemann, M. Aivado, B. Hildebrandt, and C. Aul. "Two Types of Acquired Idiopathic Sideroblastic Anemia (AISA): A Time-Tested Distinction." *British Journal of Haematology* 108 (2000): 724–28.

Gettinger, A. "Transfusion in the Perioperative Period: A Consideration of Risks and Benefits as a Guide to Determine When and Who to Transfuse." *The International Trauma Anesthesia and Critical Care Society* (Summer 2005): 158–63.

Giri, N., D. L. Batista, B. P. Alter, and C. A. Stratakis. "Endocrine Abnormalities in Patients with Fanconi Anemia." *Journal of Clinical Endocrinology & Metabolism* 92 (2007): 2624–31.

Godfrey, J. D., and J. A. Murray. "A Rapid Antibody Test Had High Specificity but Low Sensitivity for Diagnosing Coeliac Disease." *Evidence Based Medicine* 13 (2008): 118.

Gonzalez, M. I., D. Caballero, L. Vazques, C. Canizo, R. Hernandez, C. Loqez, A. Izarra, J. L. Arroyo, M. Gonzalez, R. Garcia, and J. F. San Miguel. "Allogeneic Peripheral Stem Cell Transplantation in a Case of Hereditary Sideroblastic Anemia." *British Journal of Haematology* 109 (2000): 658–60.

Good, R. A., B. Wang, N. S. El-Badri, A. Steele, and T. Verjee. "Mixed Bone Marrow or Mixed Stem Cell Transplantation for Prevention or Treatment of Lupus-Like Diseases in Mice." *Technical Seminar: Stem Cells in Kidney Diseases. Abstract.*

Goodman, A. "Abnormal Genital Tract Bleeding." *Clinical Cornerstone* 3 (2000): 25–35.

Goodnough, L., B. Skikne, and C. Brugnara. "Erythropoietin, Iron and Erythropoisis." *Blood* 96 (2000): 823–33.

Graves, R., and S. P. Weaver. "Cefdinir-Associated 'Bloody Stools' in an Infant." *Journal of the American Board of Family Medicine* 21 (2008): 246–48.

Green, R., R. Charlton, and H. Seftel. "Body Iron Excretion in Man: A Collaborative Study." *The American Journal of Medicine* 45 (1968): 336–53.

Guttmacher, A. E., D. A. Marchuk, and R. I. White. "Hereditary Hemorrhagic Telangiectasia." *New England Journal of Medicine* 333 (1995): 918–24.

Hallberg, L. "Bioavailability of Dietary Iron in Man." *Annual Review of Nutrition* 1 (1981): 123–47.

———. "Iron Balance in Pregnancy." In *Vitamins and Minerals in Pregnancy and Lactation,* edited by H. Berger, 115–27. New York: Raven Press, 1988.

Hallberg, L., and L. Hulthen. "Prediction of Dietary Iron Absorption: An Algorithm for Calculating Absorption and Bioavailability of Dietary Iron." *American Journal of Clinical Nutrition* 71 (2000): 1147–60.

Han, O., M. L. Failla, A. D. Hill, E. R. Morris, and J. C. Smith Jr. "Inositol Phosphates Inhibit Uptake and Transport of Iron and Zinc by a Human Intestinal Cell Line." *Journal of Nutrition* 124 (1994): 580–87.

Hellier, K. D., E. Hatchwell, A. S. Duncombe, J. Kew, and S. R. Hammans. "X-Linked Sideroblastic Anemia with Ataxia: Another Mitochondrial Disease?" *Journal of Neurological and Neurosurgical Psychiatry* 70 (2001): 65–69.

Hellstrom-Lindberg, E., R. Negrin, R. Stein, S. Krantz, S. Lindberg, G. Vardiman, J. Ost, and A. Greenberg. "Erythroid Response to Treatment with G-CSF Plus Erythropoietin for the Anaemia of Patients with Myelodysplastic Syndromes: Proposal for a Predictive Model." *British Journal of Haematolotgy* 99 (1997): 344–51.

Hemminki, E., and J. Merilainen. "Long-Term Follow-Up of Mothers and Their Infants in a Randomized Trial on Iron Prophylaxis During Pregnancy." *American Journal of Obstetrics and Gynecology* 173 (1995): 205–9.

Hemminki, E., and U. Rimpela. "A Randomized Comparison of Routine Versus Selective Iron Supplementation During Pregnancy." *Journal of the American College of Nutrition* 10 (1991): 3–10.

———. "A Randomized Comparison of Routine Versus Selective Iron Supplementation During Pregnancy." *Journal of the American College of Nutrition* 10 (1997): 344–51.

Heneghan, M. A., K. M. Feeley, F. M. Stevens, M. P. Little, C. F. McCarthy. "Precipitation of Iron Overload and Hereditary Hemochromatosis after Successful Treatment of Celiac Disease." *American Journal of Gastroenterology* 95 (2000): 298–300.

Herbert, V. "Everyone Should Be Tested for Iron Disorders." *Journal of the American Dietetic Association* 92 (1992): 1502–9.

Howard, D. H. "Acquisition, Transport, and Storage of Iron by Pathogenic Fungi." *Clinical Microbiology Reviews* 12 (1999): 393–404.

Hu, W. T., J. A. Murray, M. C. Greenway, J. E. Parisi, and K. A. Josephs. "Cognitive Impairment and Celiac Disease." *Archives of Neurology* 63 (2006): 1440–46.

Hudson, J. Q., and R. M. Sameri. "Darbaepoetin Alfa, A New Therapy for the Management of Anemia of Chronic Kidney Disease." *Pharmacotherapy* 9 (2002): S141–49.

Hunt, J. R., and Z. K. Roughead. "Nonheme Iron Absorption, Fecal Ferritin Excretion, and Blood Indexes on Iron Status in Women Consuming Controlled Lactoovovegetarian Diets for 8 Weeks." *American Journal of Clinical Nutrition* 69 (1999): 944–52.

Hurrell, R. F., M. B. Reddy, and J. D. Cook. "Inhibition of Non-Haem Iron Absorption in Man by Polyphenolic-Containing Beverages." *British Journal of Nutrition* 81 (1999): 289–95.

Hurrell, R. F., M. B. Reddy, J. Burri, and J. D. Cook. "An Evaluation of EDTA Compounds for Iron Fortification of Cereal-Based Foods." *British Journal of Nutrition* 84 (2000): 903–10.

Hurtado, E. K., A. H. Claussen, and K. G. Scott. "Early Childhood Anemia and Mild or Moderate Mental Retardation." *American Journal of Clinical Nutrition* 69 (1999): 115–19.

Idjradinata, P., and E. Pollitt. "Reversal of Developmental Delays in Iron-Deficient Anaemic Infants Treated with Iron." *Lancet* 341 (1993): 1–4.

Igic, P. G., E. Lee, W. Harper, and K. Roach. "Toxic Effects Associated with Consumption of Zinc." *Mayo Clinic Proceedings* 77 (2002): 713–16.

Institute of Medicine. *Nutrition During Pregnancy and Lactation: An Implementation Guide.* Washington, D.C.: National Academy Press, 1992.

Iolascon, A., V. J. Delaunay, S. N. Wickramasinghe, S. Perrotta, M. Gigante, and C. Camaschella. "Natural History of Congenital Dyserythropoietic Anemia Type II." *Blood* 98 (2001): 1258–60.

Iolascon, A., V. J. Servedio, R. Carbone, A. Totaro, M. Carella, S. Perrotta, S. N. Wickramasinghe, J. Delaunay, H. Heimpel, and P. Gasparini. "Geographic Distribution of CDA-II: Did a Founder Effect Operate in Southern Italy?" *Haematologica* 85 (2002): 470–74.

Irwing, J., and J. Kirchner. "Anemia in Children." *American Family Physician* (2001): 1379–86.

Jacobson, D. L., S. J. Gange, N. R. Rose, and N. M. Graham. "Epidemiology and Estimated Population Burden of Selected Autoimmune Diseases in the United States." *Clinical Immunology and Immunopathology* 84 (1997): 223–43.

Jaruratanasirikul, S., S. Tanchotikul, M. Wongcharnchailert, V. Laosombat, P., Sangsupavanich, and K. Leetanaporn. "A Low Dose Adrenocorticotropin Test (1 Microg ACTH) for the Evaluation of Adrenal Function in Children with Beta-Thalassemia Receiving Hypertransfusion with Suboptimal Iron-Chelating Therapy." *Journal of Pediatric Endocrinology & Metabolism* 20 (2007): 1183–88.

Johnson-Spear, M. A., and R. Yip. "Hemoglobin Difference Between Black and White Women with Comparable Iron Status: Justification for Race-Specific Anemia Criteria." *American Journal of Clinical Nutrition* 60 (1994): 117–21.

Kamao, M., N. Tsugawa, K. Nakagawa, Y. Kawamoto, K. Jukui, G. Kuwata, M. Imai, and T. Okano. "Absorption of Calcium, Magnesium, Phosphorus, Iron and Zinc in Growing Male Rats Fed Diets Containing Either Phytate-Free Soybean Protein or Soybean Protein Isolate or Cassein." *Journal of Nutritional Science and Vitaminology* 46 (2000): 34–41.

Kawanami, T., T. Kato, M. Daimon, M. Tominaga, H. Sasaki, K. Maeda, S. Arai, Y. Shikama, and T. Katagiri. "Hereditary Caeruloplasmin Deficiency: Clinicopathological Study of a Patient." *Journal of Neurology, Neurosurgery and Psychiatry* 61 (1996): 506–9.

Keller, C., and C. Langston. "Images in Clinical Medicine: Childhood Idiopathic Pulmonary Hemosiderosis." *New England Journal of Medicine* 343 (2000): 781.

Kenney, E., and S. Bowman. "Assessment of the Effect of Fat-Modified Foods on Diet Quality in Adults, 19 to 50 Years, Using Data from the Continuing Survey of Food Intake by Individuals." *Journal of the American Dietetic Association* 101 (2001): 455–60.

Kishida, T., Y. Nakai, and K. Ebihara. "Hydroxypropyl-Dispatch Phosphate from Tapioca Starch Reduces Zinc and Iron Absorption, but Not Calcium and Magnesium Absorption in Rats." *Journal of Nutrition* 131 (2001): 294–300.

Knight, S. A., E. Lesuisse, R. Stearman, R. D. Klausner, and A. Dancis. "Reductive Iron Uptake by Candida Albicans: Role of Copper, Iron and TUP1 Regulator." *Microbiology* 148 (2002): 29–40.

Koc, S., and J. W. Harris. "Sideroblastic Anemias: Variation on Imprecisions in Diagnostic Criteria, Proposal for an Extended Classification of Sideroblastic Anemias." *American Journal of Hematology* 57 (1998): 1–6.

Koklu, S., D. Ertugrul, A. M. Onat, S. Karakus, I. C. Haznedaroglu, Y. Buyukasik, N. Sayinalp, O. Ozcebe, and S. V. Dundar. "Piebaldism Associated with Congenital Dyserythropoietic Anemia Type II (HEMPAS)." *American Journal of Hematology* 69 (2002): 210–13.

Kowalski, T. E., M. Falestiny, E. Furth, and P. F. Malet. "Vitamin A Hepatoxicity: A Cautionary Note Regarding 25,000 IU Supplements." *American Journal of Medicine* 97 (1994): 523–28.

Krishnamoorthy, P. A. Alyaarubi, S. Abish, M. Gale, P. Albuquerque, and N. Jabado. "Primary Hyperparathyroidism Mimicking Vaso-Occlusive Crises in Sickle Cell Disease." *Pediatrics: Official Journal of the American Academy of Pediatrics* 118 (2006): e537–39.

Kroshner, J., M. Hatch, D. D. Hennessy, M. Fridman, and R. E. Tannous. "Anemia in Stage II and III Breast Cancer Patients Treated with Adjuvant Doxorubicin and Cyclophosphamide Chemotherapy." *Oncologist* 9 (2004): 25–32.

Lancaster, J., L. M. Sylvia, and E. Schainker. "Nonbloody, Red Stools from Coadministration of Cefdinir and Iron-Supplemented Infant Formulas." *Pharmacotherapy—The Journal of Human Pharmacology and Drug Therapy* 28 (2008): 678–81.

Layrisse, M., M. Garcia–Casal, L. Solano, M. Baron, F. Arguello, D. Llovera, J. Ramirez, I. Leets, and E. Tropper. "Iron Bioavailability in Humans from Breakfasts Enriched with Iron Bis–Glycine Chelate, Phytates and Polyphenols." *Human Nutrition and Metabolism* 9 (2000): 2195–99.

Layrisse, M., C. Martinez-Torres, M. Renzi, F. Velez, and M. Gonzalez. "Sugar as a Vehicle for Iron Fortification." *American Journal of Clinical Nutrition* 29 (1976): 8–18.

Levrat-Verny, M. A., C. Coudray, J. Bellanger, J. W. Lopez, C. Demigne, Y. Rayssiguier, and C. Remesy. "Wholewheat Flour Ensures Higher Mineral Absorption and Bioavailability than White Wheat Flour in Rats." *British Journal of Nutrition* 82 (1999): 17–21.

Leyden, J., B. Kelleher, E. Ryan, S. Barrett, J. C. O'Keane, and J. Crowe. "The Celtic Coincidence: The Frequency and Clinical

Characterisation of Hereditary Haemochromatosis in Patients with Coeliac Disease." *Irish Journal of Medical Sciences* 175 (2006): 32–36.

Lipschitz, D. A., J. D. Cook, and C. A. Finch. "A Clinical Evaluation of Serum Ferritin as an Index of Iron Stores." *New England Journal of Medicine* 290 (1974): 1213–16.

Lonnerdal, B. "Effects of Milk and Milk Components on Calcium, Magnesium, and Trace Element Absorption During Infancy." *Physiological Reviews* 77 (1997): 643–69.

Lonnerdal, B., and O. Hernell. "Iron, Zinc, Copper and Selenium Status of Breast-Fed Infants and Infants Fed Trace Element Fortified Milk-Based Infant Formula." *Acta Pediatrica* 83 (1994): 367–73.

Looker, A. C., P. R. Dallman, M. D. Carroll, E. W. Gunter, and C. L. Johnson. "Prevalence of Iron Deficiency in the United States." *Journal of the American Medical Association* 277 (1997): 973–76.

Lopez de Romana, D., M. Ruz, F. Pizarro, L. Landeta, and M. A. Olivares. "Supplementation with Zinc Between Meals Has No Effect of Subsequent Iron Absorption or on Iron Status of Chilean Women." *Nutrition* (2008): Abstract.

Lozoff, B., E. Jimenez, and A. W. Wolf. "Long–term Developmental Outcome of Infants with Iron Deficiency." *New England Journal of Medicine* 325 (1991): 687–94.

Ludwig, K., M. Bitzan, C. Bobrowski, and D. E. Muller-Wiefel. "Escherichia Coli O157 Fails to Induce a Long-Lasting Lipoploysaccharide-Specific, Measurable Humoral Immune Response in Children with Hemolytic-Uremic Syndrome." *Journal of Infectious Diseases* 186 (2002): 566–69.

Lundstrom, I. M., and F. D. Lindstrom. "Iron and Vitamin Deficiencies, Endocrine and Immune Status in Patients with Primary Sjogren's Syndrome." *Oral Diseases* 7 (2001): 144–49.

MacGregor, J. T., R. Schlegal, C. M. Wehr, P. Alperin, and B. N. Ames. "Cytogenetic Damage Induced by Folate Deficiency in Mice is Enhanced by Caffeine." *Proceedings of the National Academy of Sciences of the United States of America* 87 (1990): 9962–65.

MacPhail, A. P. "Iron Deficiency and the Developing World." *Archivos Latinoamericanos de Nutricion* 51 (2001): 2–6.

Malecki, E. A., A. G. Devenyi, J. L. Beard, and Conner Jr. "Existing and Emerging Mechanisms for Transport of Iron and Manganese to the Brain." *Journal of Neuroscience Research* 56 (1999): 113–22.

Marshall, B. M. "Helicobacter pylori." *American Journal Gastroenterology* 89 (1994): S116–28.

Massey, L. K., and M. M. Strang. "Soft Drink Consumption, Phosphorous Intake, and Osteoporosis." *Journal of the American Dietetic Association* 80 (1982): 581–83.

Mayer, B., S. Yurek, H. Kiesewetter, and A. Salama. "Mixed-type Autoimmune Hemolytic Anemia: Differential Diagnosis and a Critical Review of Reported Cases." *Transfusion* (2008): Abstract.

Means, R. T., Jr. "Clinical Application of Recombinant Erythropoietin in the Anemia of Chronic Disease." *Hematololgy/Oncology Clinics of North America* 8 (1994): 933–44.

Mehrvar, A., A. Azarkeivan, M. Faranoush, N. Mehrvar, J. Saberinedjad, R. Ghorbani, and P. Vossough. "Endocrinopathies in Patients with Transfusion-Dependent Beta-Thalassemia." *Pediatric Hematology Oncology* 25 (2008): 187–94.

Micheli, R., C. Telesca, F. Gitti, L. Giordano, and A. Perini. "Abstract: Bells' Palsy: Diagnostic and Therapeutical Trial in Childhood." *Minerva Pediatrica* 48 (1996): 245–50.

Miller, M., J. Humphrey, E. Johnson, E. Marinda, R. Brookmeyer, and J. Katz. "Why Do Children Become Vitamin A Deficient?" *Journal of Nutrition* 9 (2002): S2867–80.

Moolman, J. A. "Thyroid Hormone and the Heart." *Cardiovascular Journals of South Africa* 13 (2002): 159–63.

Morck, T. A., S. R. Lynch, and J. D. Cook. "Inhibition of Food Iron Absorption by Coffee." *American Journal of Clinical Nutrition* 37 (1983): 416–20.

Morrissey, J. A., P. H. Williams, and A. M. Cashmore. "Candida Albicans Has a Cell-Associated Ferric-Reductase Activity which Is Regulated in Response to Levels of Iron and Copper." *Microbiology* 142 (1996): 485–92.

Muretto, P., E. Angelucci, and G. Lucarelli. "Reversibility of Cirrhosis in Patients Cured of Thalassemia by Bone Marrow Transplantation." *Annals of Internal Medicine* 136 (2002): 667–72.

Myers, G., and H. Lu. "HIV and Molecular Mimicry." *Los Alamos National Laboratory Report* (1996): iv, 14–22.

Nelson, R. L. "Iron and Colorectal Cancer Risk: Human Studies." *Nutrition Reviews* 59 (2001): 140–48.

Neuwirtova, R., K. Mocikova, J. Musilova, J. Jelinek, F. Havlicek, K. Michalova, and M. Adamkov. "Mixed Myelodysplastic and Myeloproliferative Syndromes." *Leukemia Research* 20 (1996): 717–26.

Nittis, T., and J. D. Gitlin. "The Copper Iron Connection: Hereditary Aceruloplasminemia." *Seminars in Hematology* 39 (2002): 282–89.

Nordenberg, D., R. Yip, and N. J. Binkin. "The Effect of Cigarette Smoking on Hemoglobin Levels and Anemia Screening." *Journal of the American Medical Association* 264 (1990): 1556–59.

O'Brien, K. O., N. Zavaleta, J. Wen, and S. A. Abrams. "Prenatal Iron Supplements Impair Zinc Absorption in Pregnant Peruvian Women." *Journal of Nutrition* 130 (2000): 2251–55.

Obuobie, K., J. Smith, L. M. Evans, R. John, J. S. Davies, and J. H. Lazarus. "Increased Central Arterial Stiffness in Hypothyroidism." *Journal of Clinical Endocrinology and Metabolism* 87 (2002): 4662–66.

Oken, E., and C. Duggan. "Update on Micronutrients: Iron and Zinc." *Current Opinion in Pediatrics* 14 (2002): 350–53.

Olivan, Gonzalvo G. "Health and Nutritional Status of Delinquent Female Adolescents." *Anales Espanoles de Pediatrica* 56 (2002): 116–20.

Olson, J. K., J. L. Croxford, M. A. Caienoff, M. C. Dal Canto, and S. D. Miller. "A Virus-Induced Molecular Mimicry Model of Multiple Sclerosis." *Journal of Clinical Investigation* 108 (2001): 311–18.

O'Mahony, S., P. D. Howdle, and M. S. Losowsky. "Review Article: Management of Patients with Non-Responsive Coeliac Disease." *Alimentary Pharmacology & Therapeutics* 10 (1996): 671–80.

Origa, R., R. Galanello, T. Ganz, N. Giagu, L. Maccioni, G. Faa, and E. Nemeth. "Liver Iron Concentrations and Urinary Hepcidin in Betathalassenia." *Haematologica, The Hematology Journal* 92 (2007): 583–88.

Paydas, S., and Y. Gokel. "Different Renal Pathologies Associated with Hypothyroidism." *Renal Failure* 24 (2002): 595–600.

Perlmutter, M. A., and H. Lepor. "Androgen Deprivation Therapy in the Treatment of Advanced Prostate Cancer." *Reviews in Urology* 9 (2007): 1:S3–8 Abstract.

Perros, P., R. K. Singh, C. A. Ludlam, and B. M. Frier. "Prevalence of Pernicious Anaemia in Patients with Type 1 Diabetes Mellitus and Autoimmune Thyroid Disease." *Journal of the British Diabetic Association* 17 (2000): 749–51.

Perry, G. S., T. Byers, R. Yip, and S. Margen. "Iron Nutrition Does Not Account for the Hemoglobin Differences Between Blacks and Whites." *Journal of Nutrition* 122 (1992): 1417–24.

Perry, G. S., R. Yip, and C. Zyrkovoski. "Nutritional Factors Among Low-Income Pregnant U.S. Women: The Centers for Disease Control and Prevention (CDC) Pregnancy Nutrition Surveillance System, 1979 Through 1993." *Seminars in Perinatology* 19 (1995): 211–21.

Pintar, J., B. S. Skikne, and J. D. Cook. "A Screening Test for Assessing Iron Status." *Blood* 59 (1982): 110–13.

Pisacane, A., B. DeVizia, and A. Valiente. "Iron Status in Breast-fed Infants." *Journal of Pediatrics* 127 (1995): 429.

Pollitt, E. "Iron Deficiency and Cognitive Function." *Annual Review of Nutrition 13* (1993): 521–37.

Pratt, G., and S. E. Kinsey. "Remission of Severe, Intractable Autoimmune Haemolytic Anaemia Following Matched Unrelated Donor Transplantation." *Bone Marrow Transplantation* 28 (2001): 791–93.

Ramakrishnan, U., E. Kuklina, and A. D. Stein. "Iron Stores and Cardiovascular Disease Risk Factors in Women of Reproductive Age in the United States." *American Journal of Clinical Nutrition* 76 (2002): 1256–60.

Rashtak, S., M. W. Ettore, H. A. Homburger, and J. A. Murray. "Combination Testing for Antibodies in the Diagnosis of Celiac Disease: Comparison of Multiplex Immunoassay and ELISA Methods." *Alimentary Pharmacology & Therapeutics* (2008): Abstract.

Rasmussen, S. A., P. M. Fernhoff, and K. S. Scanlon. "Vitamin B_{12} Deficiency in Children and Adolescents: A Review." *Journal of Pediatrics* 138 (2001): 10–17.

Rees, M. M., and G. M. Rodgers. "Bleeding Disorders Caused by Vascular Abnormalities." In *Wintrobes' Clinical Hematology*, 10th ed., edited by G. R. Lee et al., 10–17. Baltimore: Williams and Wilkens, 1999.

Rolfs A., H. L. Bonkovsky, J. G. Kohlroser, K. McNeal, A. Sharma, U. V. Berger, and M. A. Hediger. "Intestinal Expression of Genes Involved in Iron Absorption in Humans." *American Journals Physiology. Gastrointestinal Liver Physiology* 282 (2002): G598–607.

Rotig, A., V. Cormier, S. Blanche, J. P. Bonnefont, F. Ledeist, N. Romero, J. Schultz, P. Rustin, A. Fischer, and J. M. Saudubray. "Pearson's Marrow-Pancreas Syndrome: A Multi-System Mitochondrial Disorder in Infancy." *Journal of Clinical Investigation* 86 (1990): 1601–8.

Roughead, Z. K., and J. R. Hunt. "Adaptation in Iron Absorption: Iron Supplementation Reduces Nonheme-Iron but not Heme-Iron Absorption from Food." *American Journal of Clinical Nutrition* 72 (2000): 982–89.

Rubio-Tapia, A., and J. A. Murray. "The Liver in Celiac Disease." *Journal of Hepatology* 46 (2007): 1650–58.

Rudek, M., M. M. Horne, W. D. Figg, W. Dahut, V. Dyer, J. M. Pluda, and J. M. Reed. "Reversible Sideroblastic Anemia Associated with the Tetracycline Analogue COL-3." *American Journal of Hematology* 67 (2001): 51–53.

Sakiewicz, P., and E. Paganini. "The Use of Iron in Patients on Chronic Dialysis: Mistake and Misconceptions." *Journal of Nephrology* 11 (1998): 5–15.

Salovarra, S. A., S. Sandberg, and T. Andlid. "Organic Acids Influence Iron Uptake in the Human Epithelial Cell Line Caco-2." *Journal of Agricultural and Food Chemistry* 50 (2002): 6233–38.

Sandstead, H. H. "Causes of Iron and Zinc Deficiencies and Their Effects on the Brain." *Journal of Nutrition* 130 (2000): S347S–9.

Schlammadinger, A., and Z. Boda. "Laboratory Screening and Diagnosis of von Willebrand Disease." Clinical Laboratory 48 (2002): 385–93.

Schnie, P. G., B. L. Hahn, and R. Karmarkar. "Effect of Metals on Candida Albicans Growth in the Presence of Chemical Chelators and Human Abscess Fluid." *Journal of Laboratory and Clinical Medicine* 137 (2001): 284–89.

Scholl, T. O., M. L. Hediger, R. L. Fischer, and J. W. Shearer. "Anemia Vs. Iron Deficiency: Increased Risk of Pre-Term Delivery in a Prospective Study." *American Journal of Clinical Nutrition* 55 (1992): 985–88.

Segal I., A. Otley, R. Issenman, D. Armstrong, V. Espinosa, R. Cawdron, M. G. Morshed, and K. Jacobson. "Low Prevalence of Helicobacter Pylori Infection in Canadian Children: A Cross-Sectional Analysis." *Canadian Journal of Gastroenterology* 22 (2008): 485–89.

Semba, R. D., and M. W. Bloem. "The Anemia of Vitamin A Deficiency: Epidemiology and Pathogenesis." *European Journal of Clinical Nutrition* (2002): 271–81.

Shakir, K. M., J. P. Chute, B. S. Aprill, and A. A. Lazarus. "Ferrous Sulfate-Induced Increase in Requirement for Thyroxine in a Patient with Primary Hyperthyroidism." *Southern Medical Journal* 90 (1997): 637–39.

Shapiro, M., A. J. Greenstein, J. Byrn, J. Corona, A. J. Greenstein, B. Salky, M. T. Harris, and C. M. Divino. "Surgical Management and Outcomes of Patients with Duodenal Crohn's Disease." *Journal of the American College of Surgeons* 207 (2008): 36–42.

Sherry, B., D. Bister, and R. Yip. "Continuation of Decline in Prevalence of Anemia in Low Income Children: The Vermont Experience." *Archives of Pediatrics and Adolescent Medicine* 151 (1997): 298–330.

Shovlin, C. L., A. E. Guttmacher, E. Buscarini, et al. "Diagnostic Criteria for Hereditary Hemorrhagic Telangiectasia (Rendu-Osler-Weber Syndrome)." *American Journal of Medical Geriatrics* 91 (2000): 66–67.

Siegenberg, D., R. D. Baynes, T. H. Bothwell, B. J. MacFarlane, R. D. Lamparelli, N. G. Car, P. MacPhail, U. Schmidt, A. Tal, and F. Mayet. "Ascorbic Acid Prevents the Dose-Dependent Inhibitory Effects of Polyphenols and Phytates on Nonheme-Iron Absorption." *American Journal of Clinical Nutrition* 53 (1991): 537–41.

Siimes, M. A., L. Samenpera, and J. Perheentupa, "Exclusive Breast-feeding for 9 Months: Risk of Iron Deficiency." *Journal of Pediatrics* 104 (1984): 196–99.

Silber, T. J. "Ipecac Syrup Abuse, Morbidity, and Mortality: Isn't It Time to Repeal Its Over-the-counter Status?" *Journal of Adolescent Health* 37 (2005): 256–60.

Silbergeld, E. K., M. Waalkes, and J. M. Rice. "Lead as a Carcinogen: Experimental Evidence and Mechanisms of Action." *American Journals of Internal Medicine* 38 (2000): 316–23.

Singhal, A., S. Moreea, P. D. Reynolds, and K. I. Bzeizi. "Coeliac Disease and Hereditary Haemochromatosis: Association and Implications." *European Journal of Gastroenterology & Hepatology* 16 (2004): 235–37.

Sipalphi, T. B., B. Tavil, and Y. Unver. "Neutrophil Hypersegmentation in Children with Iron Deficiency Anemia." *Pediatric Hematololgy/Oncology* 19 (2002): 235–38.

Skikne, B. S., N. Ahluwalia, B. Fergusson, A. Chomko, and J. D. Cook. "Effects of Erythropoietin Therapy on Iron Absorption in Chronic Renal Failure." *Journal of Laboratory Clinical Medicine* 135 (2000): 452–58.

Skinner, J. D., B. R. Carruth, K. S. Houck, W. Bounds, M. Morris, D. R. Cox, J. Moran III, and F. Coletta. "Longitudinal Study of Nutrient and Food Intakes of White Preschool Children Aged 24 to 60 Months." *Journal of the American Dietetic Association* 99 (1999): 1514–21.

Swenne, I. "Haematological Changes and Iron Status in Teenage Girls with Eating Disorders and Weight Loss: The Importance of Menstrual Status." *Acta Paediatrica* 96 (2007): 530–33.

Szymanski, N. "Infection and Inflammation in Dialysis Patients: Impact on Laboratory Parameters and Anemia: Case Study of the Anemic Patient." *Nephrology Nursing Journal* 28 (2001): 337–40.

Tabak, L., I. D. Mandel, D. Karlan, and H. Baumash. "Alterations in Lactoferrin in Salivary Gland Disease." *Journal of Dental Research* 57 (1978): 43–47.

Takeda, Y., H. Sawada, H. Swai, T. Matsuda, M. Tshima, M. Okuma, S. Watanabe, S. Ohmori, and M. Kondo. "Acquired Hypochromic and Microcytic Sideroblastic Anaemia Responsive to Pyridoxine with Low Value of Free Erythrocyte Protoporphyrin: A Possible Subgroup of Idiopathic Acquired Sideroblastic Anaemia (IASA)." *British Journal of Haematology* 90 (1995): 207–9.

Tam, Y. H., C. K. Yeung, K. H. Lee, J. D. Sihoe, K. W. Chan, S. T. Cheung, and J. W. Mou. "A Population-Based Study of Helicobacter Pylori Infection in Chinese Children Resident in Hong Kong: Prevalence and Potential Risk Factors." *Helicobacter* 13 (2008): 219–24.

Tanna, T., N. V. Bhanu, P. A. Oneal, S. H. Goh, P. Staker, Y. T. Lee, J. W. Noroney, et al. "High Levels of GDF15 in Thalassemia Suppress Expression of the Iron Regulatory Protein Hepcidin." *British Journal of Cancer: Nature Medicine* 13 (2007): 1096–1101.

Taylor, D. J., C. Mallen, N. McDougall, and T. Lind. "Effect of Iron Supplementation on Serum Ferritin Levels During and After Pregnancy." *British Journal of Obstetrics* 89 (1982): 1011–17.

U.S. Centers for Disease Control and Prevention. "Escherichia Coli O157:H7 Outbreak Linked to Commercially Distributed Dry-Cured Salami." *Morbidity and Mortality Weekly Report* 44 (1995): 157–60.

———. "Pulmonary Hemorrhage/Hemosiderosis Among Infants." *Morbidity and Mortality Weekly Report* 49 (2000): 180–84.

———. "Recommendations to Prevent and Control Iron Deficiency in the United States." *Morbidity and Mortality Weekly Report* 47 (1998): 1–28.

U.S. Preventive Services Task Force. "Screening for Iron Deficiency Anemia—Including Iron Prophylaxis." In *Guide to Clinical Preventative Services*, 2nd ed. Alexandria, VA: International Medical Publishing, 1993. 231–46.

Vallespi, T., M. Imbert, C. Mecucci, C. Preudhomme, and P. Fenaux. "Diagnosis, Classification, and Cytogenetics of Myelodysplastic Syndromes." *Haematologica* 83 (1998): 258–75.

van Steenbergen, W., G. Malhijs, T. Roskams, and J. Fevery. "Noniatrogenic Anaemia Type II Is Not Related to C282Y and H63D Mutation in the HFE Gene: Report on Two Brothers." *Acta Clinica Belgica* 57 (2002): 79–84.

Vichinsky, E. "Current Issues with Blood Transfusions in Sickle Cell Disease." *Seminars in Hematology* 38 (2001): 14–22.

Vichinsky, E., K. Kleman, S. Embury, B. Lubin. "The Diagnosis of Iron Deficiency Anemia in Sickle Cell Disease. *Blood* 58 (1981): 963–68.

Vogel, M., L. J. Anderson, S. Holden, J. E. Deanfield, D. J. Pennell, J. M. Walker. "Tissue Doppler Echocardiography in Patients with Thalassaemia Detects Early Myocardial Dysfunction Related to Myocardial Iron Overload." *European Heart Journal* 24 (2003): 113–19.

Waalen, J. "Haemoglobin and Ferritin Concentrations in Men and Women: Cross Sectional Study." *British Journal of Medicine* 325 (2002): 137.

Weinberg, E. D. "Iron and Susceptibility to Infectious Disease." *Science* 184 (1974): 952–56.

———. "Iron Withholding: A Defense against Viral Infections." *Biometals* 9 (1996): 393–99.

———. "The Role of Iron in Cancer." *European Journal of Cancer Prevention* 5 (1996): 19–36.

West, A. R., and P. S. Oates. "Mechanisms of Heme Iron Absorption: Current Questions and Controversies." *World Journal of Gastroenterlogy* 14 (2008): 4101–10.

———. "Subcellular Location of Heme Oxygenase 1 and 2 and Divalent Metal Transporter 1 in Relation to Endocytotic Markers During Heme Iron Absorption." *Journal of Gastroenterology and Hepatology* 23 (2008): 150–58.

Willet, Walter C. *Eat, Drink, and Be Healthy: The Harvard Medical School Guide to Healthy Eating.* New York: Simon & Schuster, 2001.

Wong, C. S., J. Srdjan, R. L. Habeeb, S. L. Watkins, and P. I. Tarr. "The Risk of the Hemolytic-Uremic Syndrome after Antibiotic Treatment of Escherichia Coli O157: H7 Infections." *New England Journal of Medicine* 342 (2000): 1930–36.

Woo, Y. L., B. White, R. Corbally, M. Byrne, N. O'Connell, E. O'Shea, B. L. Sheppard, J. Bonnar, and O. P. Smith. "von Willebrand Disease: An Important Cause of Dysfunctional Uterine Bleeding." *Blood Coagulation and Fibromyalgia* 13 (2002): 89–93.

Wood, J. C., and N. Ghugre. "Magnetic Resonance Imaging Assessment of Excess Iron in Thalassemia, Sickle Cell Disease and Other Iron Overload Diseases." *Hemoglobin* 32 (2008): 85–96.

Worwood, M. "Inborn Errors of Metabolism: Iron." *British Journal of Haematology* 55 (1999): 556–67.

Wyshak, G. "Teenaged Girls, Carbonated Beverage Consumption, and Bone Fractures." *Archives of Pediatrics & Adolescent Medicine* 15 (2000): 610–13.

Yang, T., W. Q. Dong, Y. A. Kuryshev, C. Obejero-Paz, M. N. Levy, G. M. Brittenham, S. Kiatchoosakun, D. Kirkpatrick, D. B. Hold, and A. M. Brown. "Bimodal Cardiac Dysfunction in an Animal Model of Iron Overload." *Journal of Laboratory and Clinical Medicine* 140 (2002): 263–71.

Yip, R. "Iron Supplementation: Country Level Experiences and Lessons Learned." *Journal of Nutrition* 132 (2002): S859–61.

———. "The Changing Characteristics of Childhood Iron Nutritional Status in the United States." In *Dietary Iron: Birth to Two Years*. L. J. Filer, ed. New York: Raven Press, 1989: 37–61.

Yip, R., K. M. Walsh, M. G. Goldfarb, and N. J. Binkin. "Declining Prevalence of Anemia in Childhood in a Middle-Class Setting: A Pediatric Success Story?" *Pediatrics* 80 (1987): 330–34.

Zdebska, E., E. Mendek-Czajkowska, R. Ploski, B. Woeniewicz, J. Koscielak. "Heterozygosity of CDAN II (HEMPAS) Gene May Be Detected by the Analysis of Erythrocyte Membrane Glycoconjugates from Healthy Carriers." *Haematologica* 87 (2002): 126–30.

Zhang, Z. F., R. C. Kurtz, M. Sun, M. Karpeh Jr., G. P. Yu, N. Gargon, J. S. Fein, S. K. Georgopoulos, and S. Harlap. "Adenocarcinomas of the Esophagus and Gastric Cardia: Medical Conditions, Tobacco, Alcohol, and Socioeconomic Factors in Cancer Epidemiology Biomarkers & Prevention." *A Publication of the American Association for Cancer Research & The American Society of Preventive Oncology* 5 (1996): 761–68.

Zijp, I. M., O. Korver, and L. B. Tijburg. "Effect of Tea and Other Dietary Factors on Iron Absorption." *Critical Reviews in Food Science and Nutrition* 40 (2000): 371–98.

Zubizarreta, E., E. Zapata, and A. Castiella. "Celiac Disease and Hemochromatosis." *European Journal of Gastroenterology & Hepatology* 20 (2008): 589.

Index